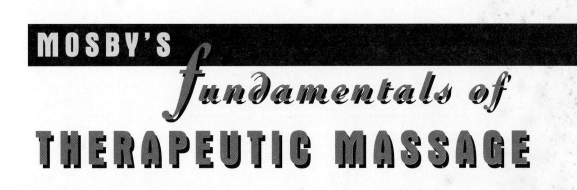

MOSBY'S
fundamentals of
THERAPEUTIC MASSAGE

MOSBY'S

fundamentals of

THERAPEUTIC MASSAGE

SANDY FRITZ

Founder, Owner, Director, & Head Instructor
Health Enrichment Center School of Therapeutic
Massage and Bodywork
Lapeer, Michigan

with 494 illustrations

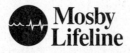

**Mosby
Lifeline**

St. Louis Baltimore Boston Carlsbad Chicago Naples New York Philadelphia Portland
London Madrid Mexico City Singapore Sydney Tokyo Toronto Wiesbaden

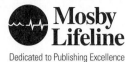

Mosby Lifeline
Dedicated to Publishing Excellence

A Times Mirror
Company

Publisher: David Dusthimer
Acquisitions Editor: Eric M. Duchinsky
Assistant Editor: Christine H. Ambrose
Project Manager: Chris Baumle
Production Editor: Stacy M. Guarracino
Design Manager: Nancy J. McDonald
Interior Design: Saki Mafundikwa
Photography: Camille Gerace, Cam–Works
Line Art: Beverley Ransom
Additional Art: Alice Chin

FIRST EDITION

Printed in the United States of America

Composition by: Clarinda
Printing/Binding by: Von Hoffmann Press

Mosby–Year Book, Inc.
11830 Westline Industrial Drive
St. Louis, Missouri 63146

Library of Congress catalog card number: 95–75933

International Standard Book Number 0–8151–3251–4
  96 97 98 99/9 8 7 6 5 4 3

To my kids Greg, Laura, Luke, and Kris for doing without me for so long. To my mother who kept the house together and worried about me. To all my dogs who spend countless hours by my side and in my lap and especially to my old bull dog, Ethan, who died quietly at my feet while I worked on rewrites. To Eric and Christine for "making it happen." To my special staff, that are my friends and family, for giving me the space to write. To all the wonderful people who teach with me. To every client and student I have had the opportunity to touch; thank you for teaching me. To all my teachers. To those who listened. To those who love me anyway.

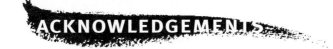

ACKNOWLEDGEMENTS

A special thank you is extended to those contributors who generously dedicated their time and talents in working with this project:

DR. LEON CHAITOW, for his support and writing the foreword for the text.

EMILY COWALL, for her contributions to the text and her extensive attention to detail in the review process.

KATHY PAHOLSKY, for her committed work on the Instructor's Manual and extensive work in helping me to revise the manuscript.

RICHARD VAN WHY, for his contributions to the historical information in the text.

My thanks to the following reviewers who have influenced the content and clarity of this text to assure the accurate presentation of information:

PATRICIA J. BENJAMIN, PH.D.
Director of Education, Connecticut Center for Massage Therapy, Newington, Connecticut

LEON K. CHAITOW, N.D., D.O.
Member of the Register of Osteopaths, Senior Lecturer, Center for Community Care & Primary Health, University of Westminster, London, England; Consultant Osteopath, The Hale Clinic, London, England

EMILY EDITH SAFRONA COWALL, REG. M.T.
Vice–Chairman (present), National Certification Board for Therapeutic Massage and Bodywork, Arlington, Virginia; Chairman (former), The College of Massage Therapists (formerly Board of Directors of Masseurs), Province of Ontario (Canada)

PETER A. GOLDBERG, DIPL. AC. (NCCA), L.M.T.
National Commission on Certification of Acupuncturists, Great Barrington, Massachusetts

LUCY LIBEN, M.S., L.M.T.
Director of Education, Swedish Institute of Massage Therapy, New York, New York

JEAN E. LOVING, B.A., L.M.T.
Director of Education, Co–owner, Seminar Network International, Inc., Lake Worth, Florida

KAREN B. NAPOLITANO, M.S.
Director of Education (Former), Potomac Massage Training Institute Washington, D.C.

KATHLEEN MAISON PAHOLSKY, M.S., PH.D.
Director of Education, Health Enrichment Center; Director, Clinical Approaches Program, Lapeer, Michigan

CHERIE MARILYN SOHNEN–MOE, B.A.
Instructor, Desert Institute of the Healing Arts, Tucson, Arizona

MARY MARGARET TUCHSCHERER, D.C., PH.D.
Doctor of Chiropractic and Associate Professor of Basic Science,
Departments of Clinical and Basic Science, Northwestern College of
Chiropractic Bloomington, Minnesota; Faculty and Chairperson of Basic
Science, Northern Lights School of Massage Therapy, Minneapolis,
Minnesota

SHERRI WILLIAMSON, L.M.T.
Founder, ABMP, Associated Bodywork & Massage Professionals (ABMP)
Evergreen, Colorado

ED WILSON, PH.D., L.M.T.
Dean of Student Development, Educator and Massage Therapist,
Educating Hands School of Massage, Miami, Florida

In addition to the contributors and reviewers, there are several people
who also deserve special recognition for their efforts in the publication
and promotion of this project:

ERIC DUCHINSKY, Acquisitions Editor: for convincing me that I was Mosby's
choice to write this text, and for having faith in me.

CHRISTINE AMBROSE, Assistant Editor: for her dedication; for being more
than an editor, and becoming my friend.

BEVERLEY RANSOM, for her terrific artwork.

CAMILLE GERACE, for the incredible photos, and her energy and enthusiasm during the photo shoots.

NANCY MCDONALD, Designer: for her innovative cover and design expertise.

STACY GUARRACINO, Production Editor: for her enthusiasm and keen
attention to detail.

MOSBY LIFELINE SALES & MARKETING DEPARTMENT: for their enthusiasm
and support of this text and product line.

It truly has been a team effort.

FOREWORD

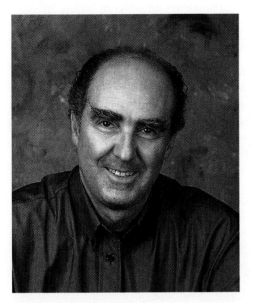

LEON CHAITOW, N.D., D.O.

Therapeutic massage, sometimes termed *structured touch,* has been a universal core healing art throughout history. This art is now demonstrating a dramatic resurgence in a variety of mainstream medical and academic settings, along with an increasing amount of pioneering research devoted to verification and explanation of the clinical results seen in daily practice. These results can be expressed most simply by saying that people, almost without exception and in almost any degree of physical or psychological distress, feel better when they receive appropriate massage therapy. The key word is *appropriate* and this word has served as the driving force behind the need for the development, writing, and publication of this excellent text.

For massage therapy to achieve its full potential, it is essential that the work of countless therapists who use these techniques should be grounded in an understanding of anatomy, physiology, and pathophysiology, the normalization or easing of which is the focus of their work. In other words, it is of little use to be skilled in a technique if that technique is applied inappropriately. Currently, there are a number of categories in which massage therapy has important applications and in all of these, the skills must be accompanied by an understanding of the mechanisms at work.

Those forms of massage therapy that aim at relaxation and easing of both physical and emotional tension require an understanding of the potency of the techniques available and the need for interdisciplinary cooperation. In more advanced applications of methods (called psychotherapeutic bodywork), where there is a focus on the intimate links between many chronic physical manifestations of tension and psychological defense mechanisms, an understanding of psychoneuroimmunologic, psychosomatic, and somaticopsychic processes can be necessary. However, often therapists working in these areas seem most reluctant to see a highly academic structure evolve for massage therapy, for fear the intuitive, compassionate side of their therapy would be lost in potentially mechanistic approaches and methods. This concern must be well understood and should not be dismissed—unless both heart and brain are involved in massage therapy, something will be lost in the provision of care for those in most distress. The truth is, no loss of compassion must occur when knowledge is acquired; no diminution of the intuitive value must take place simply because there is a greater understanding of the body's mechanisms in health and disease.

When massage therapy is used as an intervention to improve body alignment and function, there is a need for understanding of body mechanics, and employment of gait and postural, structural, and functional assessments with strategies that normalize dysfunction and deviation from the norm.

Some forms of massage therapy are concerned with enhancing sensory awareness, while others concentrate on reducing painful local and general conditions, or balance perceived energetic inequalities.

The range of therapeutic massage techniques can be enormous, whether involved in structural, psychologic, or energetic aspects of the human condition.

The limits that exist and inhibit the development of massage therapy can sometimes relate to externally applied, legal, and license-related restrictions. However, many of these limits are actually self-imposed, because the potential of the therapeutic benefits of structured touch techniques is virtually limitless—or rather limited only by gaps that exist in individual therapists' knowledge and skill base. These gaps correspond to the level of excellence or training the therapist has received. Once again, this emphasizes the value of this text, which gathers between its covers a huge range of knowledge and support for those building their resource base of assessment and therapeutic skills and filling the "tool box" from which they will choose appropriate methods.

The good news, can be summarized by stating that there are few, if any, areas of ill health that cannot be helped, to some extent, by therapeutic massage. Whether in the easing of pain, the provision of a safe space for relaxation, the restoration of suppleness and mobility to restricted tissues, the enhancement of circulatory function (both in supply and drainage), or the provision of a connecting bridge between mind and body experiences and awareness. In addition, because massage therapy enhances homeostasis, there is evidence of a preventive outcome and wellness emerging from receipt of therapeutic massage. This can also be expressed by saying that the effects of touch techniques positively and demonstrably enhance defenses, thereby reducing vulnerability and susceptibility.

However, the bad news is that prejudice against massage therapy is still widely noted among other health professionals, many academic settings, some local and national government agencies, and to some extent, specific areas of the general public. The media generally have failed to promote the positive image of therapeutic massage. Part of the blame for failing to impress these groups exists within the massage profession because of uneven and sometimes lax training standards in the past and the relatively unregulated nature of the profession. This situation is rapidly progressing as more and more schools upgrade their training standards, professional organizations lobby and educate legislative bodies, and an increasing number of therapists find themselves working in mainstream settings. A recent phenomenon has seen a large body of mainstream personnel, mainly nurses working within traditional medical settings, turn to touch therapies as a means of broadening their capacity for helping their clients and patients. The single most important aspect that encourages the acceptance of the therapeutic massage profession is, in my view, the acquisition of improved assessment and diagnostic and evaluation skills by therapists in training and in practice. This text is peppered with a great many skill-enhancing exercises which, if diligently practiced, will result in heightened palpatory awareness—the main ingredient of skillful bodywork.

Therapeutic massage should, therefore, encompass the ability to know what is being palpated, what the functions and dysfunctions of the tissues in question are, and what they feel like, to be able to feel and assess tissue and know what is wrong, what must be done and why, and to instantly provide suitable therapeutic input—whether it involves releasing fascial restrictions, easing spasm or pain, or enhancing local circulation and drainage—while simultaneously doing no harm. Without some of these skills and without the ability to discuss the procedures and their purpose, therapists will continue to be regarded with less respect than they deserve.

The only way prejudice can be overcome is through excellence in training, and a standard of professionalism in practice which breaks down barriers of ignorance toward the true value of therapeutic interventions.

It has been my privilege and pleasure to be associated with massage therapists in Europe and the United States over the past 35 years. I know exactly what they are capable of doing when given the proper tools with which to work. In this text, Sandy Fritz has diligently put together the basics for acquiring the knowledge to excellently work with structured touch techniques in any setting. Certainly, a text is no substitute for a sound and thorough training, but this text offers no less than a major contribution to that training, in a structured and orderly manner. Sandy Fritz has also examined some major areas of controversy, including the vexed question of the sexual connotations of massage. She has handled these potentially dangerous areas of debate with delicacy and directness, which can be easily recognized as her trademark. The manner in which she has presented the information will ensure that this text forms the basis for a further step forward in the progression of massage therapy to its rightful position alongside other organized health care professions.

LEON CHAITOW, N.D., D.O.

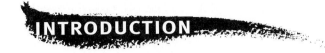

INTRODUCTION

The author, contributors, and publisher intend for **Mosby's Fundamentals of Therapeutic Massage** to be an excellent teaching and reference text. This book is designed to be used by skilled, therapeutic massage educators in the classroom setting. It can also be used as a continuing education resource by practitioners and as a reference text for health professionals and massage and bodywork practitioners.

More than 16 years ago, when I was exploring a career in therapeutic massage, there were few schools. As none of them were readily accessible to me, I taught myself. The experience I gained from clients was my teacher. I took a course of less than 100 hours, which at least provided basic skills. The rest of my massage therapy training has come from reading a multitude of books, attending hundreds of hours of workshops, apprenticeship training, college courses in related subjects, teaching over 2000 beginning students, and giving over 20,000 massage sessions. I am still learning the importance of the fundamental concepts upon which all bodywork methods are based. I learn more about the elegant simplicity of massage each time I teach and through researching and writing this textbook.

Today, the profession of therapeutic massage is in the process of standardizing and organizing. There are many highly respected schools teaching students therapeutic applications of nurturing, safe touch that stimulates the body's various physiologic processes. All massage and bodywork methods, including the very subtle techniques, are based on physical responses. A well-rounded education includes how to perform massage manipulations and bodywork techniques, the anatomy and physiology of why the methods work, and the importance of structure, intent, and purpose of touch. It is as important to touch the whole person as it is to skillfully apply techniques. The massage professional must do both. In addition, the student needs to understand the importance of sanitation, hygiene, body mechanics, business practices, and ethics to build a well-balanced, professional massage career.

The fundamentals of massage methods are relatively simple. A well-planned school curriculum, as developed in this textbook and ancillaries (Mosby's Fundamentals of Therapeutic Massage Workbook and Instructor's Manual), could teach the basics in a program of 500 to 1000 class hours. After this point, training focuses on specific evaluation of the client and application of the methods.

The days of self-teaching massage are coming to an end. Validation of a profession requires standardized, formal education. I believe that apprenticeship training is a valid and desirable way to learn. I also realize that verifiable credentials are necessary if the profession of therapeutic massage and bodywork wishes to obtain formal recognition. It is easier to standardize curriculum requirements through the formal school environment and an accepted set of teaching materials. Written and practical tests can be developed from the textbook base. These tests determine the minimum standard of practice. There is probably a better way to maintain a professional standard of expertise, but this system works. It is cost effective, simple to set in place, and easy to inspect. Massage therapy educators will find that agreement about the core body of knowledge, and standardizing of the educational process, will free them to teach the crucial, "hands on" material that a book cannot effectively teach.

Once students learn the fundamental core body of knowledge for all therapeutic massage and bodywork methods the essential learning begins. The uniqueness of our profession is not dependent upon the methods, or the technical application of massage techniques. The massage therapy profession offers skilled, structured, and safe touch in a nurturing environment. This relationship joins people in a healing partnership. A book cannot touch the student; only a teacher can.

Many massage therapy educators and practitioners learned massage the way I did, the hands on approach. It is important for these skilled people to comply with the standard body of knowledge of massage and bodywork being developed. The information in this textbook can be used to improve what is already being done well, upgrade skills and knowledge base in line with the current trends, and help current practitioners to remain competitive in today's market.

If health care providers understand the physiologic effects of therapeutic massage, they will be better able to advise their patients when massage will be beneficial. There are many claims about the effects of massage and bodywork techniques that cannot be substantiated. Current research into alternative treatment methods will reveal the physiologic process of many of these methods. Unfortunately, the conclusive results of this research may take years to become concrete. Fortunately, there is enough existing research to support the benefits of massage. The health care community is beginning to accept the effectiveness of massage as a complement to the care they currently provide. The simple physiologic effects of massage and bodywork speak for themselves. Therapeutic massage is a labor intensive therapy that requires time to perform. Other licensed health care professionals are often too busy to do this work. Our work can be effectively done at a technician level that is more cost effective.

Licensed medical professionals need a standardized basis of training proficiency before they can routinely incorporate therapeutic massage into their team healing approaches. Currently, the medical community cannot trust the expertise level of the massage profession because of the present divergence in educational standards. A program length of 500 to 1000 hours will prepare the graduate to work effectively in general applications of therapeutic massage. This level of classroom instruction may not include enough pathology, medical terminology, evaluation skills, or specific application of methods to effectively support a medical healing team approach. Ontario and British Columbia, Canada have developed therapeutic massage as part of the health care system. Their standards of education are 2200 class hours, equivalent to a typical associates degree. Many medical technicians are trained at this level. Companion textbooks in this series will become available to the massage therapist who wishes to train to this level. Few schools at this point provide the 2200 class hours. With the development of comprehensive textbooks, more schools will be better able to expand their curriculum to those who wish to pursue the more medical approach to therapeutic massage applications.

Schools that offer training programs of 500 to 1000 hours more than adequately prepare the students for the general wellness personal service approach of therapeutic massage. Everyone can benefit from massage, not just those who are under medical care. This level of education is an entry level point for those who wish to serve the general public and provide wellness and health enhancing massage and bodywork. Courses offered of less than 500 class hours provide introductory information. In my opinion, less than 500 class hours is insufficient time to cover the necessary body of knowledge to meet the emerging educational standards as set by the introduction of the National Certification Examination for Therapeutic Massage and Bodywork.

Therapeutic application of massage (structured touch) is not a new phenomenon. Very little of the information presented in this text is the author's original creation. The foundation for therapeutic massage was laid centuries ago and will not change provided the physiology of the human being remains constant. It is virtually impossible to acknowledge everyone who has contributed to the knowledge base. Our observations of the natural world are a good starting point for this basic knowledge. For example, animals know the value of rhythmic touch. Just watch a litter of puppies and observe the structured application of touch. The base of information goes beyond us to an innate need to rub an area that is hurt and to touch others to provide comfort, pleasure, and bonding.

HOW TO USE THIS BOOK

For teaching purposes, the book may be divided into two distinct sections. The first section (Chapters 1–7) teaches the "front office" material that is important for the massage practitioner to know. The second section (Chapters 8–14) presents actual applications of massage and bodywork methods. Both sections may be taught simultaneously. Appendices include Appendix A: Contraindications To Massage, Appendix B: Resource List, Appendix C: Works Consulted (includes a specific list of recommended texts to use in conjunction with **Mosby's Fundamentals of Therapeutic Massage**), and Appendix D: Massage Terminology. As the methods and techniques of therapeutic massage and bodywork are presented, the reader will learn how and why they work and when to use them to obtain the physiologic response desired. Proficiency or Think It Over exercises are provided throughout the book to enhance the reader's learning experience.

At the beginning of each chapter is a list of objectives. This list will give you a basic outline. Where possible, illustrations are used to enhance and simplify concepts. While complex terminology is defined within the body of the text, a specific massage glossary is located in Appendix D. Each discipline has its own language; disciplines share a common language so that they can communicate most effectively. This massage terminology appendix will begin to build a multi–disciplinary communication base. Sometimes the easiest way to explain a concept is with an example or a metaphor, which is done, where appropriate, throughout the text. Review questions at the end of each chapter allow students to self-test their knowledge.

Because the profession has not reached consensus on any one term, the following words are used to describe the massage and bodywork professional: massage therapist, massage practitioner, massage technician, bodyworker, touch therapist, bodywork practitioner, bodywork therapist, myomassologist, neuromuscular therapist, and massagist. All of the above terms describe a person who uses structured touch of some type to create physiologic response in the client. The use of the terms masseuse or masseur are discouraged in the United States. These terms are still used in other countries. As an educator of therapeutic massage, I prefer the terms massage practitioner, massage therapist, massage professional, or massage technician. These terms are used interchangeably.

As the author, my intent is to make reading this textbook an enjoyable learning experience; I hope my purpose is reflected in the personal, conversational tone in which I have written the text. My personal conviction is that **Mosby's Fundamentals of Therapeutic Massage** effectively presents the information and reflects both the heart and the art of therapeutic massage. After all, "No one cares how much you know, until they know how much you care."

SANDY FRITZ
Founder, Owner, Director, & Head Instructor, Health Enrichment Center, School of Therapeutic Massage and Bodywork, Lapeer, Michigan

Wellness and Massage Therapy Consultant, Center For Anxiety, Depression, and Pain Disorders, Port Huron & Metamora, Michigan

CONTENTS

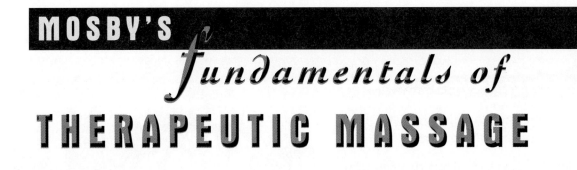

MOSBY'S *fundamentals of* THERAPEUTIC MASSAGE

CHAPTER 1

HISTORY OF MASSAGE

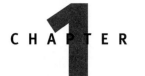

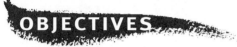

OBJECTIVES

After completing this chapter,
the student will be able to:

1 Trace the general historic progression
of massage from ancient times to
today.

2 Relate historic information to present
day events.

3 Explain the rich heritage and history of
therapeutic massage.

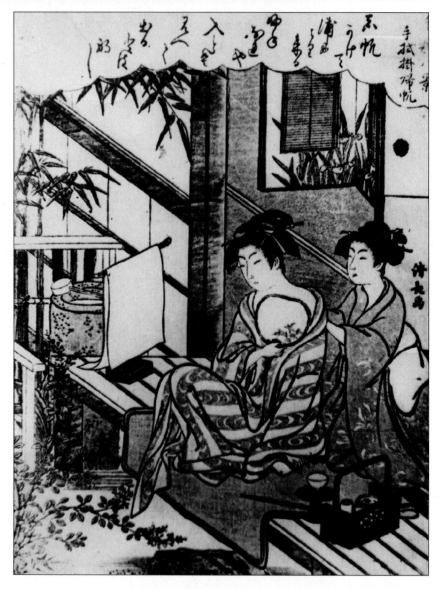

**Hygienic massage in Japan, where a massage was typically given
prior to bathing. (Bettmann Archive)**

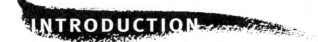

INTRODUCTION

"Why study history?" History develops professional identity. Knowledge of history helps professionals develop a sense of pride in their profession. Historic study helps a profession identify its strengths and weaknesses. If a student of massage were to obtain historic books about massage, it would be discovered that the fundamental body of knowledge has remained the same for centuries. The newest concepts in massage today were written about years ago. The history of massage is supportive and validating to the profession. Massage has stood the test of time to prove itself as a vital health enhancing and rehabilitative approach. But the history also bears a warning. The profession is at a crossroad. It has been here before and is still paying for grave mistakes that were made. As we move forward into the future, we will make mistakes as well. Let us hope someone is currently keeping a history of the profession so that fifty years from now the beginning massage professional can learn from us as well.

Numerous individuals have played an important role in compiling the historic journey of therapeutic massage and bodywork methods. Many of them are listed in Appendix C. Specific acknowledgment must be given to Richard van Why. Much of the information contained in this chapter comes from the *Bodywork Knowledgebase,* a comprehensive collection of over one hundred historic books and over four thousand research and journal articles on therapeutic massage and related modalities. If it were not for his mission, much of the history of massage would be scattered in research libraries and unknown to us today. Another who deserves mention is Fran Tappan, a true master of massage. Not only has she written respected textbooks about massage that include a historic perspective, she is a part of that history.

This chapter consolidates the historic information. Because of extensive overlapping between the references used, text citation has been kept to a minimum. With gratitude and respect to those who have devoted their lives to this work, many who are mentioned and many more who are not, let us begin the journey forward by looking to the past.

MASSAGE HISTORY

Animal behavior indicates through the application of pressure, rubbing, or licking that massage is used somewhat instinctively to either relieve pain or respond to injury. Massage probably began when cave dwellers

Box 1.1 MASSAGE	The word massage is thought to be derived from several different sources. The Latin root *massa* and Greek roots *massein* or *masso* mean to touch, handle, squeeze, or to knead. The French verb *masser* also means to knead. The Arabic root *mass* or *mass'h* and the Sanskrit root *makeh* translate to "press softly."

rubbed their bruises.[5] Massage is one of the most natural and instinctive means of relieving pain and discomfort. When a person has sore, aching muscles, abdominal pains, or a bruise or wound, it is an instinctive impulse to touch and rub that part of the body to obtain relief.

Touch as a method of healing appears to have developed from multiple cultural origins. Therapeutic massage has strong roots in Chinese folk medicine. It has many aspects in common with other healing traditions, such as Indian herbal medicine and Persian medicine. It is believed that the art of massage was first mentioned in writing about 2000 B.C.,[5] and has been written about extensively in books since about 500 B.C. Egyptian, Persian, and Japanese historic medical literature are full of references to massage. Hippocrates advocated massage and gymnastic exercise. Asclepiades, another eminent Greek physician, relied exclusively on massage.

Throughout history, many different systems and supporting theories for the management of musculoskeletal pain and dysfunction have come and gone. Scientific research has changed the philosophy of massage theory. Current ongoing research will continue to define the physical effects of therapeutic massage application. The scientific thinking of the day has provided the validation for massage. The endurance of massage throughout the years has been amazing. Current trends seem to suggest the increasing popularity of massage and body related therapies used for stress reduction, and chronic musculoskeletal problems. For more information see Chapter 6.

Massage has been considered an important part of manual medicine. Manual medicine has always been a part of the art of medicine and consists of the use of the hands in treatment of injury and disease. Its therapeutic value is gained from changes in soft tissue and structure, as opposed to surgery and pharmaceuticals.[3] Massage can be considered a part of manual medicine and throughout history has stood independently to promote health. Manual medicine has grown today to become the foundation for osteopathy, chiropractic, and physical therapy.[1]

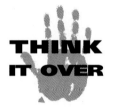

THINK IT OVER

1. **If you were going to rename massage, what would you call it?**
2. **If touch is so instinctive, why do you have to go to school to learn to do it?**
3. **Why do you think every culture has had some form of massage?**
4. **What do you think is the difference between massage and manual medicine?**

Ancient Times

According to research reports, most ancient cultures, practiced some form of healing touch. Often a ceremonial leader such as a healer, priest, or shaman was selected to perform the healing rituals. The healing methods often incorporated the use of herbs, oils, and primitive forms of hydrotherapy. Archaeologists have found many prehistoric artifacts depicting massage for healing and cosmetic purposes. It is speculated that massage was used for pain relief which incorporated concepts of counter-irritation and scraping, cutting, and burning of the skin as part of the process. Massage may have been used as a cleansing procedure along with fasting and bathing in preparation for many tribal rituals.

Massage in China has been known by two different names: *Anmo,* the more ancient name that means press-rub, and *Tui-na,* of more recent origin that means push-pull. The Chinese methods were administered by kneading or rubbing down the entire body with the hands and using a gentle pressure and traction on all the joints.[7]

The practice of acupuncture involved the stimulation of specific points along the body, usually by the insertion of tiny, solid needles, but

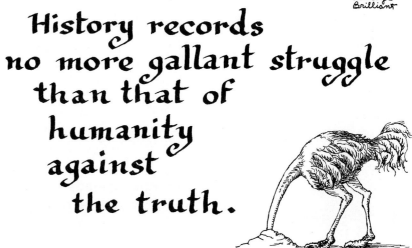

Ashleigh
Brilliant

History records
no more gallant struggle
than that of
humanity
against
the truth.

©BRILLIANT ENTERPRISES 1975.

massage and other forms of pressure were also used. Such practices were
also found in traditional Eskimo and African medicine, where sharp
stones were used to scratch the skin's surface. Today the scientific community is able to provide physiologic reasons for the value of these ancient
practices, which will be discussed in future chapters.

Knowledge of massage and its applications were already well established in medicine at the time of the Sui Dynasty, 589–617 A.D. The
Japanese came to know massage through the writings of the Chinese. The
Egyptians left art work showing foot massage. Before the Greeks took part
in the Olympic games they received friction, anointing, and rubbing with
sand. The use of touch as a mode of healing was recorded in the writings
of the Hebrew and Christian traditions. The "laying on of hands" was particularly prominent in first-century Christianity. Full body massage with
oils (anointing) goes back even further in Jewish practices. The ancient
Jews practiced anointing for its ritual, hygienic, and therapeutic benefits.
The Jewish culture honored rubbing with oils to such an extent that the
root word for rubbing with oils and for the Messiah are the same.[7] The
ancient Mayan people of Central America, the Incas of South America,
and other native people of the American continent also used methods of
joint manipulation and massage. Massage has been a part of life in India
for almost three thousand years. The Chinese introduced the methods
during trade. Like Chinese acupuncture, Hatha yoga, developed in India
with its energetic concepts of prana, chakras, and humoral balances, has
reappeared in modern forms of body therapy.

Hippocrates of Cos lived 460–377 B.C. (Fig. 1.1). He was the first in
Greek medicine to specifically describe the medical benefits of anointing and massage and the chemical properties of oils used for this purpose. He called his art *anatripsis*, which meant to rub up. Of this art he
said, "The physician must be acquainted with many things and assuredly
with anatripsis, for things that have the same name have not always the
same effects, for rubbing can bind a joint that is too loose or loosen a
joint that is too hard."[7] The Hippocratic method survived, virtually
unchanged, well into the Middle Ages. Many techniques, especially traction and stretching principles, are still being used today.[1]

Claudius Galenus, or Galen, a Greek physician who lived in the years
129–199 A.D., contributed much written material on early manual medicine, including many commentaries on Hippocrates.[1]

Massage came to the Romans from the Greeks. Julius Caesar, 100–44

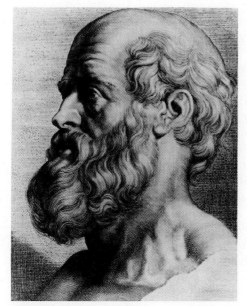

Figure 1.1
**Hippocrates. (From Donahue MP:
Nursing, the finest art—an illustrated
history, St. Louis, 1985, The CV
Mosby Co.)**

History of Massage **5**

B.C., had himself "pinched all over" daily for the relief of his neuralgia and for the prevention of epileptic attacks.[5] Aulus Cornelius Celsus was a native Roman physician who lived from 25 B.C.–50 A.D. He is credited with compiling *De Medicina,* a series of eight books covering the body of medical knowledge of the day. Seven of the books deal extensively with prevention and therapeutics using rubbing, exercise, bathing, and anointing.

This work was rediscovered during the late Middle Ages by Pope Nicholas V, 1397–1455 A.D. In 1478 *De Medicina* was one of the first medical textbooks to be published using the newly invented Guttenburg printing press. It was one of most popular medical textbooks during the Renaissance.

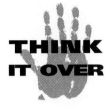

THINK IT OVER

- **Why do you think ancient people started sticking things into the skin and scratching the skin to produce healing?**

Middle Ages

Massage developed differently in the East and the West. In the East, as part of the Islamic Empire, it represented a continuation of Greco-Roman traditions. In the West, the Greco-Roman traditions disappeared, and massage was kept alive by ordinary people, to become a part of folk culture. Massage formed an important part of the healing tradition of the Slavs, Finns, and Swedes. As massage integrated with the health practices of the common people, it was often associated with supernatural experience and observances. This application alienated massage from what little scientific approach there was during this time. Practitioners of folk medicine were often objects of persecution, with the church claiming that the practitioner's healing powers were from the devil.[7]

It was not until the 16th century that one of the founders of modern surgery, Frenchman Ambrose Paré (1517–1590), began to use massage techniques again for joint stiffness and wound healing after surgery. Paré described three types of massage strokes: gentle, medium, and vigorous. His ideas were passed down to other French physicians who believed in the value of manual therapeutics.

The Nineteenth Century

Per Henrik Ling (1776–1839) is given credit for the development of Swedish massage, but it is important to realize that he did not invent it. He learned massage and, through persistent experimentation, put the information together in a workable form. The French terms *effleurage, petrissage, and tapotement* are not from Ling. Dr. John Mezger's followers from Holland began to use these names; the historic references used do not explain why French terms were chosen. So often history is confused, and who deserves credit for what becomes cloudy.[6]

Per Henrik Ling proposed an integrated program consisting of active and passive movements and massage for the treatment of disease. Legend has it that Ling's interest started when he had gout in the elbow. He developed a system of massage that used many of the positions and movements of Swedish gymnastics. By combining these strokes with exercises, he successfully healed his diseased elbow. This system was based on the newly discovered knowledge of the circulation of the blood and lymph. (It is interesting to note that the Chinese had been using these methods for centuries.) While teaching fencing, Ling observed that habitual movements interfered with the development of desired movements. Development of a skill depended on mental mastery of habit, so he began teaching bodily movements systematically. He developed his medical gymnastics in 1814, but was bitterly opposed by the Swedish medical establishment for almost twenty years. He was not trained in medicine, and his tendency to use poetic and mystic language in his writings on gymnastics was thought to intefere with wider acceptance of his ideas.[7] Current experts in massage would be wise to take notice of Ling's experience. It is essential that massage be explained in the medical and scientific terminology of the day.

With the support of influential clients, Ling was granted a license to practice and teach his method, establishing the Royal Gymnastic Central Institute. The primary focus of Ling's system, especially in his later writings, was on gymnastics applied to the treatment of disease. This position was a big shift from his earlier educational and military gymnastics, which were only appropriate for healthy people. He divided movements into active, duplicated, and passive forms. Active movements were performed by the person's own effort and correspond to what is commonly called exercise. Duplicated movements were performed by the person with the cooperation of a gymnast (therapist) and involved active effort by both parties, in which the action of the one was opposed by the action of the other. They correspond to what today is commonly called resistive exercise. Passive movements were performed for the person by active effort of the gymnast alone. They consist of passive movements of the extremities, what we today call range of motion and stretching. Movement therapy did not artificially separate massage from other kinds of movements that were considered integral to the system.

Ling taught many physicians from Germany, Austria, Russia, and England who later spread his teachings to their own native lands. Ling was recognized by his contemporaries and later followers not so much as a great innovator, but as a keen observer who adopted methods after testing them for effectiveness. He combined techniques from many times and places into one coherent system. Ling's teachings endured because he developed a school to continue teaching medical gymnastics, the Swedish Movement Cure as it became known in the United States in the late nineteenth century. By Ling's death in 1839, his system had obtained worldwide recognition.[7]

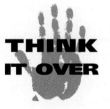

THINK IT OVER

1. **Why do you think massage developed so differently in the Eastern countries and in Europe?**
2. **Why do you think the development of a school by Ling was so important?**

Per Henrik Ling and others practicing the Swedish Movement Cure deserve the credit for the second modern revival of massage. Initially, nonprofessionals spoke to physicians in a language they did not share, making communication difficult. Later, when physicians talked to other physicians about massage, its popularity began to grow. They sought commonalities between their methods and others used throughout history, both to justify their current view of massage and to expand it. Lay magazines and medical journals published manuscripts. The successful experience and testimony of distinguished people, especially monarchs and diplomats, further bolstered the image of massage and increased public and medical acceptance. Many physicians were drawn to study massage because they had a strong scientific bent. They conducted animal studies and well-designed clinical trials, which further persuaded physicians of the value of the method and increased their interest. **This is the same situation massage is experiencing during the 1990s.** (See the works of Tiffany Field at the Touch Research Institute at the University of Miami Medical School and current studies being conducted with grants from the National Institutes of Health.) In America, the first waves of European immigration were from Northern Europe, which had earlier accepted massage because of its therapeutic benefits. The immigrants provided many great writers and teachers of massage, and they made eager, trusting patients.[7]

The Swedish Movement Cure quickly spread to the other countries of Europe, and the first institute outside Sweden was established in Denmark. In 1837, two years before Ling's death, his disciple M. LeRon brought the Movement Cure to Russia. He established a clinic in St. Petersburg. It was Charles Fayette Taylor and George Henry Taylor, two brothers, who introduced the Swedish Movements to the United States in 1856. They learned the skill from the English physician, Mathias Roth, who studied directly with Ling. Roth was also a leader in the homeopathic movement and felt that massage worked with the same principles as homeopathy: the law of similars and the concept of "like cures like."

Women also made early and important contributions to the development of massage and medical gymnastics, primarily in the United States. Two women conducted the first controlled clinical trial of the benefits of massage in the management of disease. Mary Putnam Jacobi and Victoria A. White were medical doctors and professors of medicine in New York City in 1880. Their research addressed the benefits of massage and ice packs in the management of anemia. Contemporary history has been influenced extensively by women, and a majority of practicing massage professionals today are women. Eunice Ingham formalized the system of reflexology. Dr. Janet Travell's work with myofascial pain and trigger points is unsurpassed. Bonnie Prudden popularized trigger point work. Fran Tappen's contributions to massage and physical therapy are outstanding and formalized in her text, *Healing Massage Techniques*. Sister Kenny used massage in the treatment of polio. Ida Rolf's massage system grew to become *rolfing*. Dr. Dolores Krieger has made major contributions to the more energetic approaches through her system of therapeutic touch. Because of the extensive influence of women in massage today, it is likely that when this history is written again in twenty years, many women will be listed as vital contributors to the continued development of massage.

John Harvey Kellogg, (1852–1943), founder of the Battle Creek Sanatorium, wrote dozens of articles and two textbooks on massage and hydrotherapy and edited and published a popular magazine, *Good Health*.

In 1879, Douglas Graham, in his history of massage, described the Lomi-Lomi of the Hawaiians as a hygienic measure for the relief of fatigue or for its pure pleasure. In 1889, a letter from a doctor in Kansas appeared in a New York medical journal, saying that he thought massage was but a "novel method of therapeutics" until he read a passage from Captain James Cook's diary of his third voyage around the world near the end of the eighteenth century. In it, Cook described how his pseudosciatic pain was relieved in an elegant and generous ritual by a Tahitian chief and his family, using a method called *romee*.

Dr. Johann Mezger (1839–1909) of Holland is given credit for bringing massage to the scientific community. He presented massage to fellow physicians as a form of medical treatment.

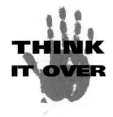

THINK IT OVER

1. **What could have helped the nonmedical massage professionals speak more effectively to the medical establishment?**
2. **How is massage a "like cures like" system?**
3. **Why do you think women are playing such prominent roles in the current development of massage?**
4. **What did Kellogg's interest in cereal and massage have in common?**

Massage was, in a very real sense, a victim of its own success. In 1886, Charles K. Mills, a prominent neurologist and massage advocate in

Philadelphia, levied sharp criticism concerning the uneven quality of lay practitioners of massage and the often unsubstantiated and unethical claims made by them. In 1889, British physicians, who were just beginning to favorably acknowledge massage because Queen Victoria supported the methods, became increasingly aware of patterns of abuse including false claims made about lay practitioners' education or skills, patient stealing, and charging high fees.

It was the massage scandals of 1894, revealed by a commission of inquiry of the British Medical Association in the British Medical Journal, which eroded the public and the medical profession's confidence in massage as a legitimate medical art during the late nineteenth century.

An inconsistent system of education included private trade schools, hospitals, and physicians who took on private students. Courses in technique, anatomy, physiology, and pathology varied immensely, as well as the experience levels and capacity of teachers. Some proposed they could teach with minimal training in massage or directly after graduation from programs of questionable quality. Students were often presented with grand expectations of career opportunities only to find a difficult job market in which many were insufficiently trained to compete.

According to Richard van Why, "many schools used improper student recruitment tactics. The worst involved young women from poor neighborhoods who were approached by recruiters claiming that extraordinary career opportunities awaited masseuses or medical gymnasts upon graduation from schools of professional training. The recruiters offered to defer payment of tuition until a reasonable time had elapsed after their graduation—so that the women could build resources to pay their living expenses and still pay the loans back. They were typically trained in short programs and then were released to a marketplace full of competent and incompetent lay practitioners. As they found no work, they could not pay the loans back. Soon the recruiters returned demanding payment. The women were told that if they did not pay, they would be thrown into debtors' prison until they did. To work off the debt, they would have to work at a clinic attached to the school or for a friend or a colleague of a school administrator. The best of these 'clinics' offered incompetently performed classical massage. The worst of the 'clinics' were pretexts for houses of prostitution. In the scandals that followed in British cities, in Chicago and New York City the 'massage parlor' caught on and the lay practice of massage became associated with vice.

Another notorious abuse concerned 'certification,' which some physician-advocates of massage considered merely a 'receipt for money paid.'

Still another concerned advertising. The medical profession and the well-trained, classical lay practitioners of massage and medical gymnastics, such as those trained at the Royal Central Gymnastics Institute, would not advertise false claims. On the other hand, many entrepreneurs and poor massagists were seeking publicity to increase the enrollment at their schools and the attendance at their clinics. Their claims flew in the face of anatomy, physiology, and pathology.

In 1894, the same year that the massage scandals were revealed in Britain, eight women who envisioned 'well-trained, properly equipped masseuses serving those in need,' formed the Society of Trained Masseuses. Before this time the quality of lay practitioners of massage was inconsistent. The founders recognized the need for rigorous standards and modeled theirs after the medical profession. They set academic prerequisites to the study of massage. Training could only be carried out in recognized schools, which were to be regularly inspected to ensure those standards were maintained. Only qualified instructors could teach classes. Examinations for teachers and graduates of basic massage training were conducted by a board, which included a physician. Examinations were to be both written and a demonstration of clinical achievement.

Problems occurred within the Society during a period of sustained growth, and another competing association was established, which weakened both of them. In 1920, the Society assembled an advisory committee to aid reorganization and reconcile the opposing parties. The two groups joined as the Chartered Society of Massage and Medical Gymnastics. In 1909, before the reorganization, the Society had six hundred members, but by 1939 membership had grown to twelve thousand. Certificates of competence were granted to persons who had passed rigorous examination. To be admitted to the association, members had to pledge not to accept patients except as referred by physicians. They were forbidden from advertising in the lay press. Members aimed to provide a Central Registry of well-trained massage practitioners and to provide referrals to inquiries from the medical profession or the lay public, based on where they lived and any special needs they had. Membership in the association was voluntary, and many ill-trained, unscrupulous practitioners continued to thrive.

Even during this difficult time, massage endured. Institutes of massage appeared in France, Germany, and Austria by the mid-nineteenth century. Between 1854 and 1918, the practice of massage developed from an obscure, unskilled trade to a field of medical health care, from which the profession of physical therapy began. Treatments consisted of massage, mineral baths, and exercise."[7]

Dr. David Gurevich, a Russian medical doctor and instructor of Russian medical massage, believes that the longstanding interest in massage and its constant developments are strong proof of its usefulness and necessity.[4] Dr. Gurevich teaches that in Russia, massage was practiced by ancient Slavic tribes, especially in combination with therapeutic bathing. Beginning in the eighteenth century, many great Russian scientists and doctors (Mudroff, Manasein, Botkin, Zakharin, and others) contributed to the development of the theory and practice of massage. I.Z. Zabludovski wrote more than one hundred books, texts, and scientific articles devoted to the methods of massage and its physiologic basis in therapy, postsurgery, and sports. An institute of massage and exercise was founded in Russia at the end of the past century. At the same time, many courses of massage were started in Russia. Massage gradually progressed from being an auxiliary method of therapy to becoming an independent therapeutic method that was used effectively with other modalities. The practice of massage in Russia is widespread. A massage room is found in all therapy clinics. Massage in conjunction with therapeutic exercises is adapted for the management of the viscera, the nervous system, gynecologic disorders, orthopedics, traumatology, and postsurgery. To be a student of massage, it is necessary to have some medical education. Currently, the recent changes in Russia's economy to a market system have made it possible for private massage clinics, which charge a fee, to open.[4]

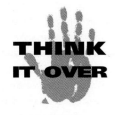

THINK IT OVER

1. **How is the success of massage today similar to the success of massage in the late 1800s?**
2. **Is it possible that an unfortunate repeat of the history of massage is happening today?**
3. **What specific current trends can be cited to support abuse and misrepresentation of massage today?**
4. **What can the profession do today to avoid a downfall similar to that which occurred in the 1800s?**

5. **In order to be a valid and respectable profession, must massage align itself with the medical community or are there other possibilities?**
6. **Why did these problems not occur in Russia? Could they begin to happen now?**

The Twentieth Century

Dr. James B. Mennell divided the effects of massage into two categories: mechanical and reflex actions. Mennell showed that massage exerts a mechanical effect in the following four ways:

1. Helping in venous return of blood to the heart
2. Aiding lymph movement out of the tissues
3. Stretching of the connective tissue (e.g., tendons, scar tissue, etc.)
4. Mechanical stimulation of the stomach, small intestine, and colon.

Mennell also maintained that certain forms of tactile stimulation (e.g., stroking, light touch, etc.) stimulated reflex arcs, causing muscles to relax or contract according to the type of stroke applied. He proposed that both smooth and skeletal muscles were under the control of such reflexes. The mechanical and reflex effects of massage that Ling, Mennell, and others observed are now supported by experimental research.

Sigmund Freud, 1856–1939, an Austrian neurologist and theorist who developed psychoanalysis, experimented with the use of massage in the treatment of hysteria, a form of mental illness common in his day. This condition is characterized by paralysis without physiologic basis. His *Studies on Hysteria*, published in 1895, explained his methods. Wilhelm Reich, an Austrian psychoanalyst, was a clinical assistant to Freud for six years. He became interested in the physiologic basis of neurosis. By the late 1920s, his radical and controversial theories concerning sexuality led to his separation from Freud. In 1934, Reich settled in the United States. He is considered by many to be the founder of psychotherapeutic body techniques. Gradually he moved the emphasis of his therapeutic approach away from the psychological and toward the realm of the physical body. Reich developed many somato-techniques to dissolve the muscular armor. He came into conflict with the medical establishment and was eventually investigated by the U.S. Food and Drug Administration. Prosecuted and convicted for fraudulent medical practices, in 1957, Reich died while serving his sentence in federal prison.

Reich's earlier ideas and therapy have greatly influenced contemporary bodywork. A popular somatotherapy that evolved directly from his system is *bioenergetics*. Bioenergetics was founded by Alexander Lowen, an American psychiatrist and a student of Reich's for twelve years.

In early 1900s, polarity therapy was created by an American physician, Randolph Stone. Stone studied many body systems, both ancient and modern: acupuncture, hatha yoga, osteopathy, chiropractic techniques, and reflexology. From his investigations, he concluded that a "magnetic field" regulated and directed the physiological systems of the body. Influenced by Eastern philosophy and medicine, Stone believed all aspects of the universe were expressed in opposite poles (e.g., male-female, positive and negative electric charges, etc.), so he called his therapeutic method "polarity."

Douglas Graham, an important contributor to literature of the nineteenth century, continued to write on massage and its use in almost every area of medicine until his death near the end of the 1920s. In 1907, Edgar Ferdinand Cyriax began a distinguished publishing career that spanned almost forty years. He was the last great proponent of Ling's Swedish movement cure, which he called mechanotherapeutics.

It was during the turn of the century that the United States and England looked to Japan for an innovation in the vocational rehabilitation of the blind. The British Institute for Massage by the Blind was established in 1900. Other nations of Europe tried to develop their own models of the Japanese and the British institutions, but they failed.

Albert Hoffa's text, published in 1900 and later revised by Max Bohm in 1913, represents the more classical massage techniques such as *effleurage, petrissage, tapotement,* and vibration. Most therapists learn these as standard massage techniques in entry-level programs. Some may disregard this type of massage, viewing it as too basic to be included in the realm of advanced manual therapy, but leaving behind traditional massage techniques can handicap even the most advanced manual therapists. Remember, it is not possible to replace the fundamentals.

The polio epidemic of 1918 renewed interest in massage, as any remedy that offered any promise at all was desperately craved. Research on the benefits of massage in the prevention of the complications of paralysis began during this time. Sister Kenny contributed extensively to the use of massage in the treatment of polio. Connective tissue massage (CTM) was developed in the 1920s by German physiotherapist Elizabeth Dicke and later expanded by Maria Ebner. CTM was first used when Dicke was suffering from a prolonged illness caused by an "impairment of the circulation" in her right leg. As with Ling, her search for self-healing added much to the development of massage.

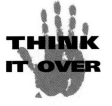

THINK IT OVER

1. **This text is only able to briefly mention names of so many important people who contributed to massage. How could you find out more about each of these people?**
2. **Why do you think people may discount the fundamental methods of massage in favor of more "advanced techniques"?**
3. **How large a part do you think exploration of self-healing played in the lives of those who made great contributions to the development of massage?**

Broad licensing for physical therapy began in the early 1940s. Louise L. Despard's book was one of a handful of textbooks about massage that was recommended as essential reading for all students of massage by the Massage Round Table of the American Physical Therapy Association in 1940. Mary McMillan was an English lay practitioner of massage who wrote an influential textbook, *Massage and Therapeutic Exercise,* in 1932. Her experience in the field was extensive. From 1911–1915, she was in charge of massage and therapeutic exercise at the Greenbank Cripple's Home in Liverpool, England, and from 1916–1918, McMillan served as Director of Massage and Remedial Gymnastics at the Children's Hospital in Portland, Maine. During World War I, she served in the military as a rehabilitation aide.[5]

After the war, Emil Vodder, a Danish physiologist, developed a technique of light massage along the course of the surface lymphatics, which he called *lymph drainage* or *manual lymphatic drainage.* It was and still is used to treat chronic lymphedema and other diseases of the lymphatic and peripheral vascular systems.

In 1943 in Chicago, The American Association of Masseurs and Masseuses was formed, subsequently to be renamed the American Massage Therapy Association. Later another professional organization, the International Myomassetics Federation, was formed through the efforts of noteworthy massage instructor Irene Gauthier and others.

James Henry Cyriax, son of Edgar Ferdinand Cyriax, became an orthopedic surgeon at St. Thomas' Hospital, a prestigious teaching institution in London. He gained fame through his development of transverse friction massage. In the late 1940s and early 1950s, Cyriax published the first edition of his now classic *Textbook of Orthopedic Medicine*. His work is of special significance in the area of massage because of its recognition, categorization, and differential diagnosis of the body's soft tissues. The fact that pain could be caused by dysfunction of soft tissues, including, but not limited to, periarticular connective tissue, is the foundation of soft-tissue manipulation today. Cyriax was also the first to introduce the concept of "end feel" in the diagnosis of soft-tissue lesions.

Dr. Herman Kabat researched neuromuscular concepts based on the work of neurophysiologists and Pavlov's conditioning of reflexes. Sherrington's law of successive induction provided the foundation for the development of rhythmic stabilization and slow reversal techniques. By 1951, research began on a new method, which was formalized in 1956 when Margaret Knott and Dorothy Voss wrote the book *Proprioceptive Neuromuscular Facilitation*. For more information see Chapter 10.

Francis Tappan and Gertrude Beard also wrote important articles and books on massage techniques during this time. Both texts are still available, and the serious student of massage would benefit from reading these classic works. As of this writing, Fran Tappan continues to influence the profession of massage in interviews, think tanks about the future of massage, and personal interaction with many leaders in the field. She has been honored by the American Massage Therapy Association for her contributions to massage.

The most recent revival of massage began around 1960 and has continued to this day. There has been increasing recognition of persistent, chronic diseases resistant to treatment by surgical and drug therapy. Neither the acute-care concept nor a single solution approach seems to work with these cases. A more complex way of envisioning and treating these diseases has had to be developed, and massage is one approach that has proven itself effective over time.

The humanistic movement that began during the 1960s spilled over into medicine and allied health. Issues about "bedside manner," "genuineness," and the benefits of touch again raised the issue of the legitimacy and value of massage for its psychic use alone. Later, the Esalen movement and Gestalt psychology inspired psychologists and psychotherapists to explore massage and other movement therapies. Many controlled clinical studies in medicine, nursing, physical therapy, and psychology inspired more academic and clinical interest.

Increased medical awareness that lack of exercise contributed to cardiovascular and other diseases led to an emphasis on physical fitness by President John F. Kennedy, beginning in 1960. This new interest grew into the physical fitness movement of the late 1960s, and led the health sciences into a movement toward preventive medicine. The benefits of sports were again discovered, and with them historic literature such as Albert Baumgartner's book *Massage in Athletics*, which discussed the relationship between massage and exercise and the value of massage in conditioning and stress control, was brought to light.

Acupressure received more attention during the 1970s and 1980s than any other bodywork modality. It was examined closely in the medical, physical therapy, and nursing literature internationally by controlled clinical trials. In the writings of nursing and rehabilitation medicine, a body of knowledge arose concerning the benefits of massage in the prevention and treatment of decubitus ulcer and in the overall management of heart rate and blood pressure in persons suffering from acute and chronic manifestations of cardiovascular disease.[7]

Again Richard van Why states: "It was in the field of pain research and pain management that the greatest gains for massage were made. Ronald Melzack, a professor of psychology in the anesthesiology department of the McGill University Medical School, and one of the initial proponents of the Gate Control Theory of Pain, published the results of several controlled clinical trials on the value of ice massage and manual massage for the relief of dental pain and low back pain. Not only were these techniques effective in preventing or reducing pain, but he proposed . . . the neural mechanisms by which they operated. Other researchers picked up on this theme and began to examine the role of massage in the liberation of endorphins, pain killing chemicals more potent than morphine and produced by the brain in response to certain stimuli, including massage. In the late 1980s Melzack proposed a theory to explain this endorphin release in the prestigious journal, *Clinics in Anesthesiology*. His theory of hyperstimulation analgesia was the first in recent decades inspired by findings concerning massage. It argued that certain intense sensory stimuli, like puncturing with a needle and exposure to extreme cold or pressure when applied near the site of an injury, sent a signal to the brain by a faster channel than the pain signal it was attempting to treat, and this signal disrupted the pain."[7] Maybe this is why ancient man scratched themselves with stones.

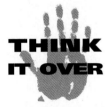

THINK IT OVER

1. **Was it inevitable that massage would split from the medical community? Do you think that this division was a good idea?**
2. **Was it possible that some massage practitioners left the tradition of natural healing to enter the medical establishment? Why would this be a possibility?**
3. **How would you classify the difference between medical massage and fitness and personal service massage?**

CURRENT APPROACHES

Modern theories and systems can be arranged into three categories: autonomic or reflexive approaches, mechanical approaches, and movement approaches. Autonomic or reflexive approaches are those that exert their therapeutic effect on the autonomic and somatic nervous system. Mechanical approaches are those that actually attempt mechanical changes in the soft tissue by direct application of force. Movement approaches are those that attempt to change abnormal movement patterns and establish more optimal ones. Ideally, the massage therapist should have a basic working knowledge of the theories or systems in all three areas, along with some application of technique from each approach. This textbook will develop these categories of massage. The student of massage will want to pay attention to Appendix C. Further study would include reading these resources.

Three areas in osteopathic medicine that are currently applicable to massage are muscle energy techniques, positional release and strain/counterstrain techniques, and neuromuscular techniques. The most noteworthy educator and author for these methods is Dr. Leon Chaitow. Dr. Chaitow emulates Ling because he is a master synthesizer of the best of many concepts. He developed a strong foundation in manual medicine working as an assistant to his uncle, Boris Chaitow, the codeveloper of neuromuscular technique with his cousin, the legendary Stanley Lief, D.C., D.O., N.D.[2] Dr.

Leon Chaitow has written many books including *Acupuncture Treatment of Pain, Soft Tissue Manipulation,* and *Palpatory Literacy.*

Other authors worthy of mention are Ida Rolf, developer of rolfing, Milton Trager, M.D., developer of Trager (®), and Dr. Janet Travell, coauthor with David Simons of the most comprehensive texts written on the subject, *Myofascial Pain and Dysfunction: The Trigger Point Manual* and *Myofascial Pain and Dysfunction: The Trigger Point Manual: The Lower Extremities,* vol 2.

Richard van Why, the developer of the *Bodywork Knowledgebase* and a prolific writer on the history of massage, deserves extraordinary credit for his work in compiling and preserving the history and research of massage. The task of compiling the *Bodywork Knowledgebase* is most likely the most important contribution to massage history in the 1990s and, without it, this textbook chapter could not have been written so efficiently.

More professional organizations have formed to establish affiliation for specific forms of bodywork. In the late 1980s, the professional organization Associated Bodywork and Massage Professionals formed to serve the needs of a growing and diverse group of bodywork therapists. It is likely that more professional organizations will form in the future.

In 1988, a proposal was spearheaded by the American Massage Therapy Association for the development of a national certification process. This proposal stirred much controversy and was hotly debated. With participation from other professional massage and bodywork sources, the National Certification Examination for Therapeutic Massage and Bodywork was created in 1992.

More states have begun to license massage, and at this point an average of five hundred hours of education is required to practice massage. European and Canadian standards vary from little or no training of massage to extensive education requirements. The University of Westminster in England offers bachelor and master degrees in massage and bodywork. This program was been developed by Dr. Patrick Peitroni, Dr. Leon Chaitow, and others. The ever increasing exchange of information from Russia, other post-Soviet Union countries, China, and other eastern countries will enrich the knowledge base for therapeutic massage.

It is likely that the Canadian provinces of British Columbia and Ontario will become the model for medical and rehabilitative massage. The educational requirements are more than twenty-two hundred class hours and focus at an educational level similar to a typical two-year allied health associate degree.

For those who have experienced this last revival of massage, the success carries with it mixed blessings. The credibility and acceptance for natural approaches to health and illness are developing, but controversy lies in the path of the profession. What the future will bring depends on our commitment to the ideals of massage.

THE FUTURE

Where the profession is headed is discussed in Chapters 2 and 6; these chapters continue the story of therapeutic massage. The future of massage hopefully will reveal that the ancient foundation and dependency on manual methods, including massage, was a valid health approach. The abundance of massage therapies will combine into a consolidated system of therapeutic massage, and the wisdom of an old Russian doctor who says "massage is massage" will bring validity and recognition to this health service.

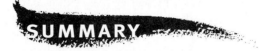

SUMMARY

As the massage profession moves forward and reclaims its heritage as an important health service, it is important to look back. In retrospect we can see the strengths and weaknesses of the professional journey. It is also important to honor those that have dedicated so much of their lives to the development of the body of knowledge of therapeutic massage. There are many today who are dedicating a significant portion of their lives for the professional advancement of therapeutic massage. When the history is written again, these names will appear along with the information they have organized and contributed. Realize that all of us are contributors to the future of massage and will become a part of its history.

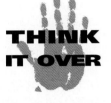

THINK IT OVER

1. **What do you want the future of massage to bring?**
2. **How are you going to assist in the development of that future?**

REVIEW QUESTIONS

1. How and where did massage originate? Why is this answer important?
2. What has provided the validation for massage?
3. What methods did the ancient Chinese massage system consist of? How are the methods of today different?
4. Why was massage associated with folk medicine and connected with supernatural experience during the Middle Ages in Europe?
5. Why is credit given to Per Henrik Ling for the development of the Swedish movement cure and Swedish massage?
6. How did problems with terminology interfere with the acceptance of Ling's work?
7. Who or what was one of the main contributors to the massage scandals in the late 1800s?
8. What aspect of massage remained active outside the medical establishment during the 1940s through to the present?
9. What research has provided the current validation for massage today?
10. How has massage brought the best of the East and West together?

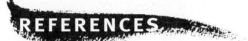

REFERENCES

1. Cantu RI and Grodin AJ: *Myofascial manipulation theory and clinical application,* Gaithersberg, Md, 1992, Aspen Publishers, Inc.
2. Chaitow L: *Soft tissue manipulation,* Rochester, Vt, 1988, Healing Arts Press.
3. Greenman PE: *Principles of manual medicine,* Baltimore, 1989, Williams and Wilkins.
4. Gurevich D: *Historical perspective,* unpublished article, 1992.
5. Tappan FM: *Healing massage techniques, holistic, classic, and emerging methods,* ed 2, Norwalk, Ct, 1988, Appleton and Lange.
6. van Why RP: *History of massage and its relevance to today's practitioner.* The bodywork knowledgebase, New York, 1992, self-published.
7. van Why RP: *Notes toward a history of massage,* ed 2, The bodywork knowledgebase, New York, 1992, self-published.

CHAPTER 2

PROFESSIONAL AND LEGAL
ISSUES

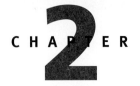

OBJECTIVES

After completing this chapter, the student will be able to:

1 Define *therapeutic massage.*

2 Define a scope of practice for therapeutic massage.

3 Develop and explain a code of ethics for *therapeutic massage.*

4 Identify legal credentialing concerns of the massage professional.

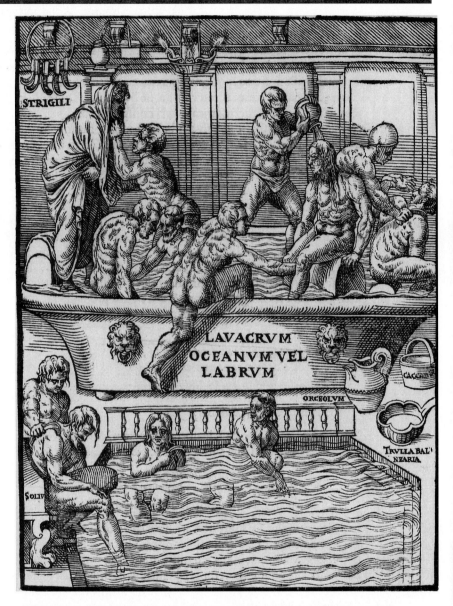

Athletic conditioning in the Roman bath, where athletes used devices called strigili to annoint themselves with oil preceding their massage. The massage aimed to stimulate circulation, cleanse the body and scrape remaining oil, dirt and dead skin from the body. (Courtesy of Brown University Library)

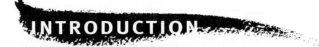

INTRODUCTION

Professional development is concerned with the definition of massage, the scope of practice, ethical conduct and standards, and credentialing, licensing, and other legal concerns of the massage professional. These issues provide the structure of any profession. The student of massage therapy needs to know what therapeutic massage is, the types of professional services a massage practitioner can legally and ethically provide, and guidelines for conduct in the professional setting. This chapter will provide the information to encourage a student to develop a standard of professionalism essential to a successful therapeutic massage practice.

ETHICS

Ethics is the discipline concerned with right and wrong conduct. It involves morals and making choices or judgments about what should or should not be done. An ethical person behaves and acts in the right way. But what is the right way?

Professional organizations create codes of ethics to serve as guidelines for respectable behavior in their profession. The code consists of rules or principles of conduct that the group members follow. In addition to standardized codes of conduct, it is important for each individual to develop a personal code of professional ethics.

One of the first things that needs to be defined in such a project is the definition and **scope of practice** for the profession. A definition includes what a professional does; a scope of practice expands on a definition to specify where, when, and how the defined professional can apply the skills.

WHAT'S IN A NAME

SECTION OBJECTIVES

Using the information presented in this section the student will be able to:

1 Explain the differences and similarities of various approaches to massage and bodywork.

2 Clarify the seven basic approaches to therapeutic massage and bodywork.

3 Classify a massage method into its fundamental physiologic basis.

In the past few years, as the popularity of therapeutic massage has increased, the profession has seen an expansion of styles and systems (Box 2.1). The term *bodywork* has been used to cover the scope of these developments. The application of systematic touch for health purposes (therapeutic massage and bodywork) has relevance. As the individual systems have emerged, a difference in the styles has developed. The overlap of these methods reveals a fundamental sameness in all of the work. The similarity should not distract from the devotion, training, and expertise of the various practitioners of specific disciplines. By carefully examining any style or system of massage or bodywork, one can see that some basic methods are being used to stimulate sensory receptors, which disrupts an existing pattern in the central nervous system control centers and results in a shift in nerve and chemical patterns to reestablish homeostasis (reflexive methods). The very same methods can be applied in a different way to change the consistency or position of connective tissue or to shift pressure in the vessel to facilitate blood and lymph circulation (mechanical methods).

Box 2.1
POPULAR METHODS
IN THE PROFESSION

Note that this list of styles, systems, founders, and developers is not meant to be all inclusive. This information is changing daily. Instead, the list is meant to show the great variety of bodywork approaches.

Oriental (Asian) Approaches: Amma, Acupressure, Shiatsu, Jin Shin Do, Do-in, Hoshino, Tuina, Watsu, Tibetan Point Holding

Amma and these other methods come from original Chinese concepts as well as from offshoots of the Chinese base. These compressive manipulations and stretches, focused to specific areas of the body, elicit responses in the nervous and the circulatory systems. Both the efficient use of the therapist's body and working over the clothing of the client have many benefits. The philosophy of the systems is grounded in ancient concepts that have stood the test of time for effectiveness. The effects are both reflexive and mechanical.

Structural and Postural Integration Approaches: Bindegewebs Massage, Rolfing, Hellerwork, Looyen, Pfrimmer, Soma, Bowen Therapy

The techniques focus more specifically on the connective tissue structure to influence posture and biomechanics. The approaches are systematic and effective because they are grounded in the fundamentals of physiology and biomechanics. The practitioners of these styles have received extensive education.

Neuromuscular Approaches: Neuromuscular Techniques, Muscle Energy Techniques, Strain/Counterstrain, Orthobionomy, Trager®, Myotherapy, Proprioceptive Neuromuscular Facilitation, Reflexology, Trigger Points

These are the European approaches based on the work of Dr. Stanley Leif and Dr. Boris Chaitow, and the Western methods based on the work of Dr. Janet Travell, Dr. John Mennell, Dr. Raymond Nimmo, Dr. Lawrence Jones, Dr. Milton Trager, Eunice Ingham, William Fitzgerald, Arthur Lincoln Pauls, Bonnie Prudden, and others. Dr. Leon Chaitow has written extensively on the concepts and currently teaches in the United States and Europe. Many of the techniques are similar to those found in Rolfing, Asian methods, and Swedish massage and gymnastics. As the name implies, the approach is a nervous or reflexive variety. Observation of the systems reveals that connective tissue is also being affected. The common thread throughout all of the styles is the basic concepts of activation of the tonus receptor mechanism, reflex arc stimulation, positional receptors, and applications of stretch and lengthening.

Manual Lymphatic Drainage: Vodder Lymph Drainage

Emile Vodder developed an excellent system that utilizes the anatomy and physiology of the mechanism of lymphatic movement with both mechanical and reflexive techniques to stimulate lymphatic fluid flow. Variations of this system exist and are sometimes called *systemic massage.*

Energetic Approaches: Polarity, Therapeutic Touch, Reiki, Rosen Method, Rubenfeld Synergy, Mariel, Zero Balancing

Box 2.1
POPULAR METHODS
IN THE PROFESSION
(continued)

These systems are based on ancient concepts of body energy patterns and recently have been formalized by Dr. Randolph Stone, Dr. Dolores Krieger, Dr. Fritz Smith, and others. Subtle energy medicine is being studied at the Menninger Foundation in Topeka, Kansas by Dr. Elmer Green as well as other researchers. Polarity and similar energetic approaches use near touch or light touch to initiate reflexive responses, often with highly effective results.

Cranial-Sacral and Myofascial Approaches: Cranial-Sacral Therapy, Myofascial Release, Soft Tissue Mobilization, Deep Tissue Massage, Connective Tissue Massage

These systems focus more specifically on the various aspects of both mechanical and reflexive connective tissue functions. Dr. Sutherland was the first to formalize the concept of minute movement of the cranium and the dura. John Upledger, D.O., and John Barnes, P.T., have expanded and formalized his work. Both light and deep touch are used depending on the method. Dr. James Cyriax's cross-fiber friction methods fall into this category.

Applied Kinesiology: Touch For Health, Applied Physiology, Educational Kinesiology, Three-In-One Concepts

Dr. George Goodheart formalized the system of applied kinesiology within the chiropractic community. The approach blends many techniques while working primarily with the reflexive mechanisms. A specific muscle testing procedure is used for evaluation purposes. Some of the corrective measures use Asian meridians and acupressure, whereas others rely on the osteopathic reflex mechanisms defined by Chapman, Bennett, and McKenzie that seem to correspond to traditional Chinese acupuncture points. Dr. John Thie and others modified these techniques for use by the massage community and general public.

Integrated Approaches: Sports Massage, Infant Massage, Equine Massage, On-Site Seated Massage, Prenatal Massage, Geriatric Massage, Massage For Abuse Survivors, Russian Massage

Many styles of bodywork, focused to a specific population, are combinations of methods rather than a physiologic intervention.

Founders and teachers of integrated methods include every massage professional who designs a massage specifically for an individual client and every devoted massage instructor who attempts to combine and explain methods to students.

Although most of the systems have developed over the centuries, a few approaches have been formalized in the past few years. The profession must begin to standardize terminology to avoid confusion about the various styles and systems of massage. Asian styles may explain the anatomy and physiology differently, but the human body is the same and the effects of these styles are the same as those developed in Polynesia, India, Europe, Africa, the United States, and all other places around the world. The study of various systems only becomes confusing when there are so many different names for methods.

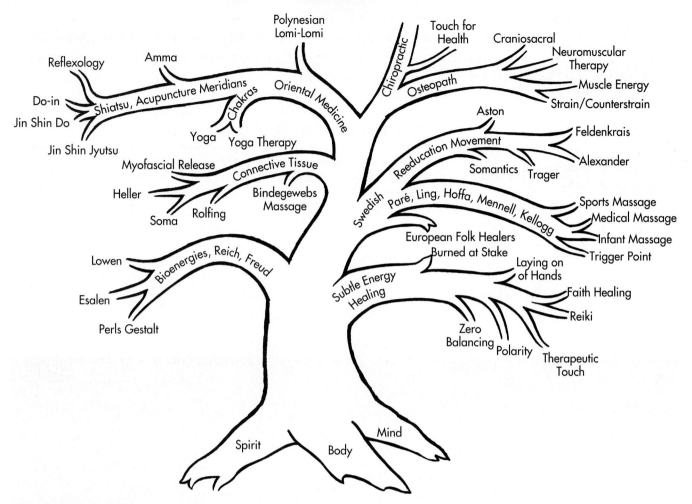

The Bodywork Tree.
Diversity as represented in the metaphor of a tree shows that all forms of therapeutic massage and related bodywork modalities stem from the same roots.

There is indeed a core body of knowledge that all massage therapists and bodyworkers use regardless of the seasoning, presentation, and environment. The expanding styles of body and mind approaches to massage and bodywork are the same concepts that focus on the homeostatic balance of the autonomic nervous system, the limbic system, and endocrine responses. Any practitioner of therapeutic massage should be proficient in all fundamental massage concepts. A skilled practitioner should be able to break down any approach into its basic components. The importance of learning the sequence of the various styles that have developed around the world speaks to one's level of expertise. To say that massage and all styles are similar is not an excuse for repetitiveness in application. All massage and bodywork has the same basis because the people it helps share similar physiology, but it is important to remember that not everyone has the same needs. Variations of applications to meet the needs of the individual and the skill levels of the professional is important. No one style of massage is better than another if the fundamental components are included, if the method serves the needs of the client, and if it is used by a trained professional with intent and purpose. It is likely that technology and research will prove that massage and bodywork methods share the same physiologic basis for their effectiveness. The different systems and styles presented in this text are variations on a theme. Learn the theme and explore the variations to become a skilled practitioner. Expect that any system can explain itself in anatomic and physiologic terminology.

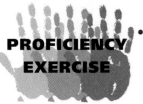

• Explore three different massage and bodywork styles from three different categories from the information presented. List the differences and similarities of each method.

DEFINITION OF MASSAGE

Using the information presented in this section, the student will be able to:

❶ Develop a definition of massage.

A definition for massage needs to be inclusive of all the methods used by the various system (Box 2.2). In addition, the scope of practice for therapeutic massage depends on individual laws and the definitions of massage included in those laws. The profession itself has not agreed on a definition. This text will offer a general definition of massage. The attempt will be made to include many definitions found in historic literature; or guidelines from state and local laws, professional organizations, and individual styles and approaches to massage and bodywork. To define massage accurately and completely becomes difficult because there are many forms of massage and bodywork currently being practiced.

Box 2.2 DEFINITION OF *THERAPEUTIC MASSAGE*	The scientific art and system of the assessment of and the manual application to the superficial soft tissue of skin, muscles, tendons, ligaments, fascia, and the structures that lie within the superficial tissue by using the hand, foot, knee, arm, elbow, and forearm through the systematic external application of touch, stroking (*effleurage*), friction, vibration, percussion, kneading (*petrissage*), stretching, compression, or passive and active joint movements within the normal physiologic range of motion. Also included are adjunctive external applications of water, heat, and cold for the purposes of establishing and maintaining good physical condition and health through normalizing and improving muscle tone, promoting relaxation, stimulating circulation, and producing therapeutic effects on the respiratory and nervous systems, and the subtle interactions between all body systems. These intended effects are accomplished through the energetic and mind/body connections in a safe, nonsexual environment that respects the client's self-determined outcome for the session.

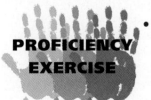

• Write a definition of therapeutic massage. Working in groups of three, combine the definitions. Continue working in different groups of three, combining until your class has developed one definition for therapeutic massage.

SCOPE OF PRACTICE

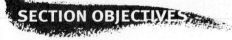

Using the information presented in this section, the student will be able to:

Currently much of the literature defines the scope of practice of massage by what cannot be done, so as to not infringe on other health and service professions' scopes of practice (Box 2.3).

The scope of practice authorized by a physician's or surgeon's certificate is broad and extensive. It authorizes the physician to use drugs and medical preparations and the surgeon to sever and penetrate human tissue during treatment. It further authorizes them to use other methods

1. Understand the scope of practice of various health and service professionals.
2. Explain what constitutes the "practice of medicine."
3. Explain the difference between medical rehabilitative massage and wellness personal service massage.
4. Develop a scope of practice for massage that respects that of other professionals.

in the treatment of disease, injuries, deformities, or other physical or mental conditions. The law grants such a broad authorization to the physician because the education and testing requirements for a physician's license assure qualification to act as a healer.

No one but the physician has the legal right to perform any act that falls within the parameters of a medical license. The principle underlying this is simple—a person may not dispense therapeutic or medicinal advice concerning the effect of his or her services on a specific disease, ailment, or condition unless he or she has adequate training, knowledge, and experience to ensure that the advice given is sound and reliable.

All these professionals have educational standards that exceed current accepted requirements for massage in most areas. Professionals with more education are allowed to do more within their specialized field. Those with less education work under supervision or with a limited scope of practice.

The scope of practice for therapeutic massage needs to fit into but not infringe on the boundaries of these professionals. Hopefully the future will provide for more flexibility and overlap of practice for the benefit of the client.

Box 2.3
OCCUPATIONAL DEFINITIONS AND SCOPE OF PRACTICE

The following are typical scope of practice regulations taken from the administrative rules of Michigan Occupational Regulations Department of Licensing and Regulation and the Occupational Regulations Section of the Michigan Public Health code for other professionals. Each state differs slightly, but the consistency of regulation is constant enough to provide for a sense of uniformity across the United States and other countries.

Chiropractic:
The discipline within the healing arts that deals with the nervous system and its relationship to the spinal column and its interrelationship with the other body systems. Chiropractic uses radiography to determine the existence of spinal subluxation or misalignment and adjustment of spinal subluxation or misalignments and related bones and tissues to establish neural integrity that uses the inherent recuperative powers of the body to restore and maintain health including the use of analytical instruments, nutritional advice, and rehabilitative exercise.

Chiropractic does not include the performance of incisive surgical procedures, the performance of any invasive procedure requiring instrumentation, or the dispensing or prescribing of drugs or medicine.

Dentistry:
The diagnosis, treatment, prescription, or surgery for a disease, pain, deformity, deficiency, injury, or physical condition of the human tooth, alveolar process, gums, jaws, or their dependent tissues.

Medicine:
The diagnosis, treatment, prevention, cure, or relieving of human disease, ailment, defect, complaint, or other physical or mental condition, by attendance, advice, device, diagnostic, test, or other means.

Nursing:
The systematic application of substantial specialized knowledge and skill derived from the biologic, physical, and

Box 2.3
OCCUPATIONAL DEFINITIONS AND
SCOPE OF PRACTICE
(continued)

behavioral sciences to the care, treatment, counsel, and health teachings of individuals who are experiencing changes in the normal health process or who require assistance in the maintenance of health and the prevention or management of illness, injury, or disability.

Osteopathic medicine:

An independent school of medicine and surgery using full methods of diagnosis and treatment in physical and mental health and disease, including the prescription and administration of drugs and biologic, operative surgery, obstetrics, radiologic and electromagnetic emission and placing special emphasis on the interrelationship of the musculoskeletal system to other body systems.

Physical therapy:

The evaluation or treatment of an individual by the use of effective properties of physical measures and the use of therapeutic exercise and rehabilitative procedures with or without devices for the purposes of preventing, correcting, or alleviating a physical or mental disability. It includes treatment planning, performance of tests and measurements, interpretation of referrals, instruction, consultative services, and supervision of personnel. Physical measures include massage, mobilization, heat, cold, air, light, water, electricity, and sound.

Podiatric medicine:

The examination, diagnosis, and treatment of abnormal nails, superficial excrescences (abnormal outgrowths or enlargements) occurring on the human hand and feet including corns, warts, callosities, bunions, and arch troubles and the treatment medically, surgically, mechanically, or by physiotherapy of ailments of the human feet or ankles and the affect the condition of the feet. It does not include amputation of the human feet or the use or administration of other than local anesthetics.

Psychology:

The rendering to individuals, groups, organizations or the public service involving the application of principles, methods and procedures of understanding, predicting, and influencing behavior for the purposes of the diagnosis, assessment related to diagnosis, prevention, amelioration (improvement), or treatment of mental or emotional disorders, disabilities or behavioral adjustment problems by means of psychotherapy, counseling, behavior modification, hypnosis, biofeedback techniques, psychologic tests, or other verbal or behavioral means. The practice of psychology shall not include the prescribing of drugs, performing of surgery, or administering of electroconvulsive therapy.

Cosmetology:

A service provided to enhance the health, condition and appearance of the skin, hair, and nails. Any external preparations intended to cleanse and beautify the skin, hair, or other part of the body. The application of beautification processes, such as makeup and skin grooming, is included.

Physical therapy is the profession most likely to be compared with the practice of massage, and care needs to be taken to respect the professional boundaries of physical therapy. In personal service wellness massage, the key is health enhancement or providing massage for individuals who are already healthy and want to maintain or improve their health. It is also important to not infringe on the cosmetology scope of practice by working with cosmetic applications to the skin through the use of oils, wraps, or other preparations. Again, with personal service wellness massage, the key is health enhancing activities.

This does not mean that massage is not important or not necessary in the medical setting, but additional training is required. Supervision by a doctor, nurse, or physical therapist is necessary, or extensive assessment procedures are needed to refer responsibility to other health care professionals. The Canadian provinces of Ontario and British Columbia have such a scope of practice for therapeutic massage. The educational standard is over twenty-two hundred class hours, and the information required to practice massage at this level is beyond the scope of this text. This book is focused to the wellness personal service level of massage, which is the entry level for all massage education, whatever the eventual level of training.

The level of education required in Ontario prepares the massage therapist to develop, maintain, rehabilitate, or augment physical function, to relieve or prevent physical dysfunction and pain, and to enhance the well-being of the client. Methods include assessment of the soft tissue and joints and treatment by soft tissue manipulation, hydrotherapy, remedial exercise programs, and client self-care programs. The ability to perform assessment and provide referral to health care practitioners is essential.

Taking all of this information into account, this text book determines the scope of practice of **wellness personal service massage** to be:

A nonspecific approach to massage with a focus on the assessment procedures to determine contraindications to massage, the need for referral to other health care professionals, and the development of a health enhancing physical state for the client. The massage session plan is developed by combining information, desired results, and directions from the client with the skills of the massage practitioner to develop an individualized massage session aimed to normalization of the body systems. This normalization is achieved through external manual stimulation of the nervous, circulatory, and respiratory systems, connective tissue, and muscle to provide generalized stress reduction, a decrease in muscle tension, symptomatic relief of pain related to soft tissue dysfunction, increased circulation, and other benefits similar to exercise or other relaxation responses produced by therapeutic massage to increase the well being of the client.

It may seem like a fine distinction between wellness personal service massage and medical rehabilitative approaches to massage, but the distinction is simple. Wellness personal service massage practitioners do not work with sick or injured people unless directly supervised by a licensed and qualified professional, such as a doctor, nurse, or physical therapist. Instead, they help most of the population, who are not sick but are stressed and uncomfortable, to feel better and cope with stress. This benefit of massage may help prevent more serious stress-induced illness.

For example, the owner's manual for a car recommends regularly scheduled maintenance. If followed, the oil and filter are changed, and the fluids are checked by a technician. Tune-ups are performed by a mechanic's assistant. Following the preventative maintenance schedule will allow the car to last a long time. It is a good idea to have a qualified mechanic do a complete evaluation of the car yearly to catch problems while they are small and can be easily corrected. If this is not done, serious problems may arise, and a skilled mechanic will have to correct them.

The wellness personal service massage practitioner is similar to the technician who keeps the car in order, changes the oil, and checks the fluids. Complete tune-ups reflect the skill levels of the massage therapist, while the skilled mechanic is the doctor or physical therapist. Lest someone think that the technician is the least important person in the chain, be reminded that if the prevention is done well, the possibility of a serious problem developing is less likely. If the car is involved in an accident, then it certainly goes straight to the mechanic and other specialists for repair. When involved in a trauma situation, a person should go to the doctor for evaluation and treatment.

When discussing scopes of practice, all professionals have specialized training, certain responsibilities, and positions where they function best. Remembering and respecting the individual's strengths is the ethical thing to do. While therapeutic massage waits for a formalized scope of practice, knowing the definition and scope of other health and service professionals helps the massage practitioner respect these professionals and maintain appropriate boundaries.

Scope of Practice — Therapeutic Massage			
	WELLNESS (Resourceful functioning with ability to respond and recover easily)	**DYSFUNCTION** (Functioning with effort with reduced ability to respond and longer recovery time)	**ILLNESS/TRAUMA** (Function Breakdown with substantially reduced ability to respond and recover)
BODY Biology—Visceral, Somatic, Anatomy/Physiology *Health (Body) care Professionals* Doctors, Physical Therapists, Acupuncturists, Exercise Specialists, Nutritionists, Chiropractors, etc.	*500+ hours Education* Wellness personal service massage without supervision from health-care professionals.	*1000+ hours Education* Therapeutic massage with consultation or indirect supervision from healthcare professionals.	*2000+ hours Education* Rehabilitation/ medical massage with direct supervision by healthcare professionals as part of multi a team.
MIND Cognitive Function— Behavior communication, coping skills, stress management, etc. *Mental Health Professionals* Psychologists, social workers, counselors, etc.	*500+ hours Education* Wellness personal service massage without supervision from mental health professionals.	*1000+ hours Education* Therapeutic massage with consultation or indirect supervision from mental health professionals.	*2000+ hours Education* Rehabilitation/medical focus with special training in mental health issues. Direct supervision by mental health professionals.
SPIRIT Purpose, Connectedness and Hope *Spiritually Based Professionals*	Wellness personal service massage to bring body/ mind connection to spiritual awareness.		
Therapeutic massage is a **BODY SYSTEM** that influences mind functions through the body/mind connection and provides an avenue for connecting with a caring professional to support spiritual awareness.			

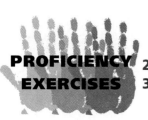

PROFICIENCY EXERCISES

1. Investigate the scope of practice defined by licensed professionals in your community for the listed health and service professions in this section. Find this information at the state department of licensing and regulation.
2. Write a scope of practice statement for therapeutic massage.
3. Share these scope of practice statements in a classroom setting and develop one scope of practice. Talk with other health professionals about this scope of practice and get their opinion as to how they would compare it with their own.

CODE OF ETHICS

SECTION OBJECTIVES

Using the information presented in this section, the student will be able to:

❶ Explore personal prejudices, fears, and limitations that may interfere with the ability to provide the best care for a client.

❷ Determine if a client can give informed consent for a massage.

❸ Help a client set and explain personal boundaries for the massage.

❹ Recognize sexual misconduct activities.

❺ Explain to clients feelings of intimacy between them and the massage professional.

❻ Defuse sexual feelings during the massage session.

❼ Develop strategies for maintaining professional space with a client.

❽ Develop a personal and professional code of ethics.

Because the massage therapy and bodywork profession is still not unified in terms of professional affiliation and techniques, it is difficult to give a code of ethics for the massage professional. Because each professional group within the massage and bodywork community has developed its own code of ethics, what is offered here is a general code of ethics based on a compilation of many existing ethical codes.

Ethics and boundaries are difficult to define; they are an individual value concept. We bring to our adulthood varying experiences that shape what we feel is correct, and define our personal boundaries. As professionals, it is essential to realize that we are responsible for finding the comfort zone of our clients. This responsibility begins with learning our personal comfort zone.

Anything that would prevent us from being able to touch a person in a respectful, nonjudgmental way must be considered so that we can decide who we may best serve as massage therapists. This includes personal prejudices such as body size, color, gender, and attitude. For example, some people do not relate well with children. It would be ethical for that person to refer children to someone else for professional care. Others may be uncomfortable with those of the opposite sex, and again it would be best to refer the client elsewhere. We may find ourselves uncomfortable with the prospects of working with people who have certain types of diseases. If this is the case, our touch will be uncomfortable for these people. A potential client may have a behavior that drives us crazy (i.e., nose snorting). The behavior interferes with our ability to be the best massage professional for that particular client. It is therefore important to begin the exploration of ethics and personal boundaries by looking honestly at our own fears, frustrations, prejudices, biases, and value systems. Massage therapists work very closely with clients. We have to be honest with ourselves and about ourselves if we are going to be able to respect the individual needs and space of our clients.

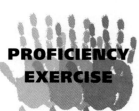

PROFICIENCY EXERCISE

The following exercise may be the most difficult you will have to do. Write a minimum of one page about your personal prejudices and fears about people, and honestly list those physical and behavioral aspects about others that are difficult for you to deal with.

Here are some examples:

- I am afraid of people with the HIV virus. I do not understand much about how it is transmitted, and I do not want to catch it.
- Old people frustrate me. I cannot make myself listen to the same stories over and over.

- **I hate ragged toe nails. I do not know if I can rub anyone's feet if the nails are not well trimmed.**
- **People who are fat are undisciplined. They should exercise more.**
- **People who are skinny are obsessed with their appearance and are exercise addicts.**
- **When someone sniffs their nose all the time it makes me crazy.**
- **I am afraid of men with mustaches because of something that happened to me when I was young.**
- **Women are so bossy; I hate it when they tell me what to do.**
- **As a man, I am uncomfortable with giving another man a massage.**

IT IS IMPORTANT THAT YOU ARE VERY HONEST WITH YOURSELF. Only by accepting that we have these areas of challenge will we be able to best serve potential clients.

RIGHT OF REFUSAL

Clients have the right to refuse the massage practitioner's services. This is called the **right of refusal.** It is a client's right to refuse or stop treatment at anytime. When this request is made during treatment, the therapist will comply despite prior consent.

Professionals do not have to work with an individual. Massage therapists may refuse to administer to, massage, or otherwise treat any person if there is just and reasonable cause. In the next few paragraphs some direction for determining what constitutes just and reasonable cause for refusing to provide professional massage services to a client will be given.

A massage therapist has the right to refuse to treat any area of the body of a client or to terminate the professional relationship if the therapist feels the client is sexualizing the relationship, or the massage professional is adversely influenced in any way by the client. At the same time, massage therapists are bound by a nondiscrimination code of conduct. The two seem to conflict. Here is the recommendation.

You may refuse to work with anyone, as long as you explain the reasons why. This is called **disclosure.**

For example, someone with multiple sclerosis wishes to be your client. Your mother had multiple sclerosis, and you have bitter feelings about how her illness interfered with your childhood. It is difficult for you to be with anyone who has this condition because of your memories. Here are your choices:

1. Tell the prospective client just what was written above and offer to refer to a therapist who can provide the work needed. Make sure that at least three different qualified individuals are given as referrals. This is so the client has a choice.
2. Be very honest with the client. Discuss your feelings and your concern that the way you feel may interfere with doing what is best. However, when explaining the situation to the prospective client, leave out all of the personal details. Knowing this up front, if the client still wants to work with you, you may decide to give it a try.

Either way, the massage therapist has taken responsibility for personal attitudes, and the client has informed choice. Remember, touch tells the truth. It is difficult to touch someone with whom you are uneasy, whatever the reasons. By honestly telling the person about the situation, the client can make the decision. If the touch seems different, the client may be able to realize that it is the practitioner's issue.

INFORMED CONSENT

Clients need enough information to make an informed choice about who they want to administer professional services, what they want the therapist to accomplish, and how the session should progress. This is **informed consent.** In this role, the massage practitioner needs to be a teacher so that massage procedures and effects can be explained to the client. Credentials and personal and professional limitations that will have an effect on the client-therapist relationship need to be disclosed and validated. This entire textbook is concerned with informed consent. As professionals, we are ethically bound to make sure that the client is making a choice based on a solid foundation and an understanding of certain information. It is the professional's responsibility to provide this information to the client.

A client must be able to understand and comprehend everything about the massage session. If there is a language barrier, if the client is under the age of eighteen, or if other circumstances prevail, it may be difficult to evaluate if comprehension is complete enough for the client to make an informed choice. Ethically, the massage professional must not work with someone without assurance of the client's informed consent.

BOUNDARIES

A **boundary** is the personal space located within an arm-length perimeter. It is also the personal emotional space designated by morals, values, and experience. Some people are not very good at defining personal boundaries or respecting others' boundaries. Certainly boundaries are defined by more than physical space, but for our purposes, a respect for personal boundaries starts with staying an arm length away from another until invited to come closer. Personal space can be defined by placing an arm directly in front of the body and turning a circle; the area within that space is your personal space. Cultural differences may change this boundary, but for massage therapy let us consider this the person's space range. No one should ever enter this space uninvited (without informed consent). It is important that students practice this policy while they are in school. First, ask if another person may be approached, then wait for their response and act accordingly. This practice may seem silly, but it will teach an awareness of boundaries. Sometimes, those who have been physically or sexually abused have not had the opportunity to define or recognize personal boundaries. It is important to be respectful in our approach and carefully explain professional boundaries to the client (Box 2.4). It is just as important for those who have boundary difficulties to learn to define their own boundaries. Setting limits during a massage session may be a safe way to begin this process.

What is acceptable for us may be offensive for someone else. We may offend someone because of differences within our value systems. It is important for the massage therapist to be able to help the client define a personal boundary. Once defined, we must respect the client's boundary. If it is too difficult for us to respect the client's boundary needs, then refer him or her to a better-suited massage practitioner.

Make sure you tell the client "I will not be offended if you share with me things that you do not like about the massage. I will be happy to refer you to someone else if you do not like my style. There are as many different ways to give a massage as there are people giving massage. I am here to serve your needs—as long as those needs do not conflict with my professional and personal standards." It is important for the client to understand the therapist's personal and professional boundaries. Therefore, the therapist must be honest in creating a personal code of ethics and must clearly communicate the professional boundaries to the client. Chapter 7 will provide more information on how this is accomplished.

CONFIDENTIALITY

Confidentiality means that client's information is private and belongs to the client. It is unethical for the massage professional to discuss anything about a client with anyone other than that client including the client's health care professional, without the client's written permission. Confidentiality is a trust.

SEXUAL MISCONDUCT

Although what constitutes **sexual misconduct** is relatively well defined, there remains a gray area regarding what is invasive (Box 2.5). A joke told between friends may be totally inappropriate in the professional setting. A statement about appearance may be taken as a compliment or could be interpreted as a sexual remark. What is appropriate with one client may not be acceptable with another. It can be overwhelming to try to second guess what is appropriate for which clients. The best defense against confusion is communication. Ask questions and provide information to clients about acceptable behavior in the professional setting.

MASSAGE THERAPY AND INTIMACY

This section addresses feelings that may develop over time for the client by the massage professional or vice versa. To dispel in advance any sexual innuendo associated with many of the terms used in the following paragraphs, definitions are included at this point for clarification.

The dictionary defines **intimacy**[4] as "the state or fact of being intimate" and, in turn, **intimate**[4] is defined as "inmost, essential, internal, most private or personal; closely acquainted or associated; very familiar." Something that is "intrinsic, fundamental, basic and inherently primary" is **essential.**[4] **Sensory**[4] is defined as "connected with the reception and transmission of sense impressions" through the nervous system.

The work of a massage practitioner is sensory stimulation; therefore, by its very definition, the body stimulation is sensual and may become intimate.

Box 2.5
GUIDELINES REGARDING
SEXUAL MISCONDUCT

The guidelines in Ontario, Canada provide the following criteria:[3]

Sexual Impropriety and Sexual Abuse:

- The therapist will respect the integrity of each person and, therefore, not engage in any sexual conduct or sexual activities involving clients
- The therapist will not date a client
- The therapist will not commit any form of sexual impropriety or sexual abuse with a client
- Whatever the behavior of the client, it is always the responsibility of the massage therapist not to engage in sexual behavior

Sexual Impropriety includes:

- Any behavior, gestures, or expressions that are seductive or sexually demeaning to a client.
- Inappropriate procedures including, but not limited to:
  - disrobing or draping practices that reflect a lack of respect for the client's privacy
  - deliberately watching a client dress or undress
- Inappropriate comments about or to the client including, but not limited to:
  - sexual comments about a client's body or underclothing
  - making sexualized or sexually demeaning comments to a client
  - criticism of the client's sexual orientation
  - discussion of the potential sexual performance
  - conversations regarding the sexual preferences or fantasies of the client or the massage therapist
  - requests to date
  - kissing of a sexual nature

Sexual Abuse includes:

- Therapist-client sex, whether initiated by the client or not. Engaging in any conduct with a client that is sexual or may reasonably be interpreted as sexual including, but not limited to:
  - genital to genital contact
  - oral to genital contact
  - oral to anal contact
  - oral to oral contact (except CPR)
  - oral to breast contact
  - touching or undraping the genitals, perineum, or anus
  - touching or undraping breasts
  - encouraging the client to masturbate in the presence of the massage therapist
  - masturbation by the massage therapist while the client is present
  - masturbation of the client by the massage therapist

The massage professional must possess an awareness of the physiologic aspects of therapeutic massage and show how the same techniques of massage that alleviate stress and promote relaxation also stimulate the entire sensory mechanism, which may include a sexual arousal response. Gaining a more thorough knowledge of the physiologic and psychologic network will lead to a better understanding of the responses by both client and practitioner. The practitioner is then better able to adjust the session to provide for proper client-practitioner boundaries and professionalism.

Within the parameters of professional ethics, it is always considered unethical for the client or the practitioner to interact on a sexual level, whether verbal or physical. However, it is essential that both client and practitioner understand why the urges and sensations of sexuality may present themselves.

The lumbar nerve plexus and sacral nerve plexus conduct sensory information to and from the abdominals, lower extremities, and buttocks, as well as to and from the genital area. Stimulation of a nerve plexus area is not confined to local perception, but is instead diffused throughout the area. When stroking the lower abdominals, the nerve signals of the genital area are being influenced. The entire sexual arousal response is part of the relaxation response via the output from the parasympathetic autonomic nervous system.

Therefore, each time a client relaxes out of the "fight or flight" responses of the sympathetic autonomic nervous system into the more relaxed response, the predisposing factors are present for sexual arousal. This reaction is not only possible for the client, but also for the practitioner as he or she begins to relax and flow with the massage.

On a physiologic level, parasympathetic stimulation activates most of the benefits of massage for stress reduction. This neurologic state is also favorable to sexual arousal. These physical responses are all connected, but it seems that the sexual response is short lived and quickly replaced by feelings of deep relaxation as the massage continues. Responses vary with every client, and the sexual response may be totally bypassed. However, it may happen, and the massage practitioner needs to understand both the physiology and how to ethically deal with this situation should it present itself.

It is the practitioner's responsibility to put the whole issue of sexuality into perspective, to understand it clearly, and to explain the "feelings" to the client on a physiologic level. It also becomes the practitioner's responsibility to monitor the client's responses and to act appropriately to adjust the physiology and change the pattern to diffuse the sexual energy. This is easily accomplished with an altered approach to the session. It is common knowledge that sexual arousal is not purely physical and depends on both psychologic and tactile responses. It is here that the practitioner can modulate the client-practitioner responses.

Intercourse[4] is defined as "connection or reciprocal action between persons or nations—the interchange of thought, feelings, products, services, communication, commerce and association." Massage becomes an intercourse in the purest sense. Essential intimacy is the circle that begins to develop between practitioner and client. People want this type of intimacy. It is this type of interaction that promotes survival and health. **Essential touch** is vital, fundamental, and crucial to well being. It is the touch of a litter of puppies, sleeping in one big pile. It is the caring, understanding look of a friend, and it can be combined with the sexual interchange between lovers. But it does not have to have sexual expression to be essential.

When a person encounters the essential touch that a sensitive and confident massage practitioner provides, that person's whole system responds. For many, the closest thing to essential touch ever experienced is sexual interaction. Because our bodies constantly react to new situations by comparison to past experience, it is understandable why a client would interpret these feelings as sexual arousal. Furthermore, for many people the only familiar routine they have for expression of these feelings is a sexual one. It is easy to see why the client would confuse the sensations and perceive the interaction of the feelings associated with massage in sexual responses and terms.

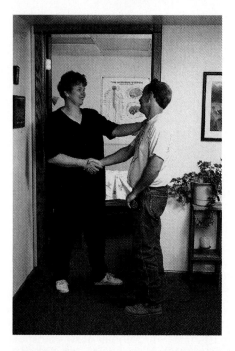

Figure 2.1
Greeting body language. When greeting a client, the massage professional leans toward the client and gently draws the client into the space of the massage session.

Remember, massage practitioners, as we touch, we are also being touched. The exchange is unavoidable, and we need to monitor our own feelings and expressions of intimacy as well (see Box 2.6).

If we do not effectively deal with these responses, the feelings associated with them could become very uncomfortable. The client may react by discontinuing the massage sessions, or the therapist may effectively detach from the client and possibly stop seeing the client altogether. In the latter case, the client may feel abandoned.

Remember, it is the intention of the touch that is the determining factor. The touch of the massage therapist is not focused toward sexual arousal and release. The psychologic aspect of this topic is another matter. Here the therapist can set the stage and monitor responses. Keep discussions light. Change the topic. This is where the interpersonal skills of the practitioner come into play. The moments of intimacy must be dealt with very carefully. Not understanding the psychologic or physiologic responses, the client may interpret this response as an indication of feelings of love or that this person is a new best friend. Clients manifest this response in different ways. What usually happens is that the clients want to bring the therapists into their lives, whether it is for lunch, a desire for more frequent sessions, or a proposal for a relationship. Do not allow this to happen. The practitioner must maintain professional space and monitor personal feelings. Keep the balance by confining the intimacy of massage to the therapy room.

As the therapist closes the session and leaves the client's space, it is important to change both physiology and body language. When greeting a client and providing the massage, the body language is open, inviting, connecting, and moving toward the client (Fig. 2.1). When it is time to close the session and for the client to leave, the body language moves away from the client, pulls in toward the massage therapist, separates, and is completed (Fig. 2.2). Separating well is a skill providing both the client and the massage therapist with a sense of closure. It often helps to establish a "time to go" ritual by always saying goodbye the same way. Clients who linger at the door may not know how to leave or recognize that it is time to leave. A "time to go" ritual helps considerably.

One example of how this can be done is to have a box labeled "A thought to take with me" containing fun, empowering quotes on some note cards. Have the client pick a card from the box. Put the next appointment information on the back, hand it to the client with a warm handshake, and say goodbye. When the session is finished, let that client go physically and emotionally as the room is prepared for the next person.

Box 2.6
STEPS TO DIFFUSE FEELINGS OF SEXUAL AROUSAL

To defuse sexual arousal feelings:

1. Recognize the physiology and interrupt it. Change what you are doing.
2. Be aware of your own psychologic state.
3. Adjust the session intent to stimulate a more sympathetic output response by using stretching, compression, joint movement, and active participation of the client.
4. Change the music, lighting, conversation, position of the client.
5. Stop working with your hands and use forearms.
6. Explain the feelings in a professional manner and clear the air by using clinical terminology.

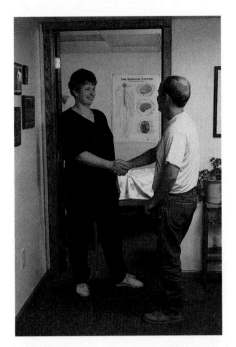

Figure 2.2
Closure body language. After the massage is complete, the massage professional will need to gently withdraw from the client by using body language that moves away from the client.

With an understanding of all of these subtle interactions, the client cannot be blamed for wanting more attention from the massage practitioner. The moments of togetherness that are shared are special and can range from a great deal of laughter to sharing work-related experiences. The session can accomplish something as simple as relieving the day's tension or as complex as overcoming years of pain. Make no more or no less of the interaction. Clients may look to the therapist for emotional support beyond the ethical scope of practice for massage. Encourage them to find the support they require from another source. If a client needs help with coping skills, refer him or her to someone who is qualified to help. There are credit counselors, ministers, rape crisis counselors, marriage counselors, counselors for sexual dysfunctions, chiropractors, therapists, physicians, and many other care givers from whom they can obtain help. The massage practitioner's job is to support and accept the client in a nonjudgmental manner, to listen, and to blend touch skills to benefit the client.

It is important to maintain professional space. Some simple ways to accomplish this include keeping a picture of family members in the reception area or the therapy room and sharing a little of the family background, such as "Laura's dance recital is next week," "Greg plays guitar," or " Luke and I are going out to dinner." This reminds the client that the massage therapist already has a personal life. Wearing a uniform or maintaining a style of dress that is professional and different from casual clothes gives visual stimulation that reflects "professionalism." The clothing does not have to be white, but must be nonrevealing and present a subtle appearance. Privacy can be preserved by using an answering machine or service and returning calls within set hours. If it is financially feasible, have a receptionist or secretary monitor phone calls.

Maintain regular appointment hours. Begin and end sessions on time. Do not spend personal time, such as lunch, with clients. If this is done, there is a risk of losing a paying client balanced by the possibility of gaining a special personal friend. It cannot be done with every client, and a choice between the two options must be made. Think carefully before setting rules about client conduct, rescheduling, and payment methods. Record this information clearly and concisely, and make sure that the client reads it. Posting it on the wall provides an additional reinforcement.

Do not be afraid of the special professional intimacy of therapeutic massage. Instead, educate clients by answering their questions intelligently, based on physiology, and encourage them to use this learning to interact more resourcefully with others. If you begin to feel physically and emotionally receptive to a client, refer to Box 2.6 on page 34 to diffuse the response. Later, review the session to evaluate personal feelings. Was it just a fleeting warm feeling? Is there just something about this particular person? Could it have been a hormonal response? Some women become more sexually responsive during certain times of their monthly cycle. Was it from feeling alone and needing to be connected? If the problem is from something lacking in life, empower yourself to search the problem out and change circumstances so that personal reactions are kept out of the therapy room. If a professional relationship cannot be maintained with a client, stop providing therapeutic massage to the client and refer the client to someone else. Provide the client with an honest and simple explanation so that the client understands that it was not something he or she said or did that prompted the referral. Professional ethics do not safeguard us from being human. Behavior becomes unethical when the problem is not acknowledged, and resourceful action is not taken to resolve the situation.

When a client refuses or is unable to alter an inappropriate response to the massage, the client must be dismissed. Explain to the client that the situation is uncomfortable, and massage therapy can no longer be provided. The dismissal must be done gently, but firmly, and the client should be told the decision is final. The client who immediately asks for sexual release is a different issue. In the event this occurs, the therapist must explain succinctly that he or she does not provide sexual release or any kind of sexual interaction, and then the person must be dismissed.

Care must be taken in situations that could become difficult, and any case where behavior could be questioned must be avoided. Some such cases would include male therapists who wish to do home calls for women who are alone in the house. A good solution is to pair up with a female therapist and do these massages as a team. It is important that a parent or legal guardian be in the room when massage services are given to a child under eighteen years. A practitioner should never work behind a locked door. Instead, a sign should be posted that indicates a massage is in session, and the room should not be entered without knocking. A therapist must be conscious of his or her appearance and make sure it is kept as nonsexual as possible.

Therapeutic/Professional Relationship for Massage Professionals

Masage Professionals
↓
caution
———————→
Countertransference

(Personal projections and feelings of the massage professional for the client.)

These professional boundaries must not be overstepped within the ethical professional relationships.

Therapeutic Relationship
————————————————→

(Professional's Responsibility)
Unidirectional = 100% Focus toward client

Specific Focus = Massage/Bodywork approaches that support body/mind connection (caution against mixing professional focuses such as providing mental or spiritual information or support)

Specific Time Frame = 15 minutes –1½ hour (caution against exceeding time limits)

Specific Environment = Professional Massage Setting (caution—avoid or limit interaction with client outside professional environment)
←————————————————

(Client's Responsibility)
Compensation for Services

Integration of Therapeutic Benefit

Client
↓
caution
←———————
Transference

Personal projection and feeling of the client for the massage professional

The Therapeutic Professional Relationship is maintained by the massage professional at all times. Countertransference issues must be observed and contained by the massage professional. Transference issues need to be contained and explained to the client by the massage professional.

Maintaining the delicate professional balance between client and practitioner is especially difficult with long-term clients. The nurturing approach of the massage therapist creates an environment where friendships can form. Regular clients do become important as people, as well as in their roles as clients. A therapist must always be honest with personal feelings and with the client.

The touch of a massage therapist is **safe touch.** What does it mean to be safe? A dictionary definition says that *safe* is not apt to cause danger or harm, or hurt, and is free from risk. Physiologically, *safe* means a state of homeostasis and not the alarm of "fight or flight" responses of the sympathetic autonomic nervous system, or the intense retreat and withdrawal of the parasympathetic autonomic nervous system responses. (See Chapter 6.) Safe is the ability to maintain well being in a situation and fluctuate easily between responses to cope resourcefully with inevitable change and demands in everyday life. The therapist must consider anything, including personal beliefs and fears, that may make touch unsafe for clients. By using this educational experience to explore these issues, more safe places can be found for the practitioner, which will influence professional touch, and make the massage room a safe place to be. The essence of this work is human touch. By dealing with personal intimacy issues, not only can the massage therapist provide essential touch for the client, but the client becomes able to establish proper boundaries. It must always be kept in mind that each individual therapist represents the entire massage therapy profession. Demonstration of respect for the self demonstrates respect for the profession as a whole.

When ethical dilemmas are difficult to resolve, massage therapists are expected to engage in a conscientious decision-making process that is explicit enough to bear public scrutiny. If the massage therapist can prove that every reasonable effort was made to apply respectable principles in the resolution of a problem, then the best possible attempt was made.

A comprehensive code of ethics for massage professionals has been compiled from codes of ethics developed by professional organizations, licenses, and standards of practice from other health professions (Box 2.7). An attempt has been made to include all points presented in the various ethical conduct codes.

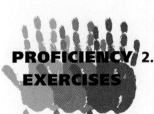

PROFICIENCY EXERCISES

1. **Select three items from your list of prejudices, fears, and behaviors, and purposely spend time with a person who triggers these responses. Risk talking with this individual about the situation in an attempt to go beyond the influences of appearance, behavior, etc. to get to know the person.**

2. **With three other students, have each person write about a specific situation where informed consent is difficult to obtain from a client. Exchange responses with a different group and role play a situation. One student is the massage practitioner, one is the client, and the other evaluates how well the situation was handled. Try different situations until each student has had a chance to play each role.**

Box 2.7
CODE OF ETHICS

Principles

A. Respect for the dignity of persons: Massage therapists will maintain respect for the interests, dignity, rights, and needs of all clients, staff, and colleagues.

B. Responsible caring: Competent, quality, client care will be provided at the highest standard possible.

C. Integrity in relationships: At all times, the therapist will behave with integrity, honesty, and diligence in practice and duties.

D. Responsibility to society: Massage therapists are responsible and accountable to society and shall conduct themselves in a manner that maintains high, ethical standards.

In compliance with the principles of the code of ethics the massage therapists will:

1. Respect all clients, colleagues, and health professionals through nondiscrimination regardless of their age, gender, race, national origin, sexual orientation, religion, socioeconomic status, body type, political affiliation, state of health, personal habits, and life-coping skills.

2. Perform only those services for which they are qualified and honestly represent their education, certification, professional affiliations, and other qualifications. The massage therapist will apply treatment only when there is a reasonable expectation that it will be advantageous to the client's condition. The therapist, in consultation with the client, will continually evaluate the effectiveness of treatment.

3. Respect the scope of practices of other health care and service professionals including medical doctors, chiropractors, physical therapists, podiatrists, orthopedists, psychotherapists, counselors, acupuncturists, nurses, exercise physiologists, athletic trainers, nutritionists, spiritual advisors, and cosmetologists.

4. Respect all ethical health care practitioners, and work together to promote heath and healing.

5. Acknowledge the limitations of their personal skills and when needed, refer clients to the appropriate qualified professional. The therapist will require consultation with other knowledgeable professionals when:
   - a client requires diagnosis and opinion beyond a therapist's capabilities of assessment
   - a client's condition is beyond the scope of practice
   - a combined health care team is required
   If referral to another health care provider is necessary, it must be done with the informed consent of the client.

6. Not work with any individual who has a specific disease process without supervision by a licensed medical professional.

7. Be adequately educated and understand the physiologic effects of the specific massage bodywork techniques used to determine if any application is contraindicated and to ensure the most beneficial techniques are applied to a given individual.

8. Not make false claims regarding the potential benefits of the techniques rendered, and actively educate the public regarding the actual benefits of massage and bodywork.

**Box 2.7
CODE OF ETHICS
(continued)**

Principles

9. Acknowledge the importance and individuality of each person including colleagues, peers, and clients.

10. Work only with the informed consent of clients, and professionally disclose to the client any situation that may interfere with the ability to provide the best care to serve the client's best interest.

11. Display respect for the client by honoring a client's process and following all recommendations by being present, listening, asking only pertinent questions, keeping agreements, being on time, draping properly, and customizing massage to fit the client's needs.

Note: Draping is covered in Chapter 9 of this text. Ontario guidelines[1] give these requirements for draping:

It is the responsibility of the massage therapist to assure the privacy and respect of the client and to find out if the client feels comfortable, safe, and secure with the draping provided.

The client may choose to be fully draped or clothed throughout the treatment.

The female client's breasts are never undraped.

The genitals, perineum, or anus are never undraped.

Consent of the client is required to work on any part of the body regardless of whether the client is fully clothed, fully draped, or partially draped.

12. Provide a safe, comfortable, and clean environment.

13. Maintain clear and honest communication with clients, and keep client communications confidential. Confidentiality is of the utmost importance. The massage professional must inform the client that the referring physician may be eligible to access client records, and records may be subpoenaed by the courts.

14. Conduct business in a professional and ethical manner in relation to clientele, business associates, acquaintances, government bodies, and the general public.

15. Follow city, county, state, national, and international requirements.

16. Charge a fair price for the session. A gift, gratuity, or benefit that is intended to influence a referral, a decision, or a treatment may not be accepted and must be immediately returned to the giver.

17. Keep accurate records and review the records with the client.

18. Never engage in any sexual conduct, sexual conversation, or any other sexual activities involving clients.

19. Not affiliate with any business that uses any form of sexual suggestiveness or explicit sexuality in advertising, promotion of services, or in the actual practice of service.

20. Practice honesty in advertising, promoting services ethically and in good taste. Advertise only those techniques for which adequate training or certification has been received.

21. Strive for professional excellence through regular assessment of personal strengths, limitations, and effectiveness by continuing education and training.

22. Accept the responsibility to self, clients, and the profession to maintain physical, mental, and emotional well being. Inform clients when the therapist is not functioning at best capacity.

continued

Box 2.7
CODE OF ETHICS
(continued)

Principles

23. Refrain from the use of any mind-altering drugs, alcohol, or intoxicants before or during professional massage bodywork sessions.
24. Maintain a professional appearance and demeanor by keeping good hygiene and dressing in a professional, modest, and nonsexual manner.
25. Undergo periodic peer review.
26. Respect all pertinent reporting requirements outlined by legislation regarding child abuse.
27. Report to the proper authorities any accurate knowledge and its supportive documentation regarding violations by massage therapists and other health or service professionals.
28. Avoid interests, activities, or influences that might conflict with the obligations to act in the best interest of clients and the massage therapy profession. Safeguard professional integrity by recognizing potential conflicts of interest and avoiding them.

3. **Using the same format as in exercise 2, write about a sexual misconduct and intimacy situation.**
4. **Develop a "time to go" ritual.**
5. **List three things you will do to maintain professional space.**
6. **Given each point of the code of ethics, answer to the following: "What does this mean to me?"**
7. **Develop a personal code of ethics.**
8. **Analyze two existing professional codes of ethics. How are they similar, and how are they different?**

CREDENTIALING AND LICENSING

SECTION OBJECTIVES

Using the information presented in this section, the student will be able to:

❶ Understand the difference between government and private credentials.
❷ Determine if a credentialing program is valid.

Credentials are designations earned by completing an educational or examination process that verifies a certain level of expertise in a given skill. Governmental and private professional credentialing processes are being developed within the massage profession. Standardization of the profession has resulted in different methods of proving skills in order to practice therapeutic massage. The massage professional should have an understanding of the various credentialing processes and what is required in order to legally practice.

The only credentials required for the practice of therapeutic massage are enacted by the government (Box 2.8). All others are voluntary. Because of some confusing and difficult local laws, special legislative concerns need to be addressed by the massage professional. Many massage and bodywork organizations have developed their own types of credentials. These credentials are only valid in so far as they indicate a level of professional achievement. A school diploma, which is received upon completion of the course work, is an example. This is a very important process for a massage professional, but it is not a legally required credential unless stipulated by the law. For instance, a diploma from a state-regulated school may be required in order to take licensing examinations in states that license massage therapists.

**Box 2.8
GOVERNMENT CREDENTIALS
AND REGULATIONS**

1. Licensing
   - Requires a state or provincial board of examiners.
   - Requires all constituents who practice the profession to be licensed.
   - Legally defines and limits the scope of practice for a profession.
   - Requires specific educational requirements or examination.
   - Provides for protection for title usage, i.e., *massage therapist*—and only those licensed can use the title.
2. Government certification (not to be confused with a private certification process)
   - Administered by an independent board.
   - Is voluntary, but would be required by anyone using the protected title, i.e. *massage therapist.* Other people can provide the service, but cannot call themselves massage therapists.
   - Requires specific educational requirements and examination.
3. Government registration (not to be confused with private registration processes)
   - Administered by the State Department of Registry or other appropriate state agency.
   - Is voluntary.
   - Does not necessarily require specific education, such as a school diploma. Often, other forms of verification of professional standards, such as years in practice, are acceptable.
   - Does not provide title protection.
4. Exemption
   - Exemption (not required to comply) from an existing local or state regulation.
   - Practitioners who meet specified educational requirements could be exempt from meeting current regulatory requirements.
   - Does not provide title protection.

Anyone can offer private certification. Given this fact, it is important to make sure that any educational program or examination you take is sanctioned and administered by a reputable, regulated, and verifiable provider. As an example, state licensed schools, recognized national and state professional organizations, and classes approved for continuing education credits for other health professionals have had to undergo a review process that validates their educational offerings. There is a National Commission for Certifying Agencies (NCCA). Approval by this agency validates certification processes.

Recently, the National Certification Examination for Therapeutic Massage and Bodywork has been developed. The test covers human anatomy, physiology, kinesiology, clinical pathology, massage and bodywork theory, assessment, adjunct techniques, business practices, and professionalism. The test was developed by a professional team through the Psychological Corporation, a recognized test development firm. The test is meant to evaluate entry-level knowledge base and skills. The educational requirement to qualify to take the examination is equivalent to five hundred hours of education. **This examination is *NOT* a government-regulated examination.** It is a voluntary, privately administered exam, unless an individual state decides to use it for a licensing examination. Passing the National Certification Examination for Therapeutic Massage and Bodywork is one concrete avenue to validate professional achievement.

LAW AND LEGISLATION

SECTION OBJECTIVES

Using the information presented in this section, the student will be able to:

❶ Understand the basic role of local and state legislation and their influence on therapeutic massage.

❷ Describe the two levels of practice for therapeutic massage.

❸ Contact local and state or provincial governments to obtain information about legislation pertinent to the practice of therapeutic massage.

State and Local Regulation

Therapeutic massage is not consistently regulated by the law anywhere. Each state in the United States, each province in Canada, and each country in Europe has different ways of dealing with massage regulation.

Because of this inconsistency, it is important for each massage professional to carefully research the government control and the laws that apply in the area where a massage business is planned. The types of legislative controls most often encountered are state or provincial controls and local controls. A province is a political unit of an empire or country such as Canada. Typically, it is a large area made up of many small local units of government. In the United States, states are the equivalent of provinces. States are further subdivided into counties, then into local townships and cities.

States (provinces) make laws that are developed to protect the public's safety and welfare. Many, but not all, health professionals are regulated at the state level through licensing. If the government feels that a particular activity could cause harm to the public, then it will seek to control and limit the individuals who can participate in the activity. Doctors, nurses, chiropractors, physical therapists, dentists, builders, electricians, cosmetologists, and plumbers are all licensed. Requirements for a knowledge base and the amount of education are determined. Tests, often called "boards," are given. The scope of practice, or what the professional is allowed to do, is described in the law that governs the licensed professional.

If the state does not choose to license a particular profession (occupational licensing), local governments (usually townships and cities) can choose to regulate activities within their jurisdiction. Again, local laws, usually called *ordinances,* are in place to protect the public's safety and welfare. Local governments are most concerned with what types of activities go on in their region and how the land is used (zoning).

If the state licenses a professional, then the local government does not feel the need to regulate the actual practice of the professional by setting educational standards and administering competency tests. The local government does regulate where the professional may work. This is done through zoning laws. Professionals such as doctors, lawyers, and accountants may have to have their place of business in a particular zone or area of land use. Land use is usually determined on a master plan that directs the way the local government wants to see their area grow and develop. It is important to designate areas as residential (living), industrial, retail business districts, (commercial) professional offices, and farming (agriculture). If this zoning is not done, a loud industrial operation could disturb the quiet living in a residential area. Local governments are also concerned with the safety of the buildings in their area. Monitoring the safety of buildings is the responsibility of the building inspector.

Many laws and local massage ordinances were written to control prostitution by preventing the practice of massage. This type of ordinance is easy to recognize because it requires finger printing, medical examinations for sexually transmitted disease, and other degrading requirements. Local ordinances of this type are still common in states where the profession of massage has not yet been licensed. Today, more than one-third of the United States has some type of state licensing for the professional practice of therapeutic massage. The trend continues in this direction. Licensing requirements in Canada, Europe, and other countries vary to such an extent that it is impossible to cover all of the information in this chapter. Overall, licensing requirements are changing quickly. To obtain the most current information, contact licensed massage therapy schools and government licensing offices in your specific area.

In states where there is licensing for massage, the massage professional must still comply with local zoning ordinances and building requirements when setting up a professional practice. When there is state licensing for massage, the local government usually treats the massage professional like any other licensed health or service professional. The business is classified as a service and the location of the business is required to comply with the proper zoning, which is usually an office or commercial zoning.

Local governments discourage any type of business operation in residential areas, but will designate, with special restriction, what types of business can be operated from a home. These home occupations are usually service orientated as opposed to retail (the sale of goods) and would limit traffic to and from the home. There may need to be a special and separate area of the home, including a separate entrance, if there is to be a home office. Another requirement is that no employees other than the family in the home may be hired. Sometimes only those with a special need, such as a disability that prevents working out of the home, are eligible for a home office permit. Usually a special permit is required to have a home office. Each local government unit is different. Many massage practitioners choose to work from a home office. The "cottage industry" or home business is growing rapidly. A massage practice is a business that fits well within these special requirements.

The main purpose for a law or ordinance is to protect the public's safety and welfare. When a governing body decides to enact regulations, it must fit this criterion. Laws and ordinances are **NOT** developed to protect the interest of a small group, also known as a special interest group. Medical massage is supposed to be supervised by licensed medical professionals, and the responsibility for the public safety falls to the supervising personnel. If proper supervision is in place, states have no reason for licensing massage professionals unless they feel the personal service massage is a public threat to safety and welfare. There could be a case for this position with the need for formal training regarding sanitation, contraindications, and necessary referrals to licensed medical personnel for suspected health problems. There may be a case for enacting massage laws to protect the massage professional from discrimination and to provide the ability to practice a professional livelihood.

Today, there are two distinct types of practices of massage and bodywork. There are the wellness personal service professionals who provide holistic approaches to massage including stress reduction and general health benefits. The second distinction is medical or rehabilitative massage that is more focused to the care of sick persons and the correction or stabilization of medical problems. Certainly, there is an overlap with all people benefiting from general wellness massage whether sick or not, and rehabilitative massage providing general beneficial effects even when focused to a particular health problem. Usually, the rehabilitative massage is provided as part of a multidisciplinary approach with a licensed medical professional in a supervisory position. Because the massage professional is working in an established medical setting, and the massage is part of the medical treatment plan, local regulation is seldom an issue.

The inherent problems include wellness personal service massage businesses being classified with massage parlors, and medical rehabilitative massage being practiced without direct medical supervision outside an established medical setting. A typical entry-level standard for the practice of massage in the United States is between five hundred and one thousand class hours of training. This is the level to which this text is focused. This level of training seems sufficient to provide the necessary knowledge to perform massage in a competent and safe manner. It does not seem to be enough time to train massage therapists in specific medical rehabilitative massage procedures. Additional pathology, medical terminology, and other requirements are needed if one is to act as a responsible massage professional within the medical community. A program more in line with the curriculum established in Ontario, Canada, of twenty-two hundred class hours, is more realistic for those wishing to pursue a career in medical and rehabilitative massage.

A more serious difficulty arises when other health professionals feel that massage practitioners are doing medical or rehabilitative massage, which is more in line with the health professionals scope of practice. This difficulty may also arise with athletic trainers and exercise physiologists, who may not be state licensed, but usually have a minimum of a bachelor degree in their chosen field. The level of education becomes an important factor. A legitimate concern of these professionals is a lack of adequate education of the massage professional regarding procedures and effects of massage in relation to a total treatment plan. There is little, if any, comprehensive massage therapy training available in the university setting. Typically, massage education is provided by the private vocational sector with the maximum training available, about two years, in areas such as British Columbia or Ontario. This training would be comparable to a two-year vocational training program at a community college resulting in an associate degree. Many medical technologists, such as respiratory therapists, physical therapy assistants, and registered nurses have graduated from associate degree programs. Massage therapy educators will need to address the issue of appropriate education to accommodate those wishing to work in the medical setting.

It is true that a written and practical test cannot measure the massage professional's gentleness, care, nonjudgmental behavior, intuition, and touch. This problem does not mean that formal tests are not valid. They are. Unfortunately, most governmental bodies are not concerned with these attributes. Local governments need to establish that the massage business is legitimate therapeutic massage and not a front for prostitution. State governments have to protect the public's health, safety, and welfare from the unregulated practice of massage. Both units of government need to protect the public from potentially dangerous acts by defining performance criteria based on education or the ability to pass a test.

Licensing, compliance with ordinances (see Box 2.9), and passing any of the nationally recognized certification exams is important in the professional practice of massage. The bottom line is to comply with the existing standards of practice, both required and voluntary. If a difficult state law or local ordinance is encountered, massage therapists must work together to change the regulation. The staff at a licensed massage school is the best resource on procedures to work with local governments to alter a nonsupportive massage ordinance.

Reciprocity

Reciprocity means the right of exchange of privileges between governing bodies. Some states have similar licensing requirements for professionals. When this happens, a state may accept a different state's license. This is not common for many professionals, and it is even less common for mas-

Box 2.9
STEPS FOR COMPLIANCE REGARDING
LICENSING REQUIREMENTS

Given this background on laws and legal issues, the steps to follow in order to be in compliance are:

1. Find out if your state or province requires licensing. Contact the Department of Licensing and Regulation, occupational licensing division, for this information. If state licensing exists, then find out what the educational requirements are to take the examination.

2. If your state does not have licensing, then contact the local government where you intend to work to inquire about local ordinances. Obtain a copy of the ordinances and read them carefully. Look especially for the educational, zoning, and facility requirements. Whether you live in a city, township, or similar government unit, it is usually the clerk's office that has this information.

     Note: Even if there is no state or local regulation, it is a good idea to only attend a licensed school or approved training program. Other states or local governments may require this type of education and without it you cannot practice in their areas.

3. Shop carefully for your school of massage training. Contact the State Department of Education and confirm that the school is licensed and in compliance with state regulations.

4. Before renting, buying, or setting up the actual massage practice, contact the local government concerning zoning requirements and building codes. If you are considering a home office, check the zoning ordinances to make sure you will be in compliance. Again, your city or township officials (usually the clerk) are your best sources of information. Zoning permits require a public hearing with your neighbors being notified by mail, and the public hearing advertised in the newspaper. Contact the zoning department to find out what action is required.

     Whether establishing a business in a home office or in a business zone, contact the neighbors to offer an explanation of your business and obtain their responses. Without their approval, or at least lack of opposition, it is unlikely that you will obtain the permit. Attend the hearing at all costs. Remember, NO PERMIT = NO BUSINESS. Zoning permits may require six to eight weeks to complete. If you start your business without proper permits you could be shut down at any time by government authorities.

5. Before you actually rent space or begin your business, contact the local government and apply for any permits or business licenses required. Make sure you meet all regulations. Plan on fees costing from $25 to $500.

sage therapists. Individual state licensing or any type of certification does not secure the right to practice massage in any other location, other than that of the government issuing the license.

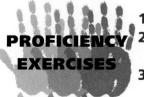

PROFICIENCY EXERCISES

1. **Investigate the legal requirements to practice massage in your area.**
2. **Collect information to develop into an educational packet about massage for government officials and the general public.**
3. **Attend a local government board meeting and observe the process.**

Regulations, standards of practice, codes of conduct, scopes of practice, and so forth are methods of setting the rules for cooperative professional relationships. All organized groups have rules that allow for effective interaction between the members. Respect is important, and working together as a team is essential in professional practice. Let us hope that the massage therapy profession is an example of cooperation, respect for other professions, and ethical standards of practice providing for internal professional regulation and compliance with external government control.

1. What are ethics?
2. What are the basic approaches to massage and bodywork?
3. Why is it difficult to develop a definition for therapeutic massage?
4. Why does the massage professional need to understand the scope of practice for other professionals?
5. How do massage practitioners keep from falling into a situation where they could be accused of practicing medicine?
6. Why is it unethical to provide massage services to a client that we do not like or with whom we are uncomfortable?
7. What is the importance of disclosure in the right of refusal?
8. Why is informed consent so important?
9. What is a way to define boundaries?
10. It is easy to determine acts that constitute sexual misconduct, but how do you decide if more subtle activities and feelings are a breach in the trust between the client and the practitioner?
11. Why could a client interpret the experience of massage as a sexual one?
12. Why is it ethical to establish rules of conduct for the client and the massage therapist and maintain professional space in the client-practitioner relationship?
13. What word sums up the code of ethics?
14. What important aspects of credentialing should the massage practitioner know?
15. Why does the massage professional need to understand legislative issues, local ordinances, and zoning?
16. What is the main purpose of a law?
17. What are the two types of massage therapy practice?
18. What difficulties arise for the wellness personal service massage professional?
19. What difficulties arise for the massage therapists who have sufficient training to work with medical rehabilitative massage?

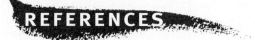

REFERENCES

1. Ontario, Canada: Therapeutic massage curriculum guidelines. Toronto, Ontario, 1867.
2. Oregon Administrative Rules, Board of Massage Technicians Chapter 334 Division 10 Massage Licensing, Oregon Board of Massage Technicians. Portland, OR, 1991.
3. Regulated Health Professions Act and the Massage Therapy Act. Ontario, Canada, 1992.
4. Webster's New Universal Unabridged Dictionary Deluxe, ed 2, New York 1983, Simon & Schuster.

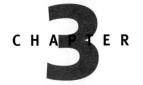

CHAPTER 3

MASSAGE AND MEDICAL
TERMINOLOGY

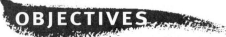

After completing this chapter, the student will be able to do the following:

1 Identify the three word elements used in medical terms.
2 Combine word elements into medical terms.
3 Translate medical terms.
4 Identify pertinent abbreviations used in health care and their meanings.
5 Review the anatomy and physiology important for the massage professional.

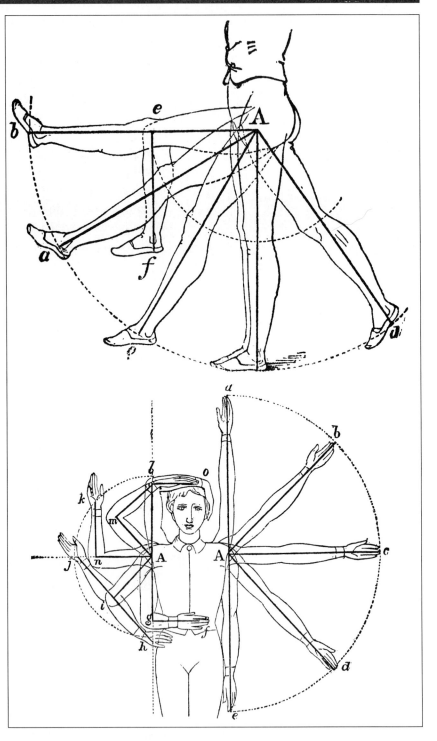

Fundamental and derivative positions of all possible therapeutic positions for applying arm movements in the exercise component of Per Henrik Ling's Swedish Movement Cure. (Courtesy of University of Pennsylvania, Special Collections Department, Van Pelt Library)

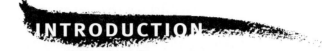

INTRODUCTION

The study of medical terminology provides a bridge to the accepted language of the sciences. As massage therapy again moves into the position of a medically valid service, it will become increasingly important for the massage professional to be able to speak and understand this language. This chapter provides an outline of the medical terminology most often encountered by the massage professional, and will assist students as they utilize medical terminology and anatomy and physiology textbooks for further study. It is recommended that the massage therapy student enroll in a medical terminology class at a local community college. Students also might be fortunate enough to attend a massage therapy school that teaches a section on medical terminology.

This chapter is dependent on the use of both a medical terminology textbook and a medical dictionary. In many cases a list of the terms most ofter encountered by the massage professional is provided for which the student is directed to look up the definitions in the medical terminology text or dictionary. This chapter will help consolidate and focus the medical terminology information specific for the massage professional as medical terminology and anatomy and physiology textbooks are used during the study of therapeutic massage.

Exploring the terminology will provide an overview of anatomy and physiology. Used with an anatomy and physiology textbook and class instruction, this section can help narrow the information into a focus that is more specific to the field of massage. The information in this chapter will be significant for understanding massage as it relates to anatomy, physiology, pathophysiology, and client records. Because the basis for medical terminology is scientific language, understanding this information will help the massage student understand massage therapy research as well as articles and books on subjects related to massage.

As a massage therapy student, you have learned or will learn the names of muscle, bones, joints, and other anatomy. This knowledge base will serve as a firm foundation for the development of an understanding and use of medical terminology.

It is important to have agreement about terminology. Without a common language we cannot communicate. It is the responsibility of massage professionals to be able to communicate with their clients in a common language. It is just as important to understand the communications of other health professionals. Currently, the terminology used in massage therapy is inconsistent. Although similar words are used, the meanings of those words do not always coincide. The definitions for massage therapy vocabulary in this textbook are based on traditional Swedish definitions, Canadian resources, available books, and common knowledge. This chapter should offer a basis of agreement for terminology for the massage profession. This must occur before others in the health profession can communicate with us as a group. As is mentioned in the history chapter (see Chapter 1), Ling had difficulty in communicating with the established authorities of his time because he did not speak their language. If those in the massage profession wish to receive the respect and understanding of other health professionals, then we must explain ourselves in their terms and patiently educate them to our language.

The information from this chapter will help you as students begin to understand the medical terminology used in this textbook, to learn the meanings of words, and to provide a foundation for further study. It is recommended that the student obtain a medical terminology textbook, an anatomy and physiology textbook, and a medical dictionary to use when studying this chapter. Appendix C lists several suggestions for these supplemental texts.

FUNDAMENTAL WORD ELEMENTS

Medical terms are made up of word elements combined together. A term can be interpreted easily by separating the word into its elements. These word elements include prefixes, roots, and suffixes.

Prefixes

A *prefix* is placed at the beginning of a word to alter its meaning. A prefix cannot stand alone; it must be combined with another word element. See Table 3.1 for a listing of common prefixes.

Table 3.1
COMMON PREFIXES

Prefix	Meaning
a-, an-	without or not
ab-	away from
ad-	toward
ante-	before, forward
anti-	against
auto-	self
bi-	double, two
circum-	around
contra-	against, opposite
de-	down, from, away from, not
dia-	across, through, apart
dis-	separation, away from
dys-	bad, difficult, abnormal
ecto-	outer, outside
en-	in, into, within
endo-	inner, inside
epi-	over, on, upon
eryth-	red
ex-	out, out of, from, away from
hemi-	half
hyper-	excessive, too much, high
hypo-	under, decreased, less than normal
in-	in, into, within, not
inter-	between
intra-	within
intro-	into, within
leuk-	white
macro-	large
mal-	bad, illness, disease
mega-	large
micro-	small
mono-	one, single

Table 3.1
COMMON PREFIXES *(continued)*

Prefix	Meaning
neo-	new
non-	not
para-	abnormal
per-	by, through
peri-	around
poly-	many, much
post-	after, behind
pre-	before, in front of, prior to
pro-	before, in front of
re-	again
retro-	backward
semi-	half
sub-	under
super-	above, over, excess
supra-	above, over
trans-	across
uni-	one

Root Words

Root words provide the fundamental meanings of words. Combined roots, prefixes, and suffixes form medical and scientific terms. A vowel, called a *combining vowel,* is often added when two roots are combined, or when a suffix is added to a root. The vowel used is usually an "o" and occasionally an "i." See Table 3.2 for a listing of common root words.

Table 3.2
COMMON ROOT WORDS

Root (combining vowel)	Meaning
abdomin (o)	abdomen
aden (o)	gland
adren (o)	adrenal gland
angi (o)	vessel
arterio (o)	artery
arthr (o)	joint
broncho (o)	bronchus, bronchi
card, cardi (o)	heart
cephal (o)	head
chondr (o)	cartilage
colo	colon
cost (o)	rib
crani (o)	skull
cyan (o)	blue
cyst (o)	bladder, cyst
cyt (o)	cell
derma	skin
duoden (o)	duodenum
encephal (o)	brain
enter (o)	intestines
fibr (o)	fiber, fibrous
gastr (o)	stomach
gyn, gyne, gyneco-	woman
hem, hema, hemo, hemat (o)	blood

continued

Table 3.2
COMMON ROOT WORDS
(continued)

Root (combining vowel)	Meaning
hepat (o)	liver
hydr (o)	water
hyster (o)	uterus
ile (o), ili (o)	ileum
laryng (o)	larynx
mamm (o)	breast, mammary gland
my (o)	muscle
myel (o)	spinal cord, bone marrow
nephr (o)	kidney
neur (o)	nerve
ocul (o)	eye
orth (o)	straight, normal, correct
oste (o)	bone
ot (o)	ear
ped (o)	child, foot
pharyng (o)	pharynx
phleb (o)	vein
pnea	breathing, respiration
pneum (o)	lung, air, gas
proct (o)	rectum
psych (o)	mind
pulmo	lung
py (o)	pus
rect (o)	rectum
rhin (o)	nose
sten (o)	narrow, constriction
stern (o)	sternum
stomat (o)	mouth
therm (o)	heat
thorac (o)	chest
thromb (o)	clot, thrombus
thyr (o)	thyroid
toxic (o)	poison, poisonous
trache (o)	trachea
ur (o)	urine, urinary tract, urination
urethr (o)	urethra
urin (o)	urine
uter (o)	uterus
vas (o)	blood vessel, vas deferens
ven (o)	vein
vertebr (o)	spine, vertebrae

Suffixes

A *suffix* is a word element that is placed at the end of a root to alter the meaning of the word. Suffixes cannot stand alone; like prefixes, they must accompany a root in order to form a word. The suffix should be the starting point when interpreting medical terms.

Roots ending with a consonant require a combining vowel. If the root ends with a vowel and the suffix begins with a vowel, the vowel at the end of the root is deleted. See Table 3.3 for a listing of common suffixes.

Combining Word Elements

Word elements are the building blocks that are combined to create medical and scientific terminology. Prefixes always precede roots and suffixes always follow roots.

Table 3.3
COMMON SUFFIXES

Suffix	Meaning
-algia	pain
-asis	condition, usually abnormal
-cele	hernia, herniation, pouching
-cyte	cell
-ectasis	dilation, stretching
-ectomy	excision, removal of
-emia	blood condition
-genesis	development, production, creation
-genic	producing, causing
-gram	record
-graph	a diagram, a recording instrument
-graphy	making a recording
-iasis	condition of
-ism	a condition
-itis	inflammation
-logy	the study of
-lysis	destruction of, decomposition
-megaly	enlargement
-oma	tumor
-osis	condition
-pathy	disease
-penia	lack, deficiency
-phasia	speaking
-phobia	an exaggerated fear
-plasty	surgical repair or reshaping
-plegia	paralysis
-rrhage, -rrhagia	excessive flow
-rrhea	profuse flow, discharge
-scope	examination instrument
-scopy	examination using a scope
-stasis	maintenance, maintaining a constant level
-stomy, -ostomy	creation of an opening
-tomy, -otomy	incision, cutting into
-uria	condition of the urine

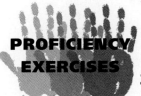

PROFICIENCY EXERCISES

1. Combine 100 words using the prefixes, root words, and suffixes listed in Tables 3.1 to 3.3. Define the words created. Look each word up in a medical dictionary to see that it exists and you have the correct meaning and spelling.
2. Find fifty medical terms in other chapters in this textbook and break them down into the prefix, root word, and suffix.

Diagnosis Terminology

It is important for the massage practitioner to understand these terms for history taking and for working within a clinical setting.

In a medical dictionary, look up each of the following terms related to the diagnosis of disease conditions of the body: acute, ambulatory, anomaly, atrophy, benign, chronic, clinic, clinical, diagnosis, malignant, metastatic, prognosis, sign, symptom, syndrome, and systemic.

Selected Terms Related to Diseases

The following terms are related to diseases: bacterial, cancer, congenital, degenerative, epidemic, exacerbation, fungal, idiopathic, infectious, trauma, and viral.

TERMINOLOGY OF LOCATION AND POSITION

It is important that the massage professional be able to use directional terminology to accurately describe a location of an area of the body. The following terms are used most often.

Directional Terms (Fig. 3.1)

Directional terms are used to describe how one body part relates to another. Consult your medical dictionary or medical terminology text to define the following terms: anterior, cephalad, caudad, deep, distal, dorsal, external, inferior, internal, lateral, medial, peripheral, plantar, posterior, proximal, superior, superficial, valgus, varus, and volar.

Positional Terms

Positional terms are used to describe the relationship of the body to the different planes.

1. Anatomic position: the stance of the body when it is erect with the arms hanging to the side, palms facing forward
2. Erect position: the body in a standing position
3. Supine position: the body lying in a horizontal position with the face up

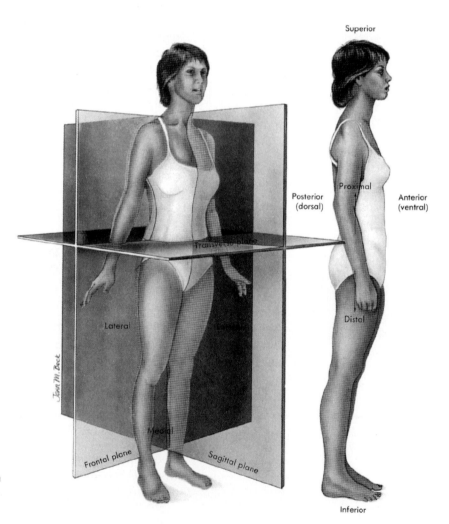

Figure 3.1
Directions and planes of the body. (From Thibodeau: Structure & function of the body, St. Louis, 1992, Mosby–Year Book, Inc.)

4. Prone position: the body lying with the face down in a horizontal position
5. Laterally recumbent position: the body lying horizontally on either the right or left side

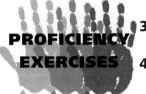

PROFICIENCY EXERCISES

1. **Act out each directional and positional term by creating a movement, a pantomine, or assuming the position.**
2. **With a partner, place each other in the postions listed above. Say each term as you position your partner.**
3. **Draw the four quadrants (Fig. 3.2) on your abdomen; palpate and list the organs in each area.**
4. **Write a story about a client who is filling out a history form and telling you about his or her condition. Use all the terms listed in this section in the story.**
5. **Refer to Chapter 4 and the indications and contraindications section in Appendix A and find all of the terms listed in Table 3.4.**

STRUCTURE OF THE BODY

The structure of the body partially consists of tissues. A *tissue* is a collection of specialized cells that perform a special function. *Histo* is a root word meaning tissue. *Histology* is the study of tissue.

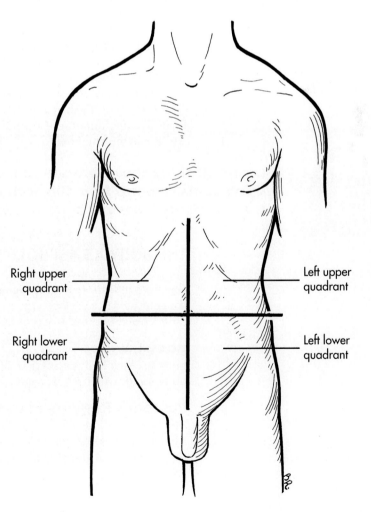

Right upper quadrant

Left upper quadrant

Right lower quadrant

Left lower quadrant

Figure 3.2
Quadrants of the abdomen.

Table 3.4

SYSTEMS OF THE BODY AND THEIR IMPORTANT ORGANS

System	Organs in the System
Musculoskeletal	Bones, ligaments, skeletal muscles, tendons, joints
Nervous	Brain, spinal cord, nerves, special sense organs
Cardiovascular	Heart, arteries, veins, capillaries
Lymphatic	Lymphatic vessels, lymph nodes, spleen, tonsils, thymus gland
Digestive	Mouth, tongue, teeth, salivary glands, esophagus, stomach, small and large intestines, liver, gallbladder, pancreas
Respiratory	Nasal cavity, larynx, trachea, bronchi, lungs, diaphragm, pharynx
Urinary	Kidneys, ureters, urinary bladder, urethra
Endocrine	Endocrine glands: hypothalamus, hypophysis (pituitary), thyroid, thymus, parathyroid, pineal, adrenal, pancreas, gonads (ovary or testis)
Reproductive	Female: ovaries, uterine tubes (oviducts), uterus, vagina; male: testes, penis, prostate gland, seminal vesicles, spermatic ducts
Integumentary	Skin, hair, nails, sebaceous glands, sweat glands, breasts

The primary tissues of the body are epithelial, connective, muscular, and nervous. Look up each of these tissues in a medical terminology book, anatomy and physiology textbook, and medical dictionary and list the function of each type.

An *organ* is of a collection of specialized tissues. An organ has a specific function(s), but does not act independently of other organs.

Organs make up systems. There are ten general systems in the body (see Table 3.4). Each system is comprised of organs that collectively perform specific functions. Consult an anatomy and physiology textbook for additional information.

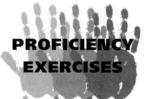

PROFICIENCY EXERCISES

1. **Locate all of the above terms in your anatomy and physiology textbook.**
2. **Using as many words from this section as possible, write a poem about the four tissue types and body systems.**

THE BODY AS A WHOLE

The body as a whole is made up of several systems. Some of the systems are concentrated in a particular part of the body (e.g., the urinary system) while others reach out to all parts of the body, as the circulatory system does.

Body Cavities

Look up each body cavity (Fig. 3.3) in your anatomy textbook and list the organs and structures each contains.

Posterior Regions of the Trunk

The back or posterior surface of the trunk is also divided into regions. The terms used to describe these regions are related to the names of the vertebrae in the spinal column (Fig. 3.4). In descending order they are as follows:

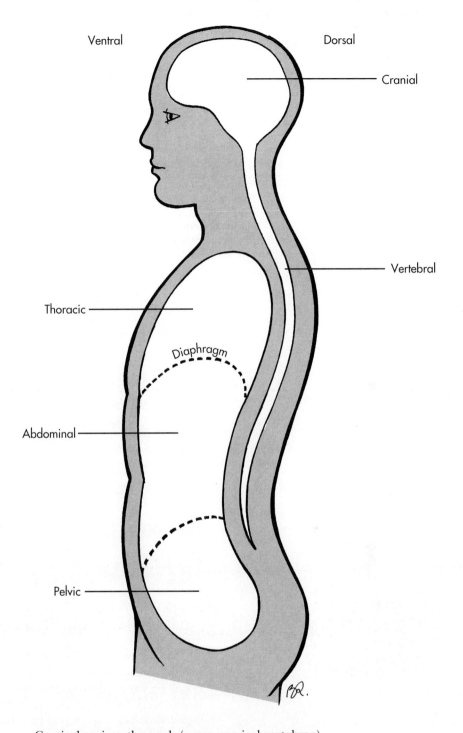

Figure 3.3
Body cavities.

Cervical region: the neck (seven cervical vertebrae)
Thoracic region: the chest (twelve thoracic vertebrae)
Lumbar region: the loin (five lumbar vertebrae)
Sacral region: the sacrum (five sacral vertebrae that are fused into one bone)
Coccyx: the tailbone (four coccygeal vertebrae that are fused into one bone)

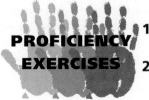

PROFICIENCY EXERCISES

1. **Using clay or some other modeling compound, build the body cavities and the regions of the posterior trunk.**
2. **With a partner palpate each area and say the names out loud.**

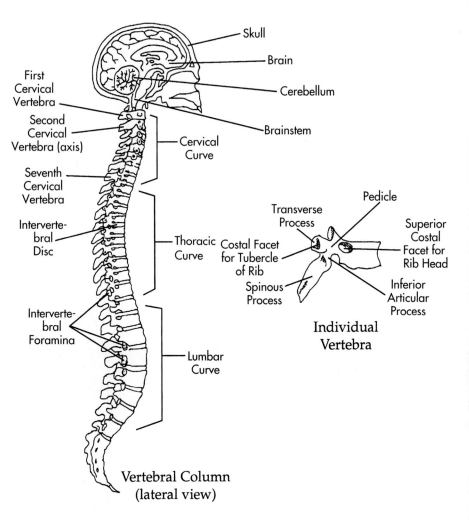

Figure 3.4
Vertebral column.

THE SKELETAL SYSTEM

The skeletal system consists of three elements: bones, cartilage, and ligaments.

Bone

Bone is a dense connective tissue compromised mostly of calcium and phosphate; os-, ossa-, oste-, and osteo- are all combining forms that mean "bone."

There are approximately 206 bones in the human skeleton. The massage professional must be familiar with all of them. Locate the following terms in your anatomy and physiology and medical terminology textbooks: cervical vertebrae, skull thoracic vertebrae, lumbar vertebrae, sacral vertebrae, coccygeal vertebrae, ribs, sternum, manubrium, body, xiphoid process, clavicle, scapula, humerus, ulna, radius, carpal, metacarpal bones, phalanges, pelvis, ilium, ischium, pubis, symphysis pubis, femur, patella, tibia, fibula, tarsal bones, metatarsal bones, phalanges, malleolus, process, crest, insertion, joint, line, olecranon, origin, spine, trochanter, tuberosity, and xiphoid (Fig. 3.5).

Cartilage

There are two types of cartilage in the skeletal system. *Hyaline cartilage,* which is very elastic, cushiony, and slippery, makes up the articular surfaces at the joints, the cartilage between the ribs, and at the nose, larynx, and trachea, and the fetal skeleton. It has a pearly, bluish color. Hyaline means "glass." *White fibrocartilage,* which is also elastic, flexible, and tough, is interarticular fibrocartilage found in joints such as the knee. The con-

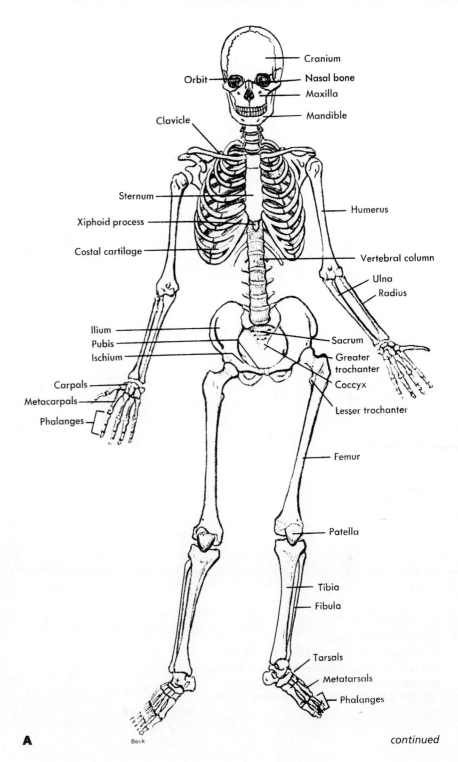

Figure 3.5
A, Skeletal system. Anterior view of skeleton.

A

Beck

continued

necting fibrocartilage is cartilage that is only slightly mobile. It is found between the vertebrae (referred to as disks) and between the pubic bones (the symphysis pubis).

Ligaments

Where the bones of the skeleton join, there is a *joint* or *articulation*. Movable joints are covered by cartilage and are held together by ligaments. Ligaments are made of white fibrous tissue. They are pliant, flexible, strong, and tough.

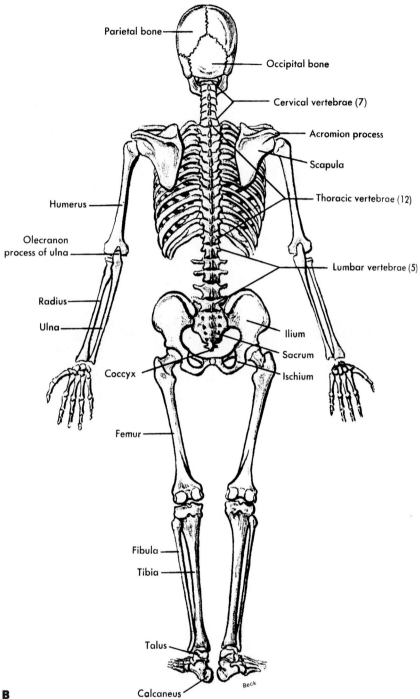

Parietal bone

Occipital bone

Cervical vertebrae (7)

Acromion process

Scapula

Thoracic vertebrae (12)

Humerus

Olecranon
process of ulna

Lumbar vertebrae (5)

Radius

Ulna

Ilium

Sacrum

Coccyx

Ischium

Femur

Fibula

Tibia

Talus

Calcaneus

Beck

Figure 3.5 *continued*
**B, Posterior view of skeleton. (From
LaFleur Brooks: Exploring medical lan-
guage—a student-directed approach
3/E, St. Louis, 1994, Mosby–Year Book,
Inc.)**

B

Selected Terms of Disease Conditions

This section is an analysis of selected terms related to disease conditions of the skeletal system. Locate each term in Appendix A for indications and contraindications to massage and in the medical dictionary: fracture, osteoarthritis, osteochondritis, osteochondrosis, osteoporosis, and spondylitis.

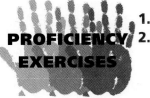

PROFICIENCY EXERCISES

1. **Palpate each bone listed and say its name out loud.**
2. **With a group of fellow students, assign each person to be a particular bone. By laying on the floor build the skeleton by having each person assume the proper bone positon. Be prepared to laugh and learn.**

THE ARTICULAR SYSTEM

Articulations are joints where two or more bones meet. The articular system concerns all of the anatomic and functional aspects of the joints.

Joints

Joints are places where bones come together, where limbs are attached, and where the motion of the skeletal system occurs. Some joints are rigid, and some allow a great degree of flexibility.

The joints function to allow motion of the musculoskeletal system, to bear weight, and to hold the skeleton together.

Look up each term related to the articular system in your anatomy and physiology and medical terminology textbooks: articulation, flexibility, synarthrodial, amphiarthrodial, diarthrodial, symphysis pubis, sacroiliac, symphysis, articular cartilage, articular disks, ligaments, synovial fluid, and tendon.

Types of Movement Permitted by Diarthrodial Joints (Fig. 3.6)

The types of movement permitted by diarthrodial joints are as follows (Fig. 3.6):

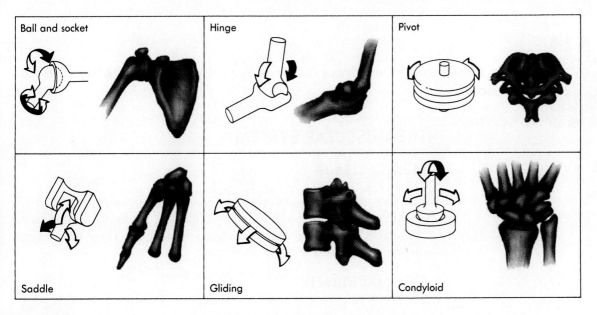

Ball and socket

Hinge

Pivot

Saddle

Gliding

Condyloid

Figure 3.6
Types of diarthrotic joints. Notice that the structure of each type dictates its function (movement). (From Thibodeau/Patton: The human body in health & disease, St. Louis, 1992, Mosby–Year Book, Inc.)

Flexion: bending that reduces the angle of a joint

Extension: straightening or stretching that increases the angle of a joint

Abduction: movement away (ab) from the midline

Adduction: movement toward (ad) the midline

Pronation: turning of the palm downward

Supination: turning of the palm upward (you can hold a bowl of soup in a supinated hand)

Eversion: turning (version) of the sole of the foot away from (e) the midline (when you evert your foot you move your little toe toward your ear)

Inversion: turning (version) of the sole of the foot inward (in)

Plantar flexion: bending of the plantar surface of the sole of the foot downward (plant your toes in the ground)

Rotation: rolling to the side (internal rotation: rolling toward the midline, external rotation: rolling away from the midline)

Circumduction: making a circle; the ability to move the limb in a circular manner

Protraction: thrusting a part of the body forward (pro)

Retraction: pulling a part of the body backward (re)

Elevation: raising a part of the body

Depression: lowering a part of the body

Opposition: the act of placing part of the body opposite another, as in placing the tip of the thumb opposite the tips of the fingers.

Bursae

Bursae are closed sacs or saclike structures (bursa) usually close to the joint cavities, with a lining similar to the synovial membrane lining of a true joint. Some bursae are continuous with the lining of a joint. The function of a bursa is to lubricate an area between tendons, ligaments, and bones where friction would otherwise develop.

Diagnostic Terms of Articular System Disease

Look up each term in the medical dictionary and in the indications/contraindications of Appendix A: diastasis, ankylosis, arthritis, bursitis, degenerative joint disease, dislocation, ganglion, genu valgum, genu varum, gout, hallux malleus, kyphosis, lordosis, rheumatoid arthritis, slipped disk, spinal curvature, scoliosis, sprain, spondylolisthesis, subluxation, tendinitis, tenosynovitis.

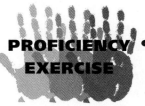

PROFICIENCY EXERCISE • **Do a dance that incorporates each of the joint movements listed in this section.**

THE MUSCULAR SYSTEM

Muscle Tissue

Tissues that are contractile make up the muscular system. There are three types of muscle tissue: cardiac muscle, smooth muscle, and skeletal muscle.

Muscle tissue is found in many organs of the body. Muscle tissue also makes up muscles, which are themselves organs. These muscles give the body shape and produce movement.

Skeletal Muscle

Each skeletal muscle is made up of sections. They have two ends, which are attached to other structures, and a belly.

Muscles cause and permit motion by the actions of contraction and relaxation. See Table 3.5 for terms used to describe movement.

Table 3.5
TERMS TO DESCRIBE MUSCLE MOVEMENT

Adductor	Muscle moving a part toward the midline
Abductor	Muscle moving a part away from the midline
Flexor	Muscle that bends a part
Extensor	Muscle that straightens a part
Levator	Muscle that raises a part
Depressor	Muscle that lowers a part
Tensor	Muscle that tightens a part

Contraction refers to the reduction in size or the shortening of a muscle. When one muscle contracts, another opposite muscle is stretched and put into a state of tension. *Relaxation* occurs when there is a reduction of tension and thus a return to the size of the resting muscle.

Muscles work in pairs of agonists and antagonists. *Agonists* are muscles responsible for the primary desired movement. The agonist is the prime mover. *Antagonists* are the muscles that oppose the action of the agonist.

Synergists are muscles that assist the agonists by holding a part of the body steady and thus giving leverage. The agonist-antagonist-synergist relationship permits the skeletal muscles to work in a purposeful manner and gives fluidity to motion. This is referred to as *coordination*. See Figure 3.7 for an anterior and posterior view of the muscular system.

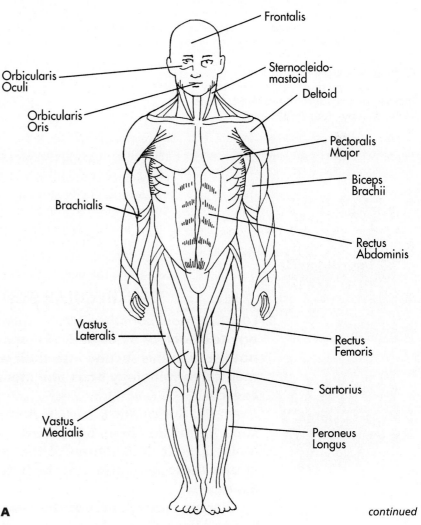

Figure 3.7
Major superficial muscles.
A, Anterior view of muscles.

A

continued

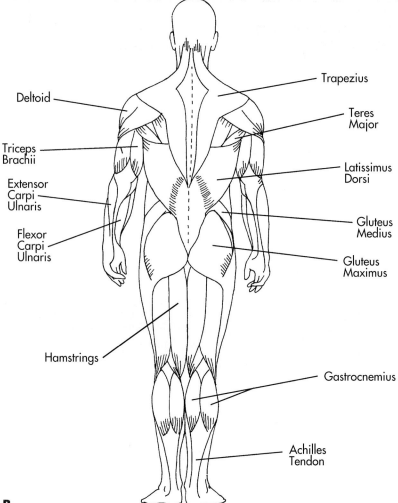

Deltoid

Triceps Brachii

Extensor Carpi Ulnaris

Flexor Carpi Ulnaris

Hamstrings

Trapezius

Teres Major

Latissimus Dorsi

Gluteus Medius

Gluteus Maximus

Gastrocnemius

Achilles Tendon

Figure 3.7 *continued*
B, Posterior view of muscles.
(From Mosby's medical terminology instructor's resource library, St. Louis, 1994, Mosby–Year Book, Inc.)

B

Use an anatomy and physiology textbook, medical dictionary, and kinesiology textbook to look up the following terms: aponeurosis, asthenia, atrophy, belly, clonus, contracture, cramp, fascia, fascicle, fasciculation, hyperkinesia, hypertrophy, insertion, musculotendinous junction, myalgia, origin, spasm, tendon, tone.

Names of muscles can be broken down into medical terminology word elements. Having a basic understanding of medical terminology can assist the student in both remembering and understanding muscle names (Table 3.6).

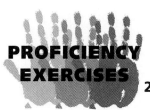

PROFICIENCY EXERCISES

1. **Locate a more complete list of muscles in your anatomy and physiology textbook or medical dictionary. Break down fifty muscle names not listed in this section into their word elements. You will need a medical terminology book and medical dictionary to complete this exercise.**
   Example: **Auricularis Superior:** *Auri* **means ear,** *ar* **means pertaining to, superior means above or upward.**
2. **Make up ridiculous sentences that explain listed muscle names. The crazier these sentences are, the better you will remember them.**
   Examples:
   Rectus femoris: part of the quadriceps muscle that is straight (rectus) and lies near the femur (femoris)

Table 3.6
MUSCLE DESCRIPTIONS USING MEDICAL TERMINOLOGY WORD ELEMENTS

The muscles listed have been chosen because they list common word elements. Once this list is learned, the student should be able to figure out the remaining six hundred muscles plus not listed.

Muscle	Description
Abductor digiti minimi pedis	Little (minimi) muscle that moves the little toe (digit) away from (abductor) the midline of the foot (pedis)
Adductor longus	Long muscle that moves the leg toward (adductor) the midline
Adductor magnus	Large (magnus) muscle that moves the leg toward (adductor) the midline
Biceps brachii	Muscle with two (bi) heads (ceps) in the arm (brachii)
Deltoid	Triangular (deltoid) muscle of the shoulder
Dilatator naris posterior	Muscle of the nose (naris) that opens (dilate) the back (posterior) portion of the nostril
External oblique	Outermost (external) muscle that is at an angle (oblique) from the ribs to the hip
Extensor hallucis longus	Long (longus) muscle that extends (extensor) the great toe (hallucis)
Extensor pollicis brevis	Short (brevis) muscle that extends the thumb (pollicis)
Flexor carpi radialis	Muscle that flexes (flexor) the wrist (carpi) toward the radius (radialis)
Flexor carpi ulnaris	Muscle attached to the ulna that flexes (flexor) the wrist (carpi) and hand
Frontalis	Muscle over the frontal bone
Gastrocnemius	Muscle that makes up the belly (gastroc) of the lower leg (nemius)
Gluteus maximus	The largest (maximus) muscle of the buttocks (gluteus)
Gluteus medius	The muscle of the buttocks (gluteus) that lies in the middle (medius) between the other gluteal muscles
Gracilis	Slender (gracilis) muscle of the thigh
Iliopsoas	Muscle that is formed from the iliacus and psoas major muscles; the iliacus extends from the iliac bone (iliacus), and the psoas major is the large (major) muscle of the loin (psoas)
Latissimus dorsi	The broadest (latissimus) muscle of the back (dorsi)
Masseter	Muscle of chewing (masseter) or mastication
Orbicularis oculi and oris	Muscles circling (orbicularis) the eye (oculi) and mouth (oris)
Palmaris longus	Long (longus) muscle of the palm (palmaris)
Pectineus	Muscle from the pubic (pectineus) bone

continued

Table 3.6
MUSCLE DESCRIPTIONS USING MEDICAL TERMINOLOGY WORD ELEMENTS *(continued)*

Muscle	Description
Pectoralis major	Large (major) muscle of the chest (pectoralis)
Peroneus longus	Long (longus) muscle attached to the fibula (peroneus)
Plantaris	Muscle that flexes the foot (plantaris) and leg
Pronator teres	Long round (teres) muscle that turns the palm downward into a prone (pronator) position
Rectus abdominis	Muscle that extends in a straight (rectus) line upward across the abdomen (abdominis); the center border of the left and right rectus abdominis muscles in the linea alba or the white (alba) line (linea) at the midline of the abdomen
Rectus femoris	Part of the quadriceps muscle that is straight (rectus) and lies near the femur (femoris)
Sartorius	Muscle of the leg that enables a person to sit in a cross-legged tailor's (sartorial) position
Semitendinosus	Muscle made up partly (semi) of tendinous tissue; this is one of the hamstring muscles
Semimembranosus	Muscle made up partly (semi) of membranous tissue; part of the hamstring group
Serratus anterior	Sawtooth-shaped (serratus) muscle in front of (anterior) the shoulder and rib-cage
Soleus	Muscle that resembles a flat fish (sole) located in the calf of the leg
Sternocleidomastoid	Muscle attached to the breastbone (sterno), the collarbone (cleido), and the mastoid (mastoid) process of the temporal bone
Temporalis	Muscle over the temporal (temporalis) bone
Tensor fascia lata	Muscle that tenses (tensor) the fascia of the thigh (lata)
Teres minor	A small (minor) round (teres) muscle that moves the arm
Tibialis anterior	Muscle in front (anterior) of the tibia (tibialis)
Trapezius	Four-sided, trapezoid-shaped (trapezius) muscle of the shoulder
Triceps brachii	Three- (tri) headed (ceps) muscle of the arm (brachii)
Vastus lateralis, medialis, intermedius	Large (vastus) lateral (lateralis), toward the midline (medialis), and middle (intermedius) muscles of the quadriceps muscle group; the quadriceps has four (quadri) heads (ceps)

Attention rectus! Straighten up and the other three of you in the quads head out to the femur.

Flexor carpi ulnaris: muscle that flexes (flexor) the wrist (carpi) and hand and is attached to the ulna

Help! There is a big carp pulling my wrist into flexion. It has my ulna in its mouth and my hand has it around the gills.

3. **Do a dance using each of the movements in Table 3.5, Terms To Describe Muscle Movement.**

THE NERVOUS SYSTEM

The nervous system is the most complex system in the body. The information included here on the workings of this system is very general but is expanded in the text where needed. Study of the nervous system is very important for the massage professional. Serious students of massage will challenge themselves to study the nervous system in comprehensive depth.

The function of the nervous system is to receive impressions from the external environment, to organize the information, and to provide appropriate responses. In other words, the nervous system allows the body to react to outside influences (environment). Outside information enters the nervous system through nerve endings in the skin and in special sense organs. These nerve endings are referred to as *receptors*. Nerve endings in the skin are sensitive to pain, touch, pressure, vibration, and temperature. Special sense nerve endings are responsible for taste, smell, vision, hearing, and sense of position and movement. Sensations from the environment are picked up by these receptors and sent to the central nervous system (CNS) by way of the peripheral nervous system (PNS). The CNS sorts out the information and sends back a message, again by way of the PNS. The nervous system and neurotransmitters, along with the endocrine system, also maintains the internal environment, or the balance of the many activities within the body (homeostasis).

The nervous system consists of all the nerve tissues in the body (see Table 3.7 for terms related to nerves). For purposes of study, terms related to the nervous system will be presented in the following three groups:

Table 3.7 TERMS RELATED TO NERVES	Afferent nerves: nerves that carry (ferent) messages to (af, variation of ad) the CNS; also known as sensory nerves because they pick up and transmit sensation (sen)
	Efferent nerves: nerves that carry (ferent) messages away (ef, variation of ex) from the brain result in motion (motor)
	Cranial nerves: the twelve pairs of nerves that arise from the brainstem in the cranium (cranial)
	Spinal nerves: the thirty-one pairs of nerves that come off the spinal cord
	Ganglion: a mass of nerve cell bodies located outside the CNS; ganglia is the plural form
	Neuro: the root word meaning "nerve"

1. the central nervous system (CNS)
2. the peripheral nervous system (PNS)
3. the autonomic nervous system (ANS)

Central Nervous System

The CNS is the center (central) of all nervous control. It consists of the brain and spinal cord, which are located in the cranial cavity and the center of the vertebrae, respectively.

Peripheral Nervous System

The PNS is comprised of cranial and spinal nerves. The term refers to a bundle of nerve fibers outside the spinal cord or brain. The PNS consists of the nerves that carry impulses between the CNS and muscles, glands, skin, and other organs that are located outside (peripheral) the CNS. The part of the PNS that has nervous control over smooth muscle, heart muscle, and glands is called the ANS. There are basically two types of nerves: sensory neurons and motor neurons.

Spinal Nerves

The thirty-one pairs of spinal nerves are attached to the spinal cord along almost its entire length. They are named for the region of the spinal column through which they exit. Many of the spinal nerves are located in groups called *somatic nerve plexuses*. The term *somatic* refers to the body wall. Thus these nerve plexuses contain nerves that are involved with the wall of the body as opposed to the organs within the body. A *plexus* is a network of intertwined (plexus) nerves. The major plexuses of spinal nerves are the cervical plexus, brachial plexus, lumbar plexus, and sacral plexus.

Autonomic Nervous System

The ANS is the part of the PNS that is an automatic or self-governing [self (auto), governing (nomic)] system. It is also called the *involuntary system* because the effects of this system are not usually under voluntary control. There are two divisions of the ANS: the sympathetic division and the parasympathetic division.

The sympathetic division controls the body's response to feelings (sympath). The nerves in this division come off the thoracic and lumbar segments of the spinal cord; thus this division is sometimes referred to as the *thoracolumbar division*. The action resulting from these nerves include the fight-or-flight and fear responses. The reaction of some organs includes an increase in the heart rate, dilation of the pupils, and an increase in adrenalin secretion. A person may sometimes exhibit great strength as a result of a sympathetic response.

The nerves in the parasympathetic division come off the cranial nerves and sacral segments of the spinal cord; thus it is sometimes called the *craniosacral division*. The parasympathetic division generally causes effects opposite (para) those caused by the sympathetic system. These effects include constriction of the pupils, the return of the heart rate to normal, and the stimulation of the lacrimal glands to produce tears.

There are also plexuses of the ANS. These intertwined nerves (plexus) are called the *autonomic plexuses*. Some examples of these plexuses are the cardiac plexus, or the intertwined nerves of the heart (cardiac) and the celiac plexus, or the intertwined nerves of the organs of the abdomen (celiac). The latter plexus is sometimes called the solar plexus because of the sun ray (solar) fashion in which the nerves come out of the plexus.

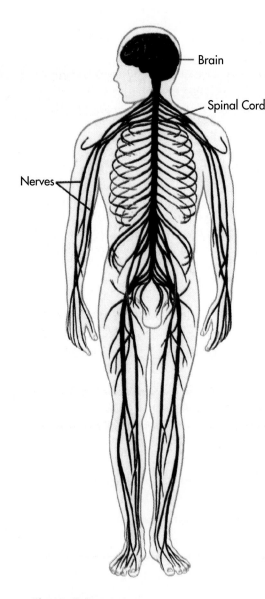

Brain

Spinal Cord

Nerves

**Figure 3.8
Nervous system. (From Thibodeau/Patton: The human body in health & disease, St. Louis, 1992, Mosby–Year Book, Inc.)**

Proprioception

Proprioception is the kinesthetic sense. Sensory receptors receive information about position, rate of movement, contraction, tension, and stretch of tissues though the distortion and pressure on the sensory receptor. Motor impulses cause the body to respond to sensory input.

Terms related to proprioception include: kinesthetic, muscle spindle cells, golgi tendon organ, and joint kinesthetic receptors.

Reflex

A *relfex* is an involuntary response to a stimulus. Important reflexes stimulated by massage are crossed, extensor thrust, flexor withdrawal, intersegmental, monosynaptic, nociceptive, optical righting, pilomotor, psychogalvanic, postural, proprioceptive, righting, startle reflex, stretch reflex, tendon reflex, vasomotor reflex, and visceromotor reflex.

It is important to note that although the divisions of the nervous system may be treated independently, they do not function independently (Fig. 3.8).

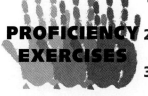
PROFICIENCY EXERCISES

1. **With a partner and washable markers, draw the four major plexus and their major nerves on your bodies.**
2. **List all the disease conditions of the nervous system described in the indications and contraindications section in Appendix A.**
3. **Look up all the reflexes listed in a medical dictionary and write down what you think are their implications for massage.**

THE CARDIOVASCULAR SYSTEM

The cardiovascular system consists of two parts, the heart and the blood vessels (Fig. 3.9).

Look up the following terms in your medical dictionary, medical terminology textbook, and anatomy and physiology textbook: angio-, artery, arteriole, blood pressure, bruise, capillary, edema, phleb-, vasoconstriction, vasodilation, vein, and venule.

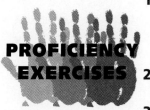
PROFICIENCY EXERCISES

1. **Choose a partner and draw the major arteries and veins on the body with washable markers. Use red for arteries and blue for veins. Notice that you can almost trace the veins because they are located near the surface of the body.**
2. **List all the disease conditions of the circulatory system described in the indications and contraindications section of Appendix A.**
3. **Look up the drug classification "anticoagulant" and list contraindications and side effects of these drugs.**

THE LYMPHATIC SYSTEM

The lymphatic system is responsible for several functions, and operates in the following ways:

1. It returns vital substances, such as plasma protein, to the bloodstream from the tissues of the body.
2. It assists in the maintenance of fluid balance by draining fluid from the body tissues.
3. It helps in the body's defense against disease-producing substances.
4. It helps in the absorption of fats from the digestive system.

The lymphatic system is a network of channels and nodes in which a substance called lymph travels (Fig. 3.10). *Lymph* is a clear, watery fluid

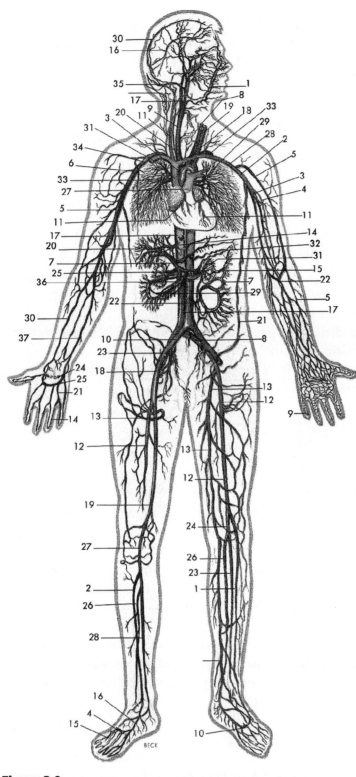

PRINCIPAL VEINS AND ARTERIES

Principal arteries

1 Angular
2 Anterior tibial
3 Aorta
4 Arcuate
5 Axillary
6 Brachial
7 Celiac
8 Common carotid, left
9 Common carotid, right
10 Common iliac, right
11 Coronary, left
12 Deep femoral
13 Deep medial circumflex femoral
14 Digital
15 Dorsal metatarsal
16 Dorsalis pedis
17 External carotid
18 External iliac
19 Femoral
20 Hepatic
21 Metacarpal
22 Inferior mesenteric
23 Internal iliac (hypogastric)
24 Palmar arch, deep
25 Palmar arch, superficial
26 Peroneal
27 Popliteal
28 Posterior tibial
29 Pulmonary
30 Radial
31 Renal
32 Splenic
33 Subclavian, left (cut)
34 Subclavian, right
35 Superficial temporal
36 Superior mesenteric
37 Ulnar

Principal veins

1 Anterior tibial
2 Axillary
3 Basilic
4 Brachial
5 Cephalic
6 Cervical plexus
7 Colic
8 Common iliac, left
9 Digital
10 Dorsal venous arch
11 External jugular
12 Femoral
13 Great saphenous
14 Hepatic
15 Inferior mesenteric
16 Inferior sagittal sinus
17 Inferior vena cava
18 Brachiocephalic, left
19 Internal jugular, left
20 Internal jugular, right
21 Lateral thoracic
22 Median cubital
23 Peroneal
24 Popliteal
25 Portal
26 Posterior tibial
27 Pulmonary
28 Subclavian, left
29 Superior mesenteric
30 Superior sagittal sinus
31 Superior vena cava

Figure 3.9
**Circulatory system. (From LaFleur
Brooks: Exploring medical language—
a student-directed approach 3/E, St.
Louis, 1994, Mosby–Year Book, Inc.)**

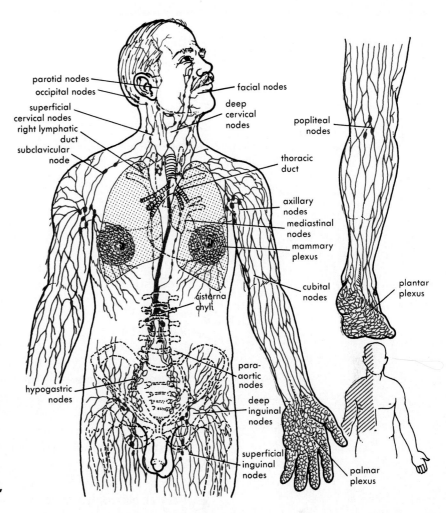

gure 3.10
Principal lymph vessels and nodes.
(From Birmingham: Medical terminology—a self-learning text 2/E, St. Louis, 1990, The C.V. Mosby Company)

Labels on figure: parotid nodes, occipital nodes, superficial cervical nodes, right lymphatic duct, subclavicular node, facial nodes, deep cervical nodes, popliteal nodes, thoracic duct, axillary nodes, mediastinal nodes, mammary plexus, cubital nodes, cisterna chyli, hypogastric nodes, para-aortic nodes, deep inguinal nodes, superficial inguinal nodes, plantar plexus, palmar plexus

similar to plasma. Contrary to the cardiovascular system, travel in the lymphatic system flows only in one direction. The system collects and drains lymph from different areas of the body and carries it through the lymphatic channels back to the venous system. There it is deposited, mixed with venous blood, and recirculated. Lymph capillaries are found close to and parallel to the veins that carry blood to the heart. The ends of the lymphatic capillaries meet to form larger lymph vessels. The lymph vessels in the right chest and right arm join the right lymphatic duct, which drains into the right subclavian vein. The lymph vessels from all other parts of the body join to meet the thoracic duct, which drains into the left subclavian vein. Throughout the lymph system are lymph nodes. *Lymph nodes* are small bodies present in the path of the lymph channels that act as filters for lymph before it returns to the bloodstream. See Table 3.8 for a description of types of lymph nodes.

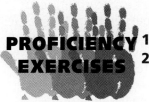

PROFICIENCY EXERCISES

1. **Palpate as many groups of lymph nodes as possible.**
2. **Draw a diagram of the lymphatic system and chart the lymphatic flow pattern.**

THE IMMUNE SYSTEM

The human body has the ability to resist organisms or toxins that tend to damage the tissues and organs that make up the body. This ability is called *immunity*. As a massage professional, you will want to explore the immune

Table 3.8
DESCRIPTION OF THE LYMPH
NODES

Nodes	Description
Parotid	The nodes around (para) or in front of the ear (otid)
Occipital	The nodes over the occipital bone at the back of the head
Superficial cervical	The nodes close to the surface (superficial) of the neck (cervic)
Subclavicular	The nodes under (sub) the collarbone (clavicular)
Hypogastric	The nodes in the area beneath (hypo) the stomach (gastric)
Facial	The nodes draining the tissue in the face
Deep cervical	Deeply (deep) situated nodes in the neck (cervic)
Axillary	Nodes in the armpit (axilla)
Mediastinal	Nodes in the mediastinal section of the thoracic cavity
Cubital	Nodes of the elbow (cubit)
Para-aortic	Nodes around (para) the aorta (aortic)
Deep inguinal	Deeply (deep) situated nodes in the groin (inguin)
Superficial inguinal	The nodes in the groin (inguin) close to the surface (superficial)
Popliteal	Nodes in back of the knee (popliteal)

There are plexuses of lymph channels throughout the body. These intertwined channels are found in the following areas:

Mammary plexus: lymphatic vessels around the breasts
Palmar plexus: lymphatic vessels in the palm (palmar) of the hand
Plantar plexus: lymphatic vessels in the sole (plantar) of the foot

Table 3.9
ANALYSIS OF SELECTED TERMS
RELATED TO IMMUNOLOGY

Term	Description
Acquired immunity	Resistance (immunity) to a particular disease developed by people who have acquired the disease
Acquired immunodeficiency syndrome (AIDS)	Group of symptoms (syndrome) caused by the transmission (acquired) of a virus that causes a breakdown (deficiency) of the immune system
Active immunity	Resistance (immunity) in which the antibodies that have been produced by a person currently exist
Allergy	State of hypersensitivity to a particular substance; the immune system overreacts [over (hyper), reacts (sensitive)] to foreign substances and physical changes occur
Antigen	Substance that stimulates the immune response
Susceptible	Said of a person who is capable (ible) of acquiring (suscept) a particular disease

system in much greater depth (see Table 3.9 for a list of terms related to immunology). Use your anatomy and physiology textbook as a place to begin, but do not stop there. Exciting research is being published in professional journals. A regular trip to your library to keep your information current is suggested.

THE RESPIRATORY SYSTEM

The respiratory system functions to supply oxygen and remove carbon dioxide from the cells of the body. There are two phases of respiration: external and internal. *External respiration* involves the absorption of oxygen from the air by the lungs and the transport of carbon dioxide from the lungs back into the air. *Internal respiration* involves the exchange of oxygen and carbon dioxide in the cells of the body. The mechanisms of breathing and its relationship to massage will be discussed.

Look up the following terms related to the respiratory system in a medical terminology textbook: alveoli, lungs, nares, nostrils, olfactory cells, pneumo-, rhino-, and trachea.

THE DIGESTIVE SYSTEM

The anatomy of the digestive system can be compared to that of a long muscular tube that travels a path through the body (Fig. 3.11). The organs of the digestive system transport food though the muscular tubes. There

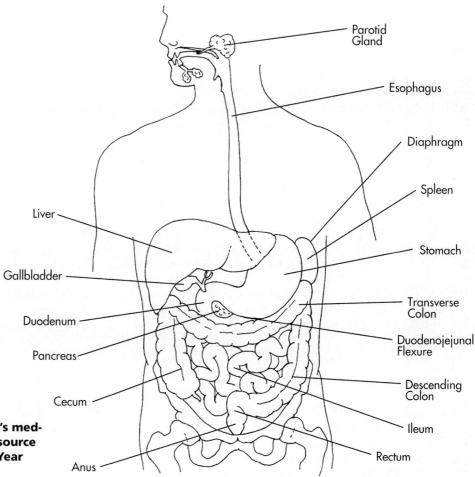

Figure 3.11
Digestive system. (From Mosby's medical terminology instructor's resource library, St. Louis, 1994, Mosby–Year Book, Inc.)

are accessory organs that carry out functions directly related to digestion and are connected to the system by way of ducts. Understanding the flow of contents through the large intestine is important for the massage professional. Investigate this process further by referring to your anatomy and physiology textbook.

THE ENDOCRINE SYSTEM

The endocrine system is comprised of glands that produce hormones which are secreted directly into the bloodstream to stimulate cells in a specific way or to set a body function in motion (Fig. 3.12). The endocrine system is very complex and very important. It is a control and regulation system of the body. As with the nervous system, you will want to commit to an in-depth study of the endocrine stytem, its relationship to the nervous system, and the connection to mind/body processes. The information from research on the mind/body phenomenon is being released too quickly to be current in any textbook. It will be important for the massage professional to read medical and scientific journals in order to remain current. The implications for massage are very important since the effects of massage are connected with the nervous system and endocrine body control functions.

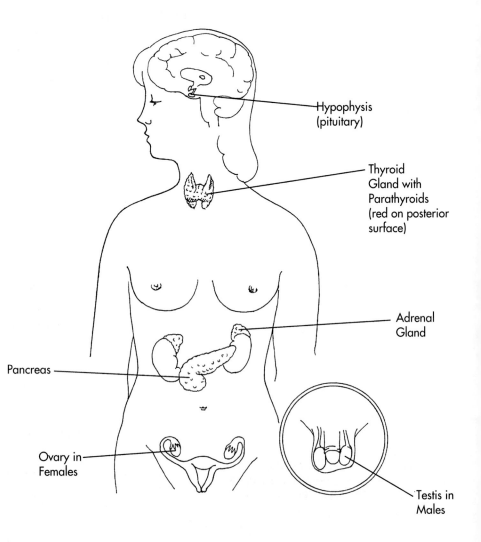

Figure 3.12
Endocrine system. (From Mosby's medical terminology instructor's resource library, St. Louis, 1994, Mosby–Year Book, Inc.)

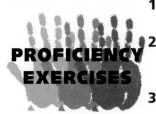

1. **Look up and read about the immune, respiratory, digestive, and endocrine systems in your anatomy and physiology textbook.**
2. **Keep a list of terms that you encounter while reading this textbook that relate to the immune, respiratory, digestive, and endocrine systems.**
3. **Visit your local library and find out to what scientific and medical journals they subscribe.**

THE INTEGUMENTARY SYSTEM

The integumentary system consists of the skin and its appendages, including hair and nails.

Skin

The skin is the largest organ in the body. It is composed of three layers of tissue (Fig. 3.13): the epidermis, dermis, and subcutaneous tissue. The *epidermis* is the outer layer of skin, which contains many layers of tissue and melanocytes, the cells that give skin color. The *dermis*, or dermal layer, lies directly under the epidermis and is often called the true skin. It is made of connective tissue. Embedded in the dermis are the blood vessels, lymphatic vessels, hair follicles, and sweat glands. *Subcutaneous tissue* attaches the dermis to the underlying structure. This fatty tissue contains varying amounts of adipose tissue, and acts as insulation for the body.

Sebaceous Glands

Sebaceous glands are located in the skin and secrete an oily substance that gives skin and hair its glossy appearance. The oily substance is called *sebum*. Most of these glands open into the walls of hair follicles. There are also sebaceous glands at the corners of the mouth and around the external sex organs that open directly upon the surface of the skin.

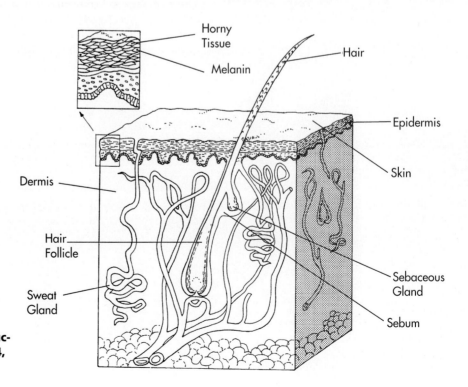

Figure 3.13
Skin structure cross section. (From Mosby's medical terminology instructor's resource library, St. Louis, 1994, Mosby–Year Book, Inc.)

Sweat Glands

Sweat glands are found in most areas of the body, and function to cool the body. The most abundant type is the eccrine sweat gland. The palms of the hands and soles of the feet contain large numbers of these glands. Sweat from these glands is odorless. Another type of sweat gland is the apocrine sweat gland, which is connected to hair follicles in the armpits and the pubic area and is also found at the navel and nipples. The secretions from these sweat glands increase in response to sexual stimulation. They function to lubricate the genital area and play a part in sexual arousal due to the mild odor.

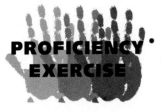

PROFICIENCY EXERCISE

- **Using the indications and contraindications list in Appendix A list all of the skin conditions and look them up in the medical dictionary.**

SUMMARY

The study of medical terminology, anatomy, physiology, and pathology must be an ongoing process for the massage professional. This basic introduction provides a study focus for you as a student. The massage professional will need this base to understand the research, books, and journal articles that relate to massage, and to understand and communicate effectively with other health care professionals. It is important to realize that many clients are not familiar with these terms, and to use the language patterns of the people with whom you speak. Often the use of technical terms with a client is not appropriate: using big words and technical language is not necessarily the way to present yourself to the public. The massage therapist will need to speak two languages and be able to translate effectively back and forth between each. When speaking with those who use this special language of the sciences, it is important to ask questions about any term you do not understand. Acting as if you understand what is being said when you do not is unprofessional.

The study of anatomy and physiology is important and fascinating. The overview of anatomy and physiology for the massage professional offered in this chapter is only the beginning. Every day, challenge yourself to learn something new about how human beings function. The more we understand about how the body works, the better we can take care of it and keep it well. That is what prevention and wellness is all about.

REVIEW QUESTIONS

1. Why study medical terminology?
2. What are the three word elements and how are they used?
3. What is the importance of additional anatomy, physiology, and pathology study to the professional practice of therapeutic massage?

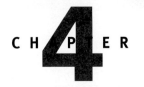

CHAPTER 4

INDICATIONS AND CONTRAINDICATIONS FOR
MASSAGE

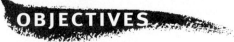

OBJECTIVES

After completing this chapter, the student will be able to do the following:

1 Discuss the physiologic mechanism of why massage therapy is beneficial.

2 Develop a basic understanding of pathology and its connection to contraindications to massage.

3 Explain the stress response, the inflammatory response, and pain.

4 Effectively refer clients to licensed medical professionals.

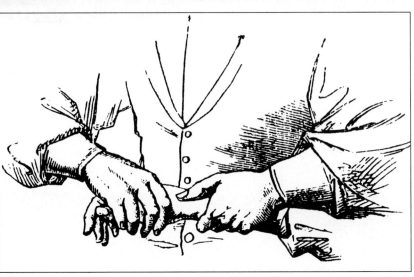

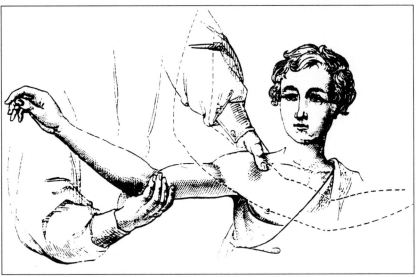

Procedure for assessing functionality and strength of injured arm muscles in preparation for therapeutic massage.

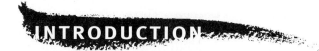

The massage professional must be able to identify the indications for massage that will benefit the client and the contraindications for when therapeutic massage should not be provided. The ability to use this information effectively is an essential part of informed consent for the client as well as for public education about the value of therapeutic massage.

WHY MASSAGE WORKS

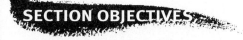

Using the information presented in this section, the student will be able to do the following:

1 Classify massage methods into five basic physiologic effects.

2 Explain a basic normalizing premise for each physiologic approach to massage.

The techniques of therapeutic massage and other types and styles of body-work are merely variations of the fundamental application of manual manipulations. The effectiveness of the techniques is a result of basic physiologic effects.

In his book, *Physician's Guide to Therapeutic Massage*, Dr. John Yates[8] lists four areas of basic physiologic effect—the neuromuscular, connective tissue, circulatory, and autonomic nervous system. This text includes a fifth—the electrical chemical aspect of the body.

BASIC PHYSIOLOGIC EFFECTS

Neuromuscular

Neuro refers to the nervous system and *muscular* refers to the muscles. The *neuromuscular effect* is the interaction between the control of the muscles by the nervous system and the response of the muscles to these nerve signals.

It is not possible to include a complete discussion of the anatomy and physiology of the nervous and muscle systems of the body in this book. There are many excellent anatomy and physiology textbooks available. See Appendix C for suggested books to accompany this chapter.

Muscles are stimulated to contract or relax (release a contraction) via nerve cells. There is a constant monitoring and protective function of specialized nerve receptors called *proprioceptors*. These proprioceptors receive and transmit information regarding muscle tension, static tone, degree of stretch, joint position, and speed of movement.

It is unusual to encounter soft tissue (muscle and connective tissue) dysfunction without proprioceptive hyperactivity. The result of proprioceptive hyperactivity is tense or spastic muscles, accompanied by hypoactivity of opposing groups of muscles. Simply, a tight muscle area results in or from a weakened muscle area and vice versa.

When working with the neuromuscular mechanism, the basic premise is to substitute a different neurologic signal stimulation through massage, to reset muscle resting length through lengthening and stretching muscles and connective tissue, and to provide re-education of the muscles involved, i.e., take the joint through its increased range of motion.

Connective Tissue

Connective tissue is the most abundant tissue of the body. Its functions include support, structure, space, stabilization, and scar formation. Connective tissue is adaptive and responsive to a variety of influences, such as injury, increased demand, and underuse or decreased demand. It is made up of various fibers and cells in a gelatinous ground matrix. In bone, this ground matrix is impregnated with minerals that harden the bone. The healing of damage to body tissues requires the formation of connective tissue. Occasionally, more tissue than necessary is formed and adhesions develop. An adhesion occurs when connective tissue binds to structures that are not directly involved with the area of injury.

During overuse, extra connective tissue is formed to provide stabilization to the musculoskeletal areas involved. In situations in which there is a chronic soft tissue problem, the connective tissue becomes fibrotic, involving areas that surround the dysfunctional area.[1] Once this occurs, any one of several conditions may exist. The connective tissue may have become thickened or thinned, or it may have dried out or become water-logged. The water-binding component of connective tissue is significant in effective connective tissue support and function. Ligaments and tendons may fail to support joint stabilization or the connective tissue may bind, restricting movement and function.

In areas of *acute* (active) dysfunction, connective tissue may not play a role in the dysfunctional pattern. Connective tissue dysfunction is usually suspected to be a factor in problems that are older than twelve weeks.[1]

With its piezoelectric properties, the collagen portion of connective tissue may be the link to energy-related forms of bodywork. *Piezoelectricity* is an electric current produced by the application of pressure to certain crystals such as mica, quartz, or Rochelle salt.[6] There seems to be a piezoelectric property to collagen. The piezoelectric phenomena in some way affects the connective tissue properties.[4]

The basic premise when working with connective tissue is to provide space and mobile stability, as opposed to the dysfunctional joint or soft tissue area, which may be "stuck" and restricted or hypermobile. This is accomplished through mechanical compression, sustained pulling and elongation of the connective tissue, and frictioning methods (see Chapter 13).

Circulation Enhancement

There are three to five basic types of circulation. All anatomy texts recognize arterial, venous, and lymphatic circulation. The remaining two types of circulation involve respiration and cerebral spinal fluid. These five systems are dependent on the pumping action of the skeletal muscles as they contract and relax. Arterial flow has the additional pumping action provided by the heart and muscle tissue in the arteries. It is important to realize that these circulatory functions are directly linked and interdependent. Massage and other forms of bodywork mimic and assist the pumping action of the muscle and respiratory pump. See Chapter 13 for additional information.

Arterial Flow

Circulation enhancement is fairly straightforward. The massage therapist must understand the anatomy and physiology of the circulation of the blood and the lymphatic systems to really grasp how circulation is affected by massage. While it is true that more body fluids are moved by taking a five-minute walk than by receiving a fifty-minute massage, for those not able to walk or even get out of bed, manual facilitation of the movement of body fluids can be a viable and significant therapeutic option.

Arteries carry blood under pressure from the pumping action of the heart. They also have a muscular component that contracts rhythmically, facilitating arterial flow. Direct compression into the area of an artery effectively crimps the artery, much like crimping a hose, and allows for some back pressure to build. When the pressure is released, the blood rushes through like a waterfall. Arteries are basically accessible to compressive pressure on the soft medial areas of the arms and legs. Compressions should begin proximal to the heart and rapidly move distal. Heavy pressure or sustained compression is not necessary. Instead, moderate pressure is used in the right location to rhythmically pump as the therapist moves distally toward the fingers or toes. In style, it resembles shiatsu or sports massage.

An increase in arterial flow is beneficial in any situation in which an increase in oxygenated blood is desirable. Such situations include sluggish circulation or increased demand such as with an athlete.

Venous Return Flow

Venous return flow is dependent on contraction of the muscles against the veins. Back flow of blood is prevented by valves. Veins usually run more superficially than arteries. Due to the valve system in the veins, and the fact that the blood is intended to flow back toward the heart, strokes to encourage venous flow move toward the heart. Short pumping, gliding, effleurage strokes are very effective.

One method that encourages venous blood flow involves starting proximal on the arms and legs and traveling distally, with the direction of the stroke toward the heart. This may prevent pooling of blood by clearing the path of the vessel. Passive and active joint movement also encourages the muscles to contract against the deeper vessels, assisting venous blood flow. If this is not possible for the client, slow meticulous mechanical work is required to drain the area. Placing the limb above the heart, allowing gravity to assist, is beneficial.

Lymphatic Drainage

The massage procedures for lymphatic drain are the same as those for venous return. Because lymph vessels are open-ended into all tissue space, the surface work is performed over the entire body instead of being focused only over the major veins. Pumping of jointed areas with passive joint movement seems to assist the movement of lymph through the areas of lymph node filtration. Deep breathing assists lymph movement in the thorax. It does not seem to be necessary to be precise about specific flow patterns. It is important to note that the lower abdomen (from umbilicus down) drains into the inguinal area and that the right side (right arm and head) drains into the right lymphatic duct. Both major vessels dump into the vena cava. No one is sure why this pattern of drainage exists; it is just the way we evolved during fetal development.

The body will retain fluids if there is a perceived fluid shortage. The best way to prevent simple edema is through moderate exercise and sufficient water intake.

Respiration

The muscular mechanism for the inhalation and exhalation of air is designed like a simple bellows system and depends on unrestricted movement of the musculoskeletal components of the thorax. The muscles of respiration include the scalenes, intercostals, anterior serratus, diaphragm, abdominals, pelvic floor muscles, and lower leg muscles (which surprises many people). This can be demonstrated by contracting any of these muscle groups and attempting to take a deep breath. You will note that the ability to breathe is restricted. Disruption of function in any of these groups will inhibit full and easy breathing. Beneficial effects of massage include enhanced breathing. Use of the breath, as outlined in Chapter 10, enhances the effectiveness of lengthening and stretching methods.

Cerebral Spinal Fluid Circulation

This subject remains a mystery. Cerebral spinal fluid cools, nourishes, and protects the brain and nerves. It also has a pumping rhythm that can be palpated. This rhythm seems to affect the phenomenon of fascial movement and is independent of the other body rhythms. Or is it? More research needs to be done. Techniques of cranial sacral therapy specifically affect cerebral spinal fluid circulation (Fig. 4.1).[2] General massage may indirectly influence this mechanism.

The basic premise when working with circulation enhancement is to provide for a sufficient, even, and unobstructed circulatory flow.

Autonomic Nervous System

The autonomic nervous system (ANS) is best known for its regulation of the sympathetic "fight/flight/fear" response and the parasympathetic "relaxation response." Sympathetic and parasympathetic systems work together to maintain homeostasis through a feedback loop system. These systems both affect and are affected by the endocrine glands. Specific muscle patterns are associated with both systems. Arm and leg muscles may be tight with sympathetic response and postural muscles tight with parasympathetic response (Fig. 4.2). See Chapter 6 for more information.

The ANS association is where the mind/body link is best understood. Emotional input registers in the body through the ANS and the endocrine system. There is a definite chemical factor to be considered in the arousal of emotion based on the body's production of endorphins, enkephalins, epinephrine, norepinephrine, hormones, and neurotransmitters. If these chemicals are released into the blood stream during bodywork, the individual may once again feel the chemical arousal of an emotion, perhaps triggering a memory.

Another aspect of the mind/body connection that interacts with the ANS is state-dependent memory. The adrenal hormones that interplay with the sympathetic responses are intimately involved with short-term memory. Norepinephrine depletion decreases memory storage and elevated levels increase memory storage. The "state" in state-dependent memory is either sympathetic or parasympathetic nervous system function. If a person has an experience while in one of these states, the memory is encoded or stored in that state. Research shows that memory is only accessible to an individual when the particular body chemistry and function are similar to when the experience first happened.[7] Because of the effects of massage on the ANS, massage may recreate these state-dependent memory patterns. This can be useful in allowing the client to resolve a past experience that was unresolvable when it occured. Often, counseling is necessary to help the person sort the memory pattern and develop strategies for resolution, integration, and coping. Again, these activities are outside the scope of practice of therapeutic massage, but, combined with effective counseling from trained professionals, massage can be very beneficial. See Chapter 12 for additional information.

Bodywork and massage primarily use mechanical stimulation to affect the ANS. It is a misconception that touch relaxes. Touch initially stimulates. All sensations initially stimulate whether they are received through visual, audio, or kinesthetic processes. Stimulation that is quick and unexpected will arouse. Sustained stimulation will eventually relax through hyperstimulation analgesia, a protective mechanism of sensory overload.[3] Examples of methods used for hyperstimulation analgesia are ice, heat, counter-irritation, topical ointments, acupressure, acupuncture, rocking, music, and repetitive massage methods.

Conservation withdrawal is another factor to be considered in a discussion of the ANS. Conservation withdrawal, which in animals is similar to "playing possum" or hibernation, may manifest in humans following

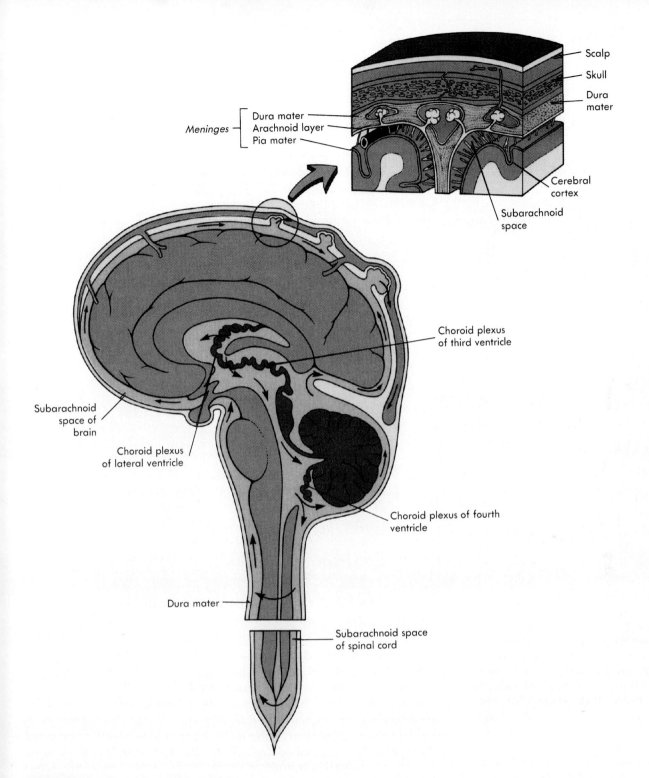

Figure 4.1
Flow of cerebrospinal fluid. The fluid produced by filtration of blood by the choroid plexus of each ventricle flows interiorly through the lateral ventricles, interventricular foramen, third ventricle, cerebral aqueduct, fourth ventricle, and subarachnoid space and to the blood. (From Thibodeau/Patton: The human body in health & disease, St. Louis, 1992, Mosby–Year Book, Inc.)

intense negative events such as abuse, neglect, or starvation. To a lesser degree, conservation withdrawal patterns play a part in depression. A massage that is more stimulating may help draw a client out of this withdrawal pattern.

Because of the generalized effect on the ANS and associated functions, massage can produce changes in mood and excitement levels, and can induce the relaxation response. Massage seems to be a gentle modulator, producing feelings of general well-being and comfort. This does not

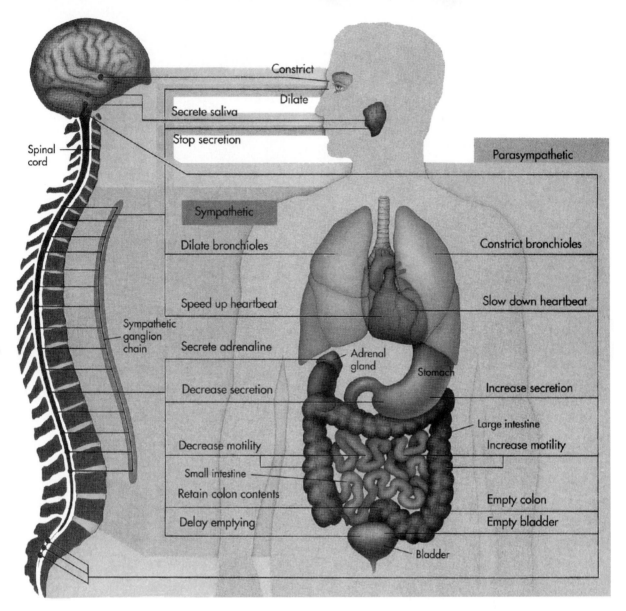

Constrict

Dilate

Secrete saliva

Stop secretion

Spinal cord

Parasympathetic

Sympathetic

Dilate bronchioles

Constrict bronchioles

Speed up heartbeat

Slow down heartbeat

Sympathetic ganglion chain

Secrete adrenaline

Adrenal gland

Stomach

Decrease secretion

Increase secretion

Large intestine

Decrease motility

Increase motility

Small intestine

Retain colon contents

Empty colon

Delay emptying

Empty bladder

Bladder

Figure 4.2
Innervation of the major target organs by the autonomic nervous system. (From Thibodeau/Patton: The human body in health & disease, St. Louis, 1992, Mosby–Year Book, Inc.)

always mean that the client responds to the massage by becoming very relaxed. The most common response is a sense that the "edge is off" and that there is less urgency or intensity of the emotional state. The client may be better able to function in a self-regulating fashion, controlling the emotional state instead of it doing the controlling. This ability to self-regulate is very important in the physiologic process. Another term for self-regulation is internal control. We tend to feel more at ease when we feel a sense of internal control.

Obviously the mind/body phenomenon could be an extensive and fascinating study. It is one that the serious student of massage is encouraged to undertake.

The basic premise of a massage focused on the ANS is to provide for a balanced mind/body state that allows for efficient self-regulation.

Electrical Chemical or Electrical Magnetic Effects

Present scientific technology is just beginning to be able to measure this subtle area. Consequently, the authenticity of the effectiveness of any modality that is based on the reaction of the electrical, chemical, or electrical magnetic component of the body is controversial. Currently, the

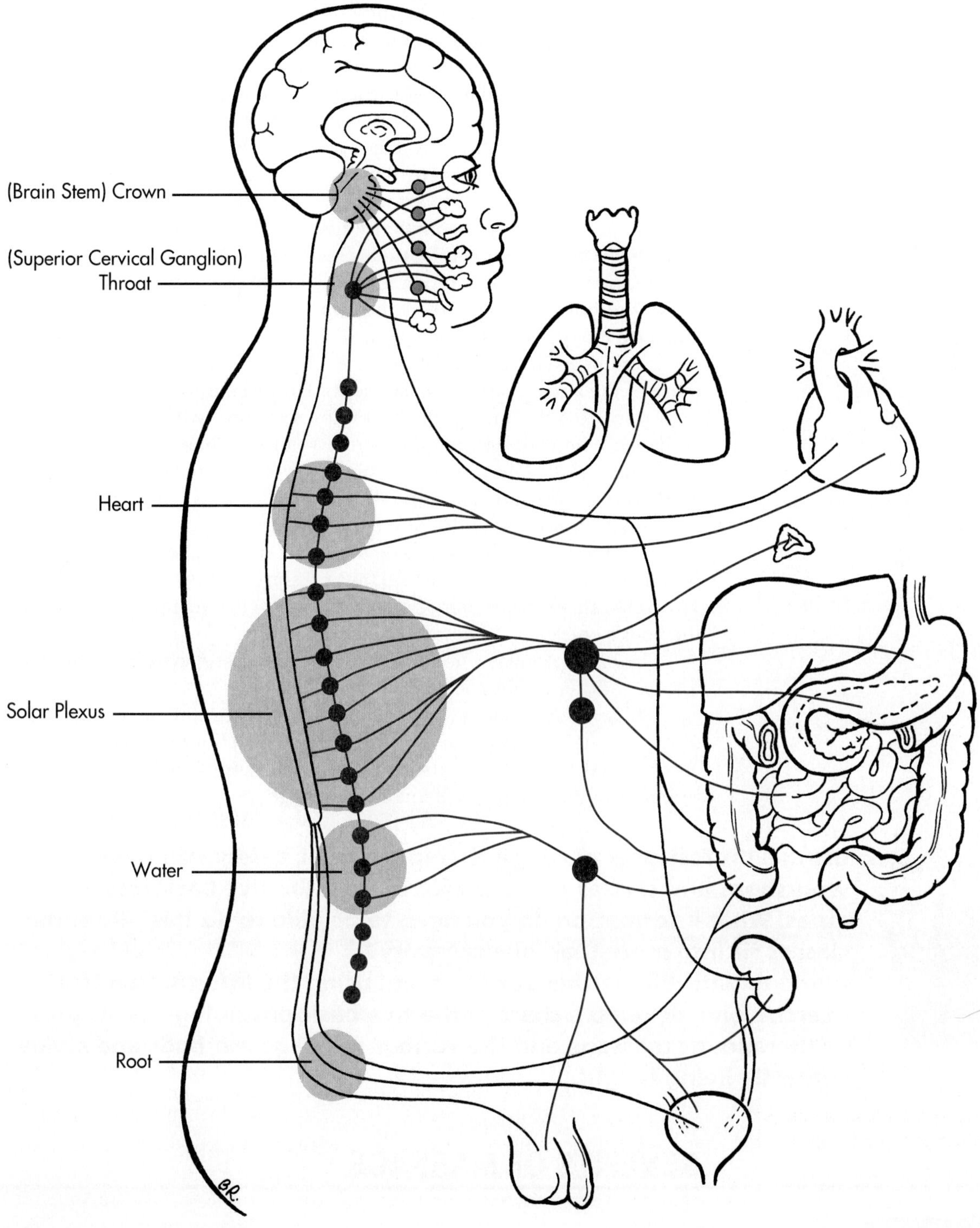
(Brain Stem) Crown
(Superior Cervical Ganglion)
Throat
Heart
Solar Plexus
Water
Root
B.R.

Figure 4.3
Comparison of the autonomic nervous system and traditional energy centers.

electrical energy generated by the body can be measured by electroencephalograms, electrocardiograms, magnetic resonance images, and other sophisticated scientific equipment. However, due to the lack of sufficient Western scientific validation of the ancient energetic flows of Chi, prana, meridians, chakras, auras, or whatever else they may be called, care must be taken to represent this area of bodywork in a legitimate manner.

Physiologically, acupuncture points and meridians can be correlated directly to the nerve tracts and motor nerve points; chakras are located over nerve plexuses; and connective tissue techniques produce a measurable electrical current via the piezoelectric properties of the connective tissue. The interrelationship of all the other body systems is sufficient to cause the body to respond to the stimulation of this innate electrical chemical energy (Fig. 4.3).

It will be exciting to watch science "discover" the validity of more and more of the ancient energetic concepts. However, until this happens, it is important to substantiate the techniques we use with the information available. When considering the wonders of the human anatomy, nothing is actually "new." Therefore, physiologically, sufficient research presently exists to demonstrate that modalities using "energy" do have an effect through ANS activity, endocrine responses, motor nerve points, and the piezoelectric properties of connective tissue fibers. Therapeutic massage stimulates the nervous system and puts pressure into the connective tissue. The generalized approach of massage may have a normalizing effect on the body's energetic processes.

The basic premise when working with the energy systems of the body is to provide an unobstructed flow of energy.

Whatever the massage or bodywork system used, the beneficial effects of therapeutic massage are elicited from the client's physiology as it adjusts to the external sensory information supplied by massage and responds to the compressive forces of massage.

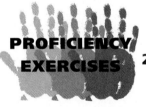

PROFICIENCY EXERCISES

1. Using a professional massage therapy journal, categorize the various workshops and classes that are offered into the five basic physiologic areas. What information do you need to be able to do this? Do some classes fit into more than one category?
2. Working with three other students and using the information from exercise one, develop a chart of the five basic physiologic principles of therapeutic massage and the various massage methods and styles currently being taught.

BENEFITS OF MASSAGE

SECTION OBJECTIVES

Using the information presented in this section, the student of massage will be able to do the following:

❶ Chart and understand the physiologic benefits of massage.
❷ Explain the difference between objective and subjective massage benefits.
❸ Explain the benefits of massage to others.

The benefits of massage therapy are both objective and subjective. That is, some results of massage can be measured accurately (objective) while others are only assumed to be effective based on observation and experience (subjective). The effects of massage are, then, both physical (objective, physically measured observation) and mental (subjective perception reporting). The dichotomy of therapeutic benefits from massage causes considerable confusion. Fortunately, this situation is changing rapidly. Researchers such as Tiffany Field at the Touch Research Institute at the University of Miami are making major advances in the understanding of the benefits and physiologic mechanisms of therapeutic massage.

Box 4.1
THE GENERAL BENEFITS OF MASSAGE THERAPY

Massage manipulations can be applied in a systematic approach or plan to influence conditions that affect physical function.

Skeletal muscles respond with direct bio-mechanical effects. Within this response, bio-mechanical effects will encourage or affect reflex reactions that involve the nervous system or chemical responses. The variety of responses is reached at many levels. The nervous system can respond through the reflex arc, secretion of endorphins and other neural chemicals, and the release of histamine and other cellular secretions. The release of chemical substances affects a structure or system of the body directly or indirectly.

The foundation for the benefits of massage therapy is understanding the nature of the effects on circulation, elimination, and nervous system control. Circulation is primarily improved by direct bio-mechanical responses to manipulations. A secondary benefit is obtained through reflex responses encouraging chemical secretion or nervous system control.

Circulation improvement delivers nutrients, oxygen, and arterial blood components to the local area being manipulated or the general circulation. The benefit of circulatory improvement is the secondary effect of improved filtration and elimination of carbon dioxide, metabolites, and bio-chemical by-products that are transported in the venous blood. Improved circulation, with its ability to affect elimination, generally enhances the abilities of the structures to benefit and support normal function.

Massage manipulations directly benefit restrictions to muscle tissue function. Mechanical benefits and reflex responses combine to help the muscular soft tissues respond through circulation improvement and elimination of by-products. Mechanical effects on the muscular tissues include influence on the stretch receptors, tendon apparatus, and direct manual stretching of the muscle fibers. The reflex effects encourage relaxation of the tissues through change in the motor nerve output and chemical secretions.

Clients receiving massage therapy report a variety of sensations, emotions, feelings, and mental perceptions that are subjective, difficult to measure, and uniquely individual. When nutrition is improved and elimination enhanced, the structures of localized areas, tissues, and systems are given the opportunity to maximize the potential for normal function.

Massage therapy benefits conditions by the method of encouraging the body through the phases involved in rehabilitation, restoration, and normalization of anatomic and physiologic function and ability. Psychologic benefits occur subjectively and individually in response to therapy with secondary effects that influence sensation and pain perception. Objective and subjective results of therapy combine to create individual responses that affect the desired health outcome.

continued

Box 4.1
THE GENERAL BENEFITS
OF MASSAGE THERAPY
(continued)

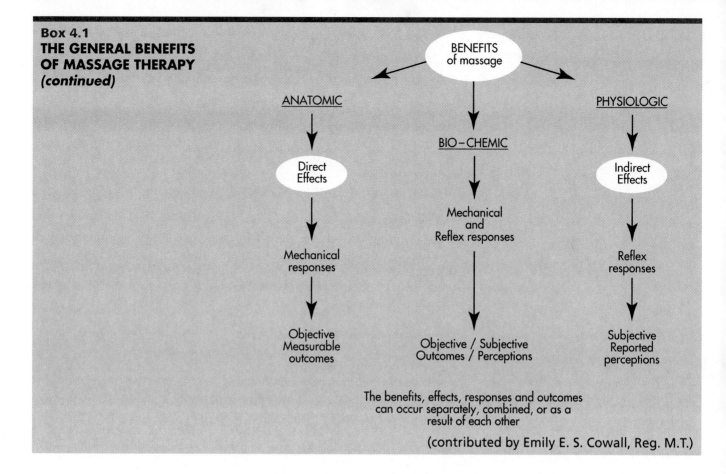

BENEFITS of massage

ANATOMIC

BIO – CHEMIC

PHYSIOLOGIC

Direct Effects

Indirect Effects

Mechanical responses

Mechanical and Reflex responses

Reflex responses

Objective Measurable outcomes

Objective / Subjective Outcomes / Perceptions

Subjective Reported perceptions

The benefits, effects, responses and outcomes can occur separately, combined, or as a result of each other

(contributed by Emily E. S. Cowall, Reg. M.T.)

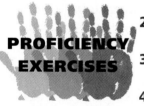

PROFICIENCY EXERCISES

1. **Write two dialogues that explain the benefits of massage. Direct one discussion to a group of medical professionals and the other to a group of business people.**
2. **After receiving a massage, write down both the objective and subjective benefits you gained and experienced from the massage.**
3. **Interview a practice client and again list the objective and subjective benefits the client received from the massage.**
4. **Using the reference section in Appendix A, choose three diseases from the Oregon Model that indicate that massage is beneficial and explain why.**

PATHOLOGY AND MASSAGE THERAPY

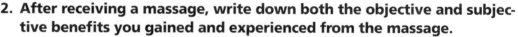

SECTION OBJECTIVES

Using the information presented in this section, the student will be able to do the following:

1 Recognize when a client's condition should be evaluated by a primary health care provider.

Because therapeutic massage has widespread effects on the physiologic functions of the body, it is necessary to understand when massage may not be desirable or may even be detrimental. It is the massage professional's responsibility, when applying bodywork techniques, to have a knowledge of pathology, contraindications, and endangerment sites. It is difficult to obtain a consensus on such information, however, since all sources do not agree.

Because most diseases have similar symptoms, it is difficult to determine the underlying causes of pathology. The massage therapist must refer clients to qualified, licensed health care providers for specific diagnosis.

2 List the mechanisms and risk factors that predispose people to disease processes.

3 Recognize the warning signs of cancer.

4 Explain the general inflammatory response.

5 Explain the mechanisms of pain and evaluate pain for referral purposes.

6 List the endangerment sites for massage.

Pathology is the study of disease. To practice safely, massage therapists need a basic understanding of pathologic processes. Although the diagnosis of disorders is not a function of massage therapy, in order to refer appropriately, the massage therapist must be able to recognize when the client's condition represents an irregularity that should be evaluated by his or her primary health care provider. There is limited published research regarding the effects of massage on various disorders. Massage students should have both a general awareness of the types of disorders that occur in each major body system and more specific knowledge of the signs and symptoms of selected disorders that could endanger the health of either the client or the practitioner. See Appendix A.

Disease conditions are usually diagnosed or identified by signs and symptoms. *Signs* are objective abnormalities that can be seen or measured by someone other than the patient. *Symptoms* are the subjective abnormalities felt only by the patient. A *syndrome* is a group of different signs and symptoms, usually with a common cause. A disease is classified as *acute* when signs and symptoms develop quickly, last a short time, then disappear. Diseases that develop slowly and last for a long time (sometimes for life) are called *chronic* diseases. *Communicable diseases* can be transmitted from one person to another. The study of communicable diseases is an important consideration for the massage therapist and is discussed in further detail in the next chapter. *Homeostasis* is the relative constancy of the body's internal environment. If homeostasis is disturbed, as occurs in a disease process, a variety of feedback mechanisms usually return the body to normal. A disease condition exists when homeostasis cannot be restored easily. In acute conditions, the body recovers its homeostatic balance quickly. In chronic diseases, a normal state of balance may never be restored.

Risk Factors

Certain predisposing conditions may make the development of a disease more likely. Usually called *risk factors*, these conditions may put an individual at risk for developing a disease, but often do not actually cause the disease. There are several major types of risk factors.

Genetic factors. There are several types of genetic risk factors. An inherited trait may sometimes put a person at a greater than normal risk for developing a specific disease. Family history of disease processes and causes of death usually can reveal the possible genetic traits. Steps can be taken to support the body against the genetic tendency toward a disease process. Changes in diet and lifestyle may be beneficial.

Age. Biologic and behavioral factors increase the risk for developing certain diseases at certain times in life. For example, musculoskeletal problems are common between ages of thirty and fifty years.

Lifestyle. The way we live and work can put us at risk for some diseases. Some researchers believe that the high-fat, low-fiber diet common among people in developed nations actually increases their risk of developing certain types of cancer and cardiovascular diseases.

Stress. Stress may be defined as any substantial change in routine, or any activity that forces the body to adapt. Stress will place demands on mental and emotional resources. Research has shown that as stresses accumulate, the individual becomes increasingly susceptible to physical illness, mental and emotional problems, and accidental injuries.

Long-term stress produces many difficulties. The normal adrenal cortex responds to stressful conditions by quickly increasing its secretion of glucocorticoid. This action is only one of many ways in which the body responds to stress, and it elicits many other stress responses.

Selye labeled the body's response to stress as the *general adaptation syndrome* (GAS),[5] which involves three stages. The first stage is alarm, or the "fight or flight" response, which is the body's initial reaction to the perceived stressor. The second stage is known as the resistance reaction. This stage, through the secretion of regulating hormones, allows the body to continue fighting a stressor long after the effects of the alarm reaction have dissipated. The third stage is exhaustion, which occurs if the stress response continues without relief. General adaptation is a uniform, consistent, general response to the perceived stimuli.

The term GAS is often used to describe how the body mobilizes different defense mechanisms when threatened by harmful (actual or perceived) stimuli. In generalized stress conditions the hypothalamus acts on the anterior pituitary gland to cause the release of adrenocorticotropic hormone, which stimulates the adrenal cortex to secrete glucocorticoid. In addition, the sympathetic subdivision of the ANS is stimulated by the adrenal medulla, so the release of epinephrine and norepinephrine occurs to assist the body in responding to the stressful stimulus. Unfortunately, during periods of prolonged stress, glucocorticosteroids may have harmful side effects, including a decreased immune response, decreased blood glucose levels, altered protein and fat metabolism, and decreased resistance to stress.

Considering the variety and number of organs and glands innervated by the ANS, it is no wonder that autonomic disorders have varied and broad consequences. This is especially true of stress-induced diseases. A prolonged or excessive physiologic response to stress, the fight-or-flight response, can disrupt normal functioning throughout the body. Stress has been cited as an indirect cause or an important risk factor in many conditions.

Environment. Some environmental situations put us at greater risk for contracting certain diseases. For example, living in an area with high concentrations of air pollution may increase the risk for development of respiratory problems.

Preexisting conditions. A primary (preexisting) condition can put a person at risk of developing a secondary condition. For example, a viral infection can compromise the immune system, rendering the individual more susceptible to bacterial infection.

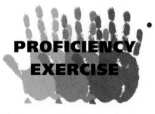

PROFICIENCY EXERCISE

• **Do a self-evaluation listing all your predisposing risk factors for disease. Pick one area and research a wellness plan to provide support for your body to prevent or lessen the possibility of the development of the pathologic condition.**

Tumors and Cancer

Benign tumors remain localized within the tissue from which they arose and usually grow very slowly. Malignant tumors (cancer) tend to spread to other regions of the body. The cells migrate by way of lymphatic or blood vessels. This manner of spreading is called *metastasis.* Cells that do not metastasize can also spread by growing rapidly and extending the tumor into nearby tissues. Malignant tumors may replace part of a vital organ with abnormal tissues, which is a life-threatening situation.

Cancer specialists, or oncologists, have summarized some major signs of the early stages of cancer. Early detection of cancer is important because it is in the early stages of primary tumor development, before metastasis and the development of secondary tumors have begun, that cancer is most treatable.

The following are warning signs of cancer:
• Sores that do not heal
• Unusual bleeding

- A change in appearance or size of a wart or mole
- A lump or thickening in any tissue
- Persistent hoarseness or cough
- Chronic indigestion
- A change in bowel or bladder function

It is possible that the massage therapist may be the first to recognize these early warning signs. Although it is important to refer the client for proper evaluation to find out if a cancer process is developing, the massage therapist is cautioned never to suggest to the client that cancer is evident. Instead, the practitioner should simply point out the changes, and explain that it is important that the changes be evaluated by a qualified professional.

INFLAMMATORY RESPONSE

Inflammation may occur as a response to any tissue injury. The inflammatory response is a combination of processes that attempts to minimize injury to tissues, thus maintaining homeostasis. Inflammation may also accompany specific immune system reactions. The inflammatory response has four primary signs—redness, heat, swelling, and pain.

Heat and Redness

As tissue cells are damaged, they release inflammation mediators such as histamine, prostaglandins, and compounds called kinins. Some inflammation mediators cause blood vessels to dilate, increasing blood volume in the tissue. Increased blood volume produces the redness and heat of inflammation. This response is important because it allows immune system cells (white blood cells) in the blood to travel quickly and easily to the site of injury.

Swelling and Pain

Some inflammation mediators increase the permeability of blood vessel walls. When water leaks out of the vessel, tissue swelling or edema results. The pressure caused by edema triggers pain receptors. The fluid that accumulates in inflamed tissue is called *inflammatory exudate* and has the beneficial effect of diluting the irritant. Inflammatory exudate is removed slowly by lymphatic vessels. Bacteria and damaged cells are held in the lymph nodes and are destroyed by white blood cells. Occasionally, lymph nodes enlarge when they process a large amount of infectious material.

Sometimes the inflammatory response is more intense or prolonged than desirable. Inflammation can be suppressed by antihistamines, which block the action of histamine, and aspirin, which disrupts the body's synthesis of prostaglandins. Therapeutic massage seems to be beneficial in cases of prolonged inflammation. Possible theories include the following:

1. The stimulation from massage induces a release of the body's own anti-inflammatory agents.
2. Certain types of massage increase the inflammatory process to a small degree, triggering the body to complete the process.
3. Massage may facilitate the dilution and removal of the irritant by increasing lymphatic flow.

The processes of inflammation eventually eliminate the irritant, and tissue repair can begin. Tissue repair is the replacement of dead cells with living cells. In a type of tissue repair called *regeneration,* the new cells are similar to those they replace. Another type of tissue repair is *replacement.* In replacement, the new cells are formed from connective tissue, and are different from those they replace, resulting in a scar. Often, fibrous connective tissue replaces the damaged tissue, resulting in a condition called *fibro-*

sis. Most tissue repairs are a combination of regeneration and replacement. A goal in the healing process is to promote regeneration and keep replacement to a minimum. Massage has been shown to slow the formation of scar tissue and keep scar tissue pliable when it does form.

Inflammatory Disease

Local inflammation occurs in a limited area, as in a small cut that becomes infected. Systemic inflammation occurs when the irritant spreads through the body or when inflammation mediators cause changes throughout the body. Conditions involving chronic inflammation are classified as *inflammatory diseases.* Inflammatory conditions such as arthritis, asthma, eczema, and chronic bronchitis are among the most common in the world.

PAIN

The massage therapist especially needs to understand the mechanisms of pain. Chapter 6 provides additional research and information on the reasons why massage is beneficial for the symptomatic reduction of pain perception. Here we will consider the types of pain and how massage can be beneficial or contraindicated for pain. Understanding the various types of pain helps the massage practitioner know when to refer the client to a physician.

Pain is a complex, private, abstract experience that is difficult to explain or describe. It is the main symptom or complaint that causes people to seek health care. Its effective management is a major challenge. Defining pain in descriptive and measurable terms is not easy since pain has physiologic, psychologic, and social aspects. The massage professional needs to recognize that pain is what the client says it is and exists when the client says it does. Mosby's *Medical, Nursing, & Allied Health Dictionary, (ed 4),* defines pain as "an unpleasant sensation caused by noxious stimulation of the sensory nerve endings. It is a subjective feeling and an individual response to the cause."

Pain Sensations

Pain provides information about tissue-damaging stimuli, and thus often enables us to protect ourselves from greater damage. It is pain that initiates our search for medical assistance. It is the subjective description and indication of the location of the pain that helps to pinpoint the underlying cause of disease.

The receptors for pain, called *nociceptors,* are simply the branching ends of the dendrites of certain sensory neurons. Pain receptors are found in almost every tissue of the body, and may respond to any type of stimulus. When stimuli for other sensations, such as touch, pressure, heat, and cold, reach a certain intensity, they stimulate the sensation of pain as well. Injured tissue may release prostaglandins, making peripheral nociceptors more sensitive to the normal pain response (hyperalgesia). Aspirin and other nonsteroidal anti-inflammatory drugs inhibit the action of prostaglandins and relieve pain.

As stated previously, excessive stimulation of a sensory organ causes pain. Additional stimuli for pain receptors include excessive distention or dilation of a structure, prolonged muscular contractions, muscle spasms, inadequate blood flow to an organ, or the presence of certain chemical substances. Because of their sensitivity to all stimuli, pain receptors perform a protective function by identifying changes that may endanger the body. Pain receptors adapt only slightly or not at all. *Adaptation* is the decrease or disappearance of the perception of a sensation even though the stimulus is still present. (An example is how we get used to our clothes soon after dressing.) If there were adaptation to pain, pain would cease to be sensed and irreparable damage could result. Sensory impulses for pain are conducted by the central nervous system along spinal and cranial nerves to the thalamus. From here the impulses may be relayed to the parietal lobe. Recognition of the type and intensity of most pain is localized ultimately in the cerebral cortex. Some awareness of pain occurs at subcortical levels. Pain may be classified as acute, chronic, or intractable.

Acute Pain

Acute pain is either a symptom of a disease condition or a temporary aspect of medical treatment. It acts as a warning signal since it can activate the sympathetic nervous system. Acute pain is usually temporary, of sudden onset, and easily localized. The client frequently can describe the pain, which often subsides with or without treatment.

Chronic Pain

Chronic pain is a major health problem for approximately 25% of the population affected. Chronic pain is pain that persists or recurs for indefinite periods, usually for longer than six months. It frequently has an obscure onset, and the character and quality of the pain changes over time. Chronic pain is usually diffuse, poorly localized, and often requires the efforts of a multidisciplinary health care team, which may include a massage therapist for its effective management.

Intractable Pain

When chronic pain persists even when treatment is provided, or when it exists without demonstrable disease, it is called *intractable pain.* Intractable pain represents the greatest challenge to all health care providers. Short, temporary, symptomatic relief of this type of pain may be provided by massage. The flooding of the sensory receptors may distract the client temporarily from the perception of pain.

Phantom Pain

A type of pain frequently experienced by clients who have had a limb amputated is called *phantom pain*. These clients still experience pain or other sensations in the area of the amputated extremity as if the limb were still there. This pain probably occurs because the remaining proximal portions of the sensory nerves that previously received impulses from the limb are being stimulated by the trauma of the amputation. Stimuli from these nerves are interpreted by the brain as coming from the nonexistent (phantom) limb.

Because pain is a primary indicator in the disease process, the massage practitioner must have a basic evaluation protocol of pain in order to refer his or her clients to the appropriate health care provider. The following guideline for evaluating pain will help in this process.

Evaluation of Pain

The massage therapist should observe clients as they move by noticing their general mobility level and range of pain-free movement, and should ask specific questions for a subjective evaluation of pain.

There are many characteristics of pain. **Location** can be divided into four categories. Localized pain is pain confined to the site of origin. Projected pain is typically a result of proximal nerve compression. This pain is perceived in the tissue supplied by the nerve. Radiating pain is dif-

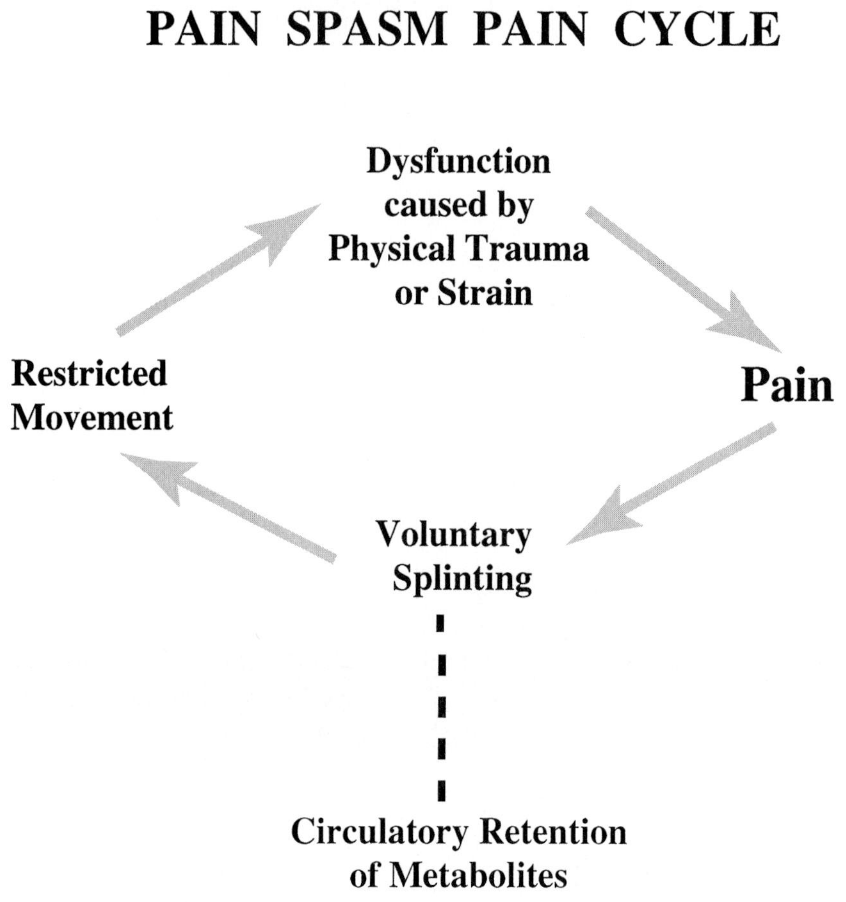

PAIN SPASM PAIN CYCLE

Dysfunction caused by Physical Trauma or Strain

Restricted Movement

Pain

Voluntary Splinting

Circulatory Retention of Metabolites

Figure 4.4
Pain-spasm-pain cycle.

fuse pain around the site of origin that is not well localized. Referred pain is felt in an area distant from the site of the painful stimulus.

There are five types of pain.

1. *Pricking or bright pain.* This type of pain, which is experienced when the skin is cut or jabbed with a sharp object, is short-lived but intense and easily localized.

2. *Burning pain.* This type, which is slower to develop, lasts longer, and is less accurately localized, is experienced when the skin is burned. It often stimulates cardiac and respiratory activity.

3. *Aching pain.* Aching pain occurs when the visceral organs are stimulated. It is constant, not well localized, and is often referred to areas of the body far from where the damage is occurring. This type of pain is important because it may be a sign of a life-threatening disorder of a vital organ.

4. *Deep pain.* The main difference between superficial and deep sensibility is the different nature of the pain evoked by noxious stimuli. Unlike superficial pain, deep pain is poorly localized, nauseating, and frequently associated with sweating and changes in blood pressure. Deep pain can be elicited experimentally from the periosteum and ligaments by injecting them with hypertonic saline. Pain produced in this fashion initiates reflex contraction of nearby skeletal muscles. This reflex contraction is similar to the muscle spasm associated with injuries to bones, tendons, and joints. The steadily contracting muscles become ischemic, and ischemia stimulates the pain receptors in the muscles. The pain, in turn, initiates more spasms, creating a vicious circle. (Fig. 4.4)

5. *Muscle pain.* If a muscle contracts rhythmically in the presence of an adequate blood supply, pain does not usually result. However, if the

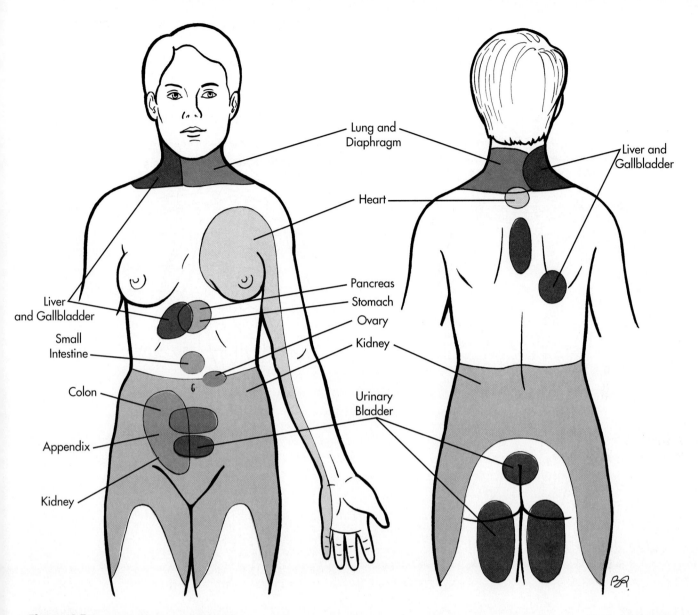

Lung and Diaphragm

Heart

Liver and Gallbladder

Pancreas

Stomach

Ovary

Kidney

Liver and Gallbladder

Small Intestine

Colon

Appendix

Kidney

Urinary Bladder

Figure 4.5
Referred pain. The diagram indicates cutaneous areas to which visceral pains may be referred. The massage professional encountering pain in these areas needs to refer the client for diagnosis to rule out visceral dysfunction.

blood supply to a muscle is occluded (closed off), contraction soon causes pain. The pain persists after the contraction until blood flow is reestablished. If a muscle with a normal blood supply is made to contract continuously without periods of relaxation, it also begins to ache because the maintained contraction compresses the blood vessels supplying the muscle.

The origins of pain can be divided into two types: somatic and visceral. *Somatic pain* arises from stimulation of receptors in the skin (called superficial somatic pain), or from stimulation of receptors in skeletal muscles, joints, tendons, and fascia (called deep somatic pain). *Visceral pain* results from stimulation of receptors in the viscera (internal organs).

The ability of the cerebral cortex to locate the origin of pain is related to past experience. In most instances of somatic pain and in some instances of visceral pain, the cortex accurately projects the pain back to the stimulated area.

The pain may also be felt in a surface area far from the stimulated organ. This phenomenon is called *referred pain*. In general, the area to which the pain is referred and the visceral organ involved receive their innervation from the same segment of the spinal cord. Figure 4.5 illus-

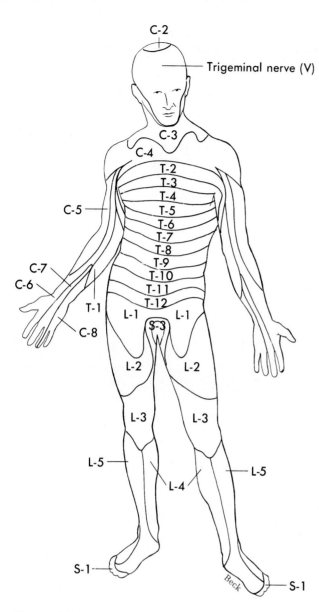

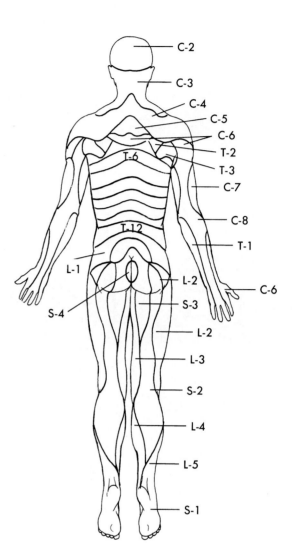

Figure 4.6
Dermatomes. Segmented dermatome distribution of spinal nerves to the front and back of the body. C, Cervical segments; T, thoracic segments; L, lumbar segments; S, sacral segments. (From Thibodeau/Patton: The human body in health & disease, St. Louis, 1992, Mosby–Year Book, Inc.)

trates cutaneous regions to which visceral pain may be referred. If the client has a reoccurring pain pattern that resembles patterns on the chart, he or she should be referred to a physician for an accurate diagnosis.

As already stated, irritation of the viscera frequently produces pain that is felt not in the viscera but in some somatic structure that may be located at a considerable distance. Such pain is said to be referred to the somatic structure. Deep somatic pain may also be referred, but superficial pain is not. When visceral pain is both local and referred, it sometimes seems to spread (radiate) from the local to the distant site. Visceral pain, like deep somatic pain, initiates reflex contraction of nearby skeletal muscle. Since somatic pain is much more common than visceral pain, the brain has "learned" to project the pain to the somatic area.

Obviously, a knowledge of referred pain and the common sites of pain referral from each of the viscera are very important to massage therapists and other health care professionals. However, sites of reference are not stereotyped, and unusual reference sites occur with considerable frequency. Heart pain, for instance, may be experienced as purely abdominal, may be referred to the right arm, and may even be referred to the neck.

Any client with a referred or unexplained pain pattern should be referred to a physician, especially if the pattern is similar to visceral referred pain patterns (Fig. 4.5). When pain is referred, it is usually to a structure that developed from the same embryonic segment or dermatome as the structure in which the pain originates (Fig. 4.6).

Pain may be brought on by mechanical, electrical, thermal, or chemical stimuli. We do not appear to adapt to pain or to accommodate it. We may be distracted from it or ignore it, but it recurs unchanged if we pay attention to it. Subjective measurements of pain intensity are more reliable than observable ones. Only the client in pain can determine the amount of severity experienced. Pain is rarely the same at all times. It is felt (perceived) differently over time and differs with various precipitating and aggravating factors. Pain can range from excruciating to mild and may be difficult for the client to verbalize.

Pain is a complex problem with physical, psychologic, social, and financial components. There are many ways to alleviate pain. The massage therapist, as part of a health care team, can contribute valuable manual therapy in various pain conditions using direct tissue manipulation and reflex stimulation of the nervous system and the circulation. As a therapeutic intervention, massage may help reduce the need for pain medication, thus reducing the side effects of medication. All medications, including over-the-counter medication available without a prescription, have some side effects. Obviously, clients in extreme pain must have their therapy monitored by a doctor or other appropriate health care professional. Most people experience less extreme pain occasionally throughout life. Massage may provide temporary symptomatic relief for moderate pain brought on by daily stress, replacing over-the-counter pain medications or reducing their use.

ENDANGERMENT SITES

Endangerment sites are areas in which nerves and blood vessels surface close to the skin and are not well protected by muscle or connective tissue. Consequently, deep sustained pressure into these areas could damage these vessels and nerves. The kidney area is included as such a site because the kidneys are loosely suspended in fat and connective tissue. Heavy pounding is contraindicated in that area. The following areas are commonly considered endangerment sites for the massage therapist. Refer to Fig. 4.7 to locate the specific sites; the listed areas correspond to the letters as labelled.

A Anterior triangle of the neck—carotid artery, jugular vein, and vagus nerve, which are located deep to the sternocleidomastoid

B Posterior triangle of the neck—specifically, the nerves of the brachial plexus; the brachiocephalic artery and vein superior to the clavicle; and the subclavian arteries and vein

C Axillary area—the brachial artery, axillary vein and artery, cephalic vein; nerves of the brachial plexus

D Medial epicondyle of the humerus—the ulnar nerve

E Lateral epicondyle—the radial nerve

F Area of the sternal notch and anterior throat—nerves and vessels to the thyroid gland; vagus nerve

G Umbilicus area—to either side; descending aorta and abdominal aorta

H Twelfth rib, dorsal body—location of the kidney

I Sciatic notch—sciatic nerve (the sciatic nerve passes out of the pelvis through the greater sciatic foramen, under cover of piriformis muscle)

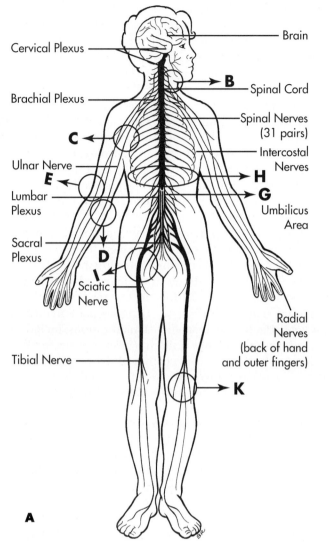

Cervical Plexus

Brain

Brachial Plexus

B Spinal Cord

Spinal Nerves (31 pairs)

C

Intercostal Nerves

Ulnar Nerve

E

Lumbar Plexus

H

G

Umbilicus Area

Sacral Plexus

D

Sciatic Nerve

Radial Nerves (back of hand and outer fingers)

Tibial Nerve

K

A

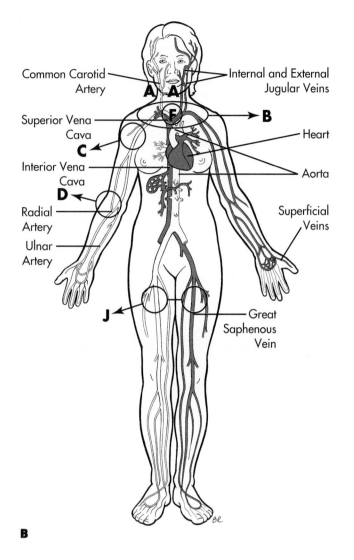

Common Carotid Artery

Internal and External Jugular Veins

A **A**

Superior Vena Cava

F

B

C

Heart

Interior Vena Cava

D

Aorta

Radial Artery

Ulnar Artery

Superficial Veins

J

Great Saphenous Vein

B

Figure 4.7
Endangerment sites of A, the nervous system. B, the cardiovascular system.

J Inguinal triangle located lateral and inferior to the pubis—medial to the sartorius; external iliac artery; femoral artery; great saphenous vein; femoral vein; femoral nerve

K Popliteal fossa—popliteal artery and vein; tibial nerve

Deep stripping over a vein in a direction away from the heart is contraindicated due to possible damage to the valve system.

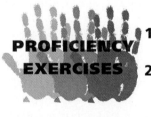

PROFICIENCY EXERCISES

1. **Using your anatomy and physiology textbook, list the pages that provide similar information to that presented in this section.**
2. **Locate all endangerment sites on a fellow student.**

CONTRAINDICATIONS TO MASSAGE THERAPY

SECTION OBJECTIVES

Using the information presented in this section, the student will be able to do the following:

❶ **Evaluate a client's status to determine if massage is contraindicated.**

A *contraindication* is any condition that renders a particular treatment improper or undesirable. Contraindications to massage concern both responsible physicians and massage therapists.

Massage therapists should not rely on lists of specific contraindications but rather on a set of medical and therapeutic guidelines pertinent to clinical applications and recent research developments. Such guidelines are not consistent in current literature. Contraindications are unique to each client, as well as to each region of the body. It is important to

2 Effectively refer a client to a primary health care provider.

3 Interpret the reference list of indications and contraindications provided in Appendix A.

understand when to refer a client for diagnosis and when to obtain assistance in modifying the approach to the massage session so that it will best serve the client. A medical professional must always be consulted if there is any doubt concerning the advisability of therapy. When in doubt, refer!

Contraindications are separated into regional and general types. *Regional contraindications* are those that relate to a specific area of the body. For our purposes, regional contraindication means that massage may be provided but not to the problematic area. However, the client should be referred to a physician to obtain a diagnosis of the condition and to rule out underlying conditions. *General contraindications* are those that require a physician's evaluation to rule out serious underlying conditions before any massage is indicated. If massage is recommended by the physician, then the physician will need to help the therapist develop a comprehensive treatment plan. Therapeutic massage is often beneficial for clients who are receiving treatment for a specific medical condition. The general effects of stress and pain reduction, increased circulation, and physical comfort complement most other medical treatment modalities. However, when other therapies, including medication, are being used, the physician must be able to evaluate accurately the effectiveness of each treatment the client is receiving. If the physician is not aware that the client is receiving massage, the effects of other therapy may be misinterpreted.

The massage practitioner must remember to work as part of a team for the benefit of the client. In general, massage is indicated for musculoskeletal discomfort, circulation enhancement, relaxation, and pain control as well as in situations in which analgesics, anti-inflammatories, and muscle relaxants may be prescribed.

Immediately refer patients with any vague symptoms of fatigue, muscle weakness, and general aches and pains to a physician. Many disease processes share these symptoms. This recommendation may seem overly cautious, but in the early stages of some very serious illnesses, the symptoms are not well defined. If the physician is able to detect a disease process early in its development, there is often a more successful outcome. A specific diagnosis is essential for effective treatment. Massage should be avoided in all infectious diseases suggested by fever, nausea, and lethargy until a diagnosis is received and recommendations given by a physician can be followed.

The massage therapist is not expected to diagnose any condition, but should learn the client's particular condition by taking a thorough history. The massage professional must be able to recognize the indications and contraindications to these conditions and be aware of the client's medications. The massage therapist should have a current *Physician's Desk Reference* or similar book so that all medications the client lists on the client information form can be studied. The client may also be able to provide information about each drug being taken. The massage therapist should be able to assess the effects of the medications and discover how massage may interface with these effects. Massage practitioners will need to be specifically aware of anti-inflammatories, muscle relaxants, anticoagulants (blood thinners), analgesics (pain reduction), or any other medications that alter sensation, muscle tone, standard reflex reactions, cardiovascular function, kidney or liver function, or personality. If a client is taking medication, it is important to contact the physician for recommendations about the advisability of massage therapy.

For example, one side effect of some medications is anxiety. The massage may either help the client by reducing anxiety, or may be the cause of an adverse reaction. If the doctor is using the level of anxiety to monitor the correct drug dose, and anxiety levels are lowered through massage, there may be a possibility that the dose could be too high.

It is also recommended that the massage therapist have available a current medical dictionary so that unfamiliar terms and names of pathologic conditions can be looked up. A massage practitioner is not a physician, and is not expected to know the symptoms of all diseases, but resources must be available to locate specific information as needed.

REFERRALS

Referral is a method by which a client is sent to a health care professional for diagnosis and treatment of a disease. When a client is ill, he or she is aware of it. If the client is very sick, it shows. Common sense should be the guide. Although massage cannot cure anything, it can assist in the client's healing process. Massage therapists may pick up subtle changes in the tissue before the client consciously recognizes that something is out of balance. When this happens, the client should be referred to a qualified professional for specific diagnosis.

Massage therapists are advised to become familiar with the health professionals in their area, including medical doctors, osteopathic doctors, podiatrists, chiropractors, physical therapists, psychologists, licensed counselors, and dentists. There may also be health care providers that provide alternative therapy such as acupuncture and homeopathy. Clients trust the practitioner. Before referring a client to a specific health professional, the therapist should take the time to get to know that professional. This can be done by calling that person's office and making an appointment for a short visit, during which the professional's feelings about massage would be discussed. Information about massage should be left for reference.

Clients must always be referred to their personal health care professionals. The therapist should make no attempt to direct them to different health care professionals. If the client does not have a doctor, chiropractor, or counselor, then a list of the professionals who have been contacted and educated about massage therapy should be provided. The practitioner can simply explain to the client why a referral to a health care professional is being recommended by stating that the observed set of signs or symptoms should be evaluated by someone who has more specific training. No specific condition should be named. The client should be given a business card or brochure from the massage therapist to give to the health care professional so that he or she can be contacted easily.

For example, a therapist named Sandy has been seeing Ms. Jones for massage every other week for about one year. Ms. Jones has a mole on her left shoulder. During the last two visits Sandy notices that the mole has started to change shape and looks different, and feels that these signs should be evaluated by someone who has more specific training. She says to Ms. Jones, "The mole you have on your left shoulder looks a little different to me. Have you noticed any change? It is important to have your doctor look at any changes in a mole. Will you please make an appointment with your personal physician to have the mole examined? Have your doctor give you a written statement that you were seen, and that massage may be continued, along with any special instructions. It is important for you to do this before we schedule the next massage. Once I feel it is a good idea to refer a client, and I put that on your record, I need the written verification from the doctor to see you again." If the client does not have a personal physician, Sandy could say, "I have talked with various health care professionals in our area and have developed a referral list. I am sure one of the doctors listed will be able to help you, or you can ask a family member or friend for a recommendation." Ms. Jones may say, "What do you think the change in the mole is?" Sandy replies, "I am trained to notice changes in the body and when to refer a client, but I am not trained to be able to diagnose what any specific condition is. That is the

Box 4.2
INDICATIONS
FOR REFERRAL

- Pain—local, sharp, dull, achy, deep surface
- Fatigue
- Inflammation
- Lumps and tissue changes
- Rashes and changes in the skin
- Edema
- Mood alterations—e.g., depression, anxiety
- Infection—local or general
- Changes in habits, such as in appetite, elimination, or sleep
- Bleeding and bruising
- Nausea, vomiting, or diarrhea
- Temperature—hot (fever) or cold

role of a physician. It is best for you to go and have it checked by someone who has much more training in this area."

If the therapist feels it is necessary to refer a client for diagnosis, some sort of written permission from the doctor will be needed to continue to see the client. The client should obtain the written documentation and bring it to the next massage session. This information is kept in the client's file. If the doctor or other health care professional has given any specific directions or recommendations, they must be followed exactly. The care plan of the physician must never be interfered with or contradicted, nor should the massage therapist assume the role of counselor. If it is necessary to contact the health care professional directly, the therapist should always work through the receptionist. Leave whatever information is needed with the front desk and if the doctor feels it is necessary to speak with the massage therapist directly, he or she will call.

The referral and the date must be noted on the client's record, along with the signs and symptoms. If the client responds in any unusual way, such as by panicking or refusing to go to the doctor, then this must be indicated on the client record as well. The written permission for continuation of the massage from the health professional must then be placed in the client's file.

There are only a few basic symptoms to most disease processes. See Appendix A for more comprehensive information. Always refer for diagnosis when the symptoms listed in Box 4.2 do not have a logical explanation (i.e., if the client has been up late or working long hours, naturally they will display the symptom of fatigue). Use common sense. Remember, a gentle spirit, holding a client's hand, a hug, and listening is never contraindicated.

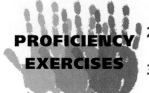

PROFICIENCY EXERCISES

1. **Using the reference section in Appendix A, list five regional contraindications to massage that you have encountered with practice clients. Also list five general contraindications that you think you will encounter most often.**
2. **Using the Oregon Model in Appendix A, list two specific disease conditions that correspond to the twelve basic symptoms listed in Box 4.2.**
3. **Research three pathologic conditions from Appendix A and expand on the symptoms and specific indications for which massage would be beneficial with supervision. Refer to the section on the benefits of massage in this chapter to provide a physiologic rationale for your recommendation.**

4. **Develop a class project that combines each of the research projects from the above exercise and develop an indications manual.**

5. **Choose a condition from each of the categories in the Oregon Model in Appendix A. Pretend that clients display symptoms of that condition or actually role play in the classroom, having a fellow student act out the signs and symptoms of the conditions. Write down what things you would notice about each condition that would make you want to refer. Write down or act out a referral process with the pretend client.**

6. **Develop a list of health care providers in your area who you would like to place on a referral list. Since they need to support your work, set up a plan to meet and interview each one. Write down a list of questions to be asked, and information that you must provide about your skills. Have at least three professionals from each category so the client has a choice. If time permits, contact these people while you are still a student.**

SUMMARY

This chapter has discussed the physiologic effects of therapeutic massage. Indications for massage are based on the physiologic effects that provide the benefits of massage. Massage is beneficial for most people, yet contraindications do exist. The responsible massage professional will always refer a client for diagnosis and treatment by a qualified health professional, without delay, as soon as any condition is noticed that may suggest an underlying physical or mental health problem. Once a condition has been diagnosed, and appropriate treatment established, the massage professional may provide massage under the supervision of the medical professional. Massage may prove beneficial and supportive to the interventions of the health care professional, and may enhance the healing process by temporarily reducing pain, relaxing the client and reducing stress responses, increasing circulation, and much more. In addition, the client's subjective experience with the one-on-one contact given by the massage professional may provide support and gentle touch during a difficult time, thereby reducing feelings of frustration, isolation, anxiety, and depression that often accompany illness.

REVIEW QUESTIONS

1. Why are the effects of massage sometimes difficult to measure?
2. Why do massage methods work?
3. What are the five basic physiologic effects of massage?
4. What is the basic premise when working with each of the physiologic areas?
5. What information is necessary to understand the functional operation of the neuromuscular mechanism?
6. What happens to the connective tissue in chronic problems?
7. What are the five types of circulation?
8. What words describe the sympathetic ANS functions?
9. What words are used to describe the parasympathetic functions?
10. Of what importance is state-dependent memory to the massage therapist?
11. What is hyperstimulation analgesia?
12. How does massage promote the body's ability to effectively maintain self-regulation and structural and functional balance?
13. What seems to be the physiology of the energy approaches to massage?
14. Define health.
15. How do acute and chronic conditions affect homeostasis?
16. Why would a massage practitioner need to be aware of risk factors?
17. Why does the massage practitioner need to understand tumor pathology?
18. Why does the massage therapist need to understand the inflammatory response?
19. Why is describing pain difficult?
20. What would be the benefits of massage for acute pain, chronic pain, and intractable pain?
21. What is the difference between localized pain, radiating pain, referred pain, and projected pain?

22. What is the difference between somatic and visceral pain?

23. Why is the knowledge of referred pain patterns important?

24. What role do dermatomes play in pain pattern?

25. What is phantom pain?

26. What are endangerment sites?

27. What is an indication for massage?

28. What is a contraindication to massage? What are the two main types of contraindications?

29. What are some important warning signs that indicate that the client should be referred to a medical doctor for specific diagnosis?

30. What resource material should the massage practitioner have available to help understand medications and terminology?

31. Why should the massage therapist understand the action of medications?

32. How do you refer a client to a health care professional?

33. What is the purpose for the listings of contraindications, indications, and pathologic states?

REFERENCES

1. Cantu RI and Grodin AJ: *Myofascial manipulation theory and clinical application,* Gaithersburg, Maryland, 1992, Aspen Publishers, Inc.
2. Greenman PE: *Principles of Manual Medicine,* Baltimore, 1989, Williams and Wilkins.
3. Melzack R: TP relationship to mechanisms of pain, *Arch Phys Med Rehabil.* 62, March 1981.
4. Nimmi ME, ed: *Collagen Vol I biochemistry,* Boca Raton, 1988, CRC Press.
5. Selye H: *The stress of life,* ed. 2, New York, 1978, McGraw-Hill.
6. Thomas, CL, ed: *Taber's cyclopedic medical dictionary,* Philadelphia, 1985, F. A. Davis.
7. Waites EA: *Trauma and survival: post-traumatic and dissociative disorders in women,* New York, 1993, Norton.
8. Yates J: *Physiological effects of therapeutic massage and their application to treatment,* British Columbia, 1989, Massage Therapist Association of British Columbia.

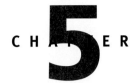

C H A P 5 E R

HYGIENE, SANITATION, AND
SAFETY

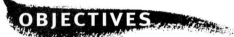
After completing this chapter, the student will be able to do the following:

❶ Identify good health and personal hygiene practices.

❷ Explain the major disease-causing agents.

❸ Describe methods for prevention and control of disease.

❹ Give specific recommendations for sanitary practices for massage businesses.

❺ Implement universal precautions.

❻ Provide information about HIV, AIDS, and hepatitis.

❼ Develop a safe and hazard-free massage environment.

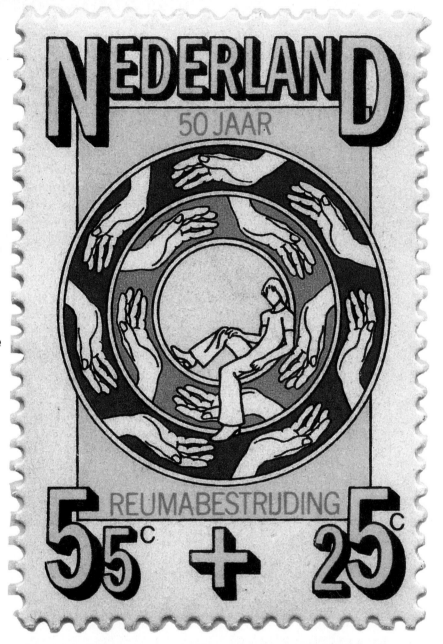

Schema of a patient surrounded by a circle of caring hands. This stamp was issued in 1976 to partially fund contributions to the Dutch Rheumatism Society and to celebrate the use of manual methods to treat rheumatic disease. (Courtesy of Holland)

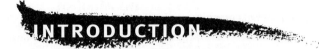

INTRODUCTION

This chapter deals with hygiene and sanitation practices in a professional setting. Most of the information presented is common sense, yet a reminder and review of sanitation and safety rules is beneficial. Many local and state laws governing massage deal extensively with sanitary procedures. The health code requirements for the state of Oregon, the legislation of which has been used as a model for part of this chapter, are both typical and well defined.

There is much concern, misunderstanding, and misinformation about the spread of hepatitis, the human immunodeficiency virus (HIV) and the acquired immune deficiency syndrome (AIDS). In the hopes of providing accurate information on HIV and AIDS, and detailing the responsibilities of the massage practitioner, an extensive section devoted to these topics is included in this chapter. Because new information is being dispensed almost daily, it is important to stay current. The Centers for Disease Control (CDC) standards and guidelines for communicable diseases may change as new information becomes available. It is the responsibility of the massage practitioner to update information biyearly regarding changes in CDC recommendations and to follow the most current standards and guidelines.

Besides a sanitary environment, the massage therapist must provide a safe environment. It is important to consider fire and accident prevention for both the client and the therapist. This discussion about hygiene, sanitation, and safety begins with the personal care of the massage practitioner.

PERSONAL HEALTH, HYGIENE, AND APPEARANCE

SECTION OBJECTIVE

Using the information presented in this section, the student will be able to do the following:

❶ Identify the hygienic procedures important to a professional environment.

One of the best ways to control disease is to stay healthy. If our bodies are strong, and our immune systems are functioning properly, we do not become sick easily. If injured, we heal better if we are healthy. Diet, sleep, rest, body mechanics (how we use our body), exercise, and lifestyle need to be considered in the overall health picture.

Smoking

Smoking is considered one of the leading causes of disease. It is directly linked to cardiovascular disease and is the leading cause of lung cancer.[3] Exposure to secondary smoke has been determined to cause cancer and other heath problems in nonsmokers. Besides the dangerous health effects, smoking is offensive to many people. Smoke odors linger in the air and on hands, hair, and clothing. Many nonsmokers find this smell obnoxious. The smell of smoke can cause reactions in sensitive individuals. Because the massage therapist works physically closely to the client, any smoke odors from the therapist are reason for concern.

The massage therapist should never smoke in the massage therapy room, even when clients are not present because the smell of smoke lingers in carpets, draperies, and other furniture. If the practitioner must smoke during business hours, it should be done outside, away from any access doors or windows. Hands should be washed carefully before touching a client. If the therapist is a smoker, he or she must inform any client when an appointment is made. If the client is bothered by the smoke odors, referral to a different massage therapist is appropriate.

Drugs and Alcohol

Drugs and alcohol interfere with the ability to function as a massage therapist. Because they affect thinking, feeling, behavior, and functioning, the therapist must never be under the influence of alcohol or drugs when working with a client. This includes any prescription drugs that affect mental or physical abilities. Use of these substances by the massage therapist can place the client in danger. At least twelve hours should elapse from the time of the last drink of alcohol before working with a client, since it takes this long for the direct effects of alcohol to wear off. For the next twenty-four hours the therapist will be affected indirectly by the alcohol consumption. Often called a hangover, the body is exhausted and toxic. This is not a good condition to be in while giving a massage. Clients should be referred or rescheduled if the therapist's ability to function is affected.

Hygiene

The massage therapist must pay careful attention to personal hygiene. Preventing breath and body odor, without the use of chemical cover-ups, is essential. The massage therapist should not wear perfume, aftershave, or perfumed hair products since many clients are sensitive to these odors.

The massage therapist should bathe or shower at the beginning of each work day. Using soap or a similar cleaning agent, the armpit, genital, and foot regions should be washed carefully. During menstruation, female therapists must be especially mindful of odor.

Because breath odor is offensive, careful brushing and flossing of the teeth after each meal is important. During work hours, any food that may cause breath odor should be avoided. Gum chewing is unprofessional and irritating to many people, and is ineffective in covering breath odors. Using breath mints helps to combat breath odor.

Hair should be clean. The use of any chemicals such as hair sprays and gels must be avoided since they may cause an allergic reaction in sensitive people. Hair must not fall onto the face of the therapist or drag on the client. If long, it should be kept pulled back.

Proper care of the hands is especially important. Nails should be short and well manicured, and should not extend over the tip of the fingers. Care must be taken to keep the space under the nails clean which is best accomplished with a nail brush. Any hangnails, breaks, or cracks in the skin of the hands must be kept clean and covered during a massage. Nail polish and synthetic nails promote bacterial growth. Therefore, avoid their use.

Massage uniforms should be loose and made of cotton or a cotton blend. Since body temperature increases while giving a massage, clothing will need to breathe and wick off perspiration. Sleeves should be above the elbow, but sleeveless uniforms should not be worn. All clothing should be opaque and modest. T-shirts and shorts are usually inappropriate. If skirts or shorts are worn, they must be knee-length or longer. Loose pants are preferred. (White clothing is not necessary or even desirable since lubricant stains show less on colors.) Clothing should be laundered in a disinfectant, usually a bleach. Whatever uniform is chosen must be able to withstand this type of laundering. If perspiration is heavy, or the clothing becomes stained, it may be necessary to change clothes. A spare uniform

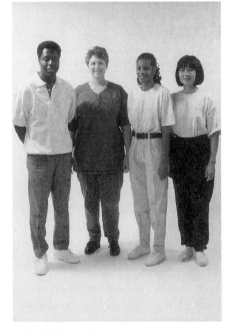

Figure 5.1
Properly groomed massage professionals.

should be kept available. Underclothing must be changed daily, and possibly more frequently if perspiration is heavy.

Comfortable and clean shoes should be worn while giving a massage. It is not sanitary or professional to be barefoot. Changing socks daily will help to prevent foot odor.

Make-up should be modest to avoid a painted and severe appearance; heavy make-up is never appropriate. Jewelry should not be worn while giving a massage. Necklaces and bracelets can become tangled or drag on the client, and rings can scratch the client (Fig. 5.1).

If the client or therapist is ill, and there is any concern that the condition is contagious, the massage therapist should refer or reschedule the client until the condition changes.

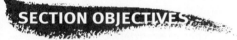

PROFICIENCY EXERCISES

1. **Design your ideal uniform and ask three massage professionals what they think of your idea.**
2. **Develop a class project where anonymous evaluations of fellow students' personal hygiene and professional appearance are given.**
3. **Ask honest trusted family or friends if you have breath or body odor.**

SANITATION

Sanitary massage methods promote conditions that are conducive to health. This means that pathogenic organisms must be eliminated or controlled.

Pathogenic Organisms

Pathogenic organisms cause the development of many disease processes. They include viruses, bacteria, fungi, protozoa, and pathogenic animals.

Viruses

Viruses invade cells and insert their own genetic code into the host cell's genetic code. They use the host cell's nutrients and organelles to produce more virus particles. New viruses may leave the cell to infect other cells by bursting the cell membrane.

Bacteria

Bacteria are primitive cells without nuclei. They produce disease by secreting toxic substances that damage human tissues, by becoming parasites inside human cells, or by forming colonies in the body that disrupt normal human function. Because bacteria can produce resistant forms called *spores* under adverse environmental conditions, it is difficult for humans to destroy pathogenic bacteria.

Fungi

Fungi are a group of simple parasitic organisms similar to plants but without chlorophyll (green pigment). Most pathogenic fungi live on tissue on or near the skin or mucous membranes, e.g., athletes' foot and vaginal yeast infections. Yeasts are small, single-celled fungi, and molds are large, multicellular fungi. Fungal or mycotic infections often resist treatment, so they can become quite serious.

Protozoa and Pathogenic Animals

Protozoa are one-celled organisms, larger than bacteria, that can infest human fluids and cause disease by parasitizing (living off) or directly destroying cells. Pathogenic animals, sometimes called metazoa, are large, multicellular organisms. Most are worms that feed off human tissue or cause other disease processes.

DISORDERS OF THE SKIN

The massage professional spends much time working directly with skin. Because skin integrity prevents infection, it is important for the massage professional to obtain additional information concerning pathology. See Appendix C for the list of recommended texts for Chapter 5.

PREVENTION AND CONTROL

The key to preventing many diseases caused by pathogenic organisms is to stop the organisms from entering the human body. This sounds simple enough, but is often very difficult to accomplish. The following is a partial list of the ways in which pathogens can spread:

1. *Environmental contact.* Many pathogens are found in the environment in food, water, soil, and on assorted surfaces. Diseases caused by environmental pathogens can often be prevented by avoiding contact with certain materials and by maintaining safe sanitation practices.

2. *Opportunistic invasion.* Some potentially pathogenic organisms are found on the skin and mucous membranes of nearly everyone. They do not cause disease until they have the opportunity. Preventing opportunistic infection involves avoiding conditions that could promote infections. Changes in the pH (acidity), moisture, temperature, or other characteristics of skin and mucous membranes often promote these infections. Cleansing and aseptic treatment of wounds can prevent them.

3. *Person-to-person contact.* Small pathogens can often be carried in the air from one person to another. Direct contact with an infected person, or with contaminated materials handled by the infected person, is a familiar mode of transmission. The rhinovirus that causes the common cold is often transmitted in these ways. Some viruses, such as those causing hepatitis B virus (HBV), are transmitted when infected blood, semen, or other body fluids enter a person's bloodstream.

Aseptic technique involves killing or disabling pathogens on surfaces before they can spread to other people (see Box 5.1).

Most massage conditions require disinfection. Protective apparel is necessary occasionally. In rare instances, the use of gloves, masks, and

---

Box 5.1
COMMON ASEPTIC TECHNIQUES THAT PREVENT THE SPREAD OF PATHOGENS

1. Method: Sterilization
   Action: Destruction of all living organisms
   Example: Pressurized steam bath, extreme temperature, or radiation
2. Method: Disinfection
   Action: Destruction of most or all pathogens (but not necessarily all microbes) on inanimate objects
   Example: Chemicals such as iodine, chlorine, alcohol, and soaps
3. Method: Isolation
   Action: Separation of potentially infectious people or materials from noninfected people
   Example: Quarantine of affected patients; protective apparel worn while giving treatments; sanitary transport, storage, and disposal of body fluids, tissues, and other materials

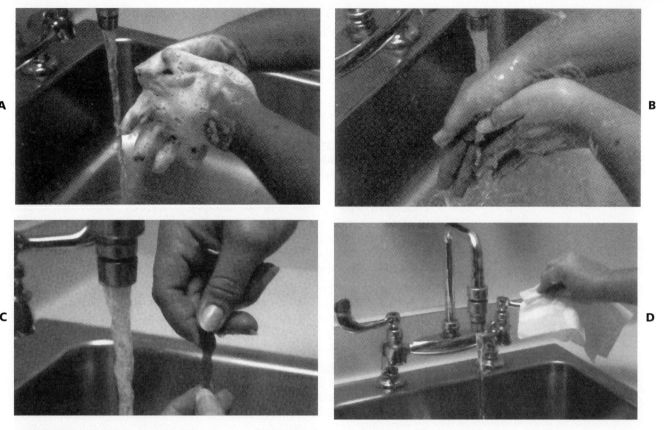

Figure 5.2
Handwashing technique.
A, Interlace the fingers to wash between them. Create a lather with the soap. Keep hands pointed down.
B, Rinse hands well, keeping fingers pointed down.
C, Use the blunt edge of an orange-wood stick to clean under the fingernails.
D, After drying your hands, turn water faucet off, using a dry paper towel. (From Zakus: Clinical procedures for medical assistants, St. Louis, 1995, Mosby–Year Book, Inc.)

gowns may be appropriate to protect the massage therapist or the client. Such cases are discussed later in the chapter.

Hand Washing

Proper hand washing is the single most effective deterrent to the spread of disease (Fig. 5.2). Hands must be washed before and after each massage, after nose-blowing or coughing into the hands, and after using the toilet. Hands and forearms need to be washed in hot running water to remove any infectious organisms. Soap or another hand washing product must be used. A clean towel must be used to dry the hands and forearms. Faucets and door handles are contaminated and should not be touched after hand washing. The towel should be used to open the door and turn off the water. Since frequent washing may dry and chap the skin, a lotion used after washing helps replace the natural oils. Using the clean towel to hold the lotion bottle will avoid contamination of the hands.

Suggested Sanitation Requirements

The following sanitation requirements for the practicing massage therapist have been developed from the State of Oregon Model.[2]

The massage therapist must clean and wash his or her hands and forearms thoroughly with an antibacterial/antiviral agent before contacting each client. Any therapist known to be infected with any communicable disease, or to be a carrier of such disease, or who has an infected wound or open lesion on any exposed portions of the body, will be excluded from practicing massage until the communicable condition is alleviated. The therapist must wear clean clothing. If at all possible, lockers or closets for personnel should be maintained apart from the massage room for the storage of personal clothing and effects.

All doors and windows opening to the outside must be tight-fitting and provide for the exclusion of flies, insects, rodents, or other vermin. All floors, walks, and furniture must be kept clean, well maintained, and in good repair.

All rooms in which massage is practiced must have 1) the capability of heating and maintaining room air to a temperature of 75°F; 2) adequate ventilation to remove objectionable odors; and 3) lighting fixtures capable of providing a minimum of five foot candles of light at floor level, which should be used during cleaning.

All sewage and liquid waste must be disposed of in a municipal sewage system or approved septic system. All interior water distribution piping should be installed and maintained in conformity with the state plumbing code. The water supply must be adequate, deemed safe by the health department, and sanitary. Drinking fountains of an approved type or individual paper drinking cups should be provided for the convenience of employees and patrons.

Every massage business must have a sanitary toilet facility with an adequate supply of hot and cold water under pressure that must be conveniently located for use by the employees and patrons. Bathroom doors must be tight-fitting and the rooms kept clean, in good repair, and free from flies, insects, and vermin. A supply of soap in a covered dispenser and single-use sanitary towels in a dispenser must be provided at each lavatory installation with a covered waste receptacle for proper disposal; a supply of toilet paper on a dispenser must be available for each toilet.

Lavatory and toilet rooms must be equipped with fly-tight containers for garbage and refuse, which should be easily cleanable, well maintained, and in good repair. Such refuse must be disposed of in a sanitary manner.

Massage lubricants, including but not limited to oil, alcohol, powders, and lotions, should be dispensed from suitable containers to be used and stored in such a manner as to prevent contamination. The bulk lubricant must not come in contact with the massage therapist. It should be poured, squeezed, or shook into a separate container or the massage therapist's hand. Any unused lubricant coming into physical contact with the client or the massage therapist must be disposed of.

The use of unclean linen is prohibited. Only freshly laundered sheets and linens should be used for massage. All single-service materials and clean linens should be stored at least four inches off the floor in shelves, compartments, or cabinets used for that purpose only. All soiled linens must be placed immediately in a covered receptacle until washed in a washing machine that provides a hot water temperature of at least 140° F and is subject to antiviral agents (10% bleach solution, i.e., nine parts water to one part bleach).

Massage tables must be covered with impervious material that is cleanable and must be kept clean and in good repair. Equipment coming into contact with the client must be cleansed thoroughly with soap (or other suitable detergent) and water followed by adequate sanitation prior to use on each individual client. (Again, a 10% bleach solution made up daily is recommended.) All equipment must be clean, well maintained, and in good repair.

When cleaning the massage area:
1. Avoid shaking linen and dust with a damp cloth to minimize the movement of dust.
2. Clean from the cleanest area to the dirtiest. This prevents soiling a clean area.
3. Clean away from your body and uniform. If you dust, brush, or wipe toward yourself, microorganisms will be transmitted to your skin, hair, and uniform.

4. Used linens must be stored in closed bag or container while in the massage room or during transport.
5. Floors are dirty. Any object that falls on the floor should not be used with a client.

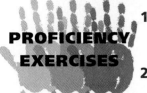

PROFICIENCY EXERCISES

1. **Contact your local health department and find out what information they have on disease control, health practices, and sanitation requirements.**
2. **Review your local and state laws concerning sanitation requirements.**

UNIVERSAL PRECAUTIONS

Universal precautions, issued by the CDC in 1987, prevent the spread of both bacterial and viral infections.

Under normal circumstances, the massage therapist should not come in contact with blood, body fluid, or body substances (urine, feces, vomit, etc.) of a client. Very rarely, an accident may occur in which such contact is possible. With additional training and under medical supervision, the massage therapist may work with a client who has a contagious condition. In these instances, knowledge of universal precautions is essential. In these special situations it is important to remember the importance of the massage therapist's gentle nurturing touch. The human connection becomes difficult through layers of protective coverings. We need to remember that for any immune-suppressed (sick) client, our normal germs can be very dangerous. We need to use universal precautions to protect the client from viruses and bacteria. Extra effort is required to carry out universal precautions, but this extra effort should not hinder the safety of both clients and therapists. Clients who are considered contagious may feel isolated and "unclean." We do not want to make such clients feel ashamed and guilty for having a contagious disease. Many of them desperately need to be touched in a supportive and nonjudgmental way. It is the pathogen that is undesirable, not the client, and people should always be treated with respect, kindness, and dignity. The therapist must remember to touch the person and not the disease, to see and listen to the person first, and not the disease. These are *people* who are sick—not sick people.

The massage therapist may need to wear gloves (Fig. 5.3) in special situations, e.g., if a client is infected with a contagious, transmittable disease, or if a client is in an immune-suppressed state and must be protected from germs. In these situations, the massage therapist would be working under the supervision of a medical professional. It is important to follow all of his or her directions carefully.

Any person touching a spill of blood or other bodily substances, such as vomit, urine, or feces, should wear single-use, disposable gloves. Such contact could conceivably happen during a massage. The most common blood exposure would be menstrual blood if the client's protective product was inadequate. On rare occasions, men who have a history of premature ejaculation could be stimulated indirectly from the general massage and ejaculate or leak fluid. An incontinent client could leak urine or feces, or a client could suddenly become sick and vomit. Universal precautions should be taken during any clean-up.

To clean up spills of bodily fluids, a 10% bleach solution (one part bleach, nine parts water) should be used. The spill should be surrounded with solution, and then mopped or wiped, working slowly and carefully inward to avoid splashes or aerosols (airborne particles). Stronger bleach solutions should be used if excessive amounts of blood or other substances are present. Afterward, the mop head or cloth should be soaked in the

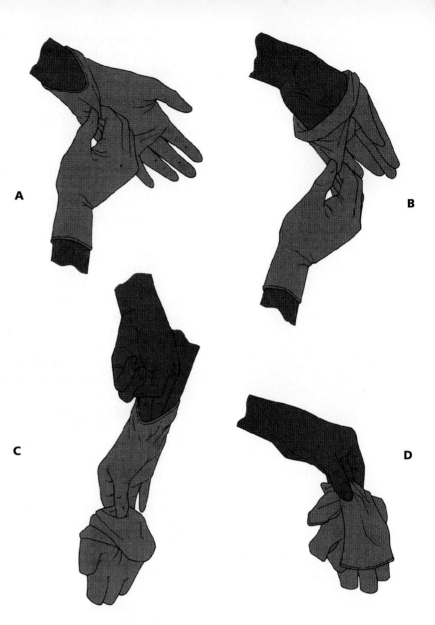

Figure 5.3
Removing gloves. A, The glove is grasped below the cuff.
B, The glove is pulled down over the hand. The glove is inside out.
C, The fingers of the ungloved hand are inserted inside the glove.
D, The glove is pulled down and over the hand and glove. The glove is inside out. (From Sorrentino: Mosby's textbook for nursing assistants 3/E, St. Louis, 1992, Mosby–Year Book, Inc.)

bleach solution. The mop head should be agitated carefully to ensure that all mopped surfaces are exposed to the cleaning fluid. All linens should be rolled away and bagged separately from other soiled linens. A double-plastic bag should be used and marked "contaminated with body fluids." The table should be washed with a strong disinfectant solution and air-dried. Latex gloves should be worn during the clean-up process.

If a contaminated substance comes into contact with human skin, the skin should be washed off immediately with soap and water and an antiviral agent such as 10% bleach solution. If an open wound is exposed to a contaminated substance, it should be flushed immediately with large amounts of hydrogen peroxide or a 10% bleach solution. Hydrogen peroxide should *not* be placed on mucous membrane surfaces or into any bodily orifice (e.g., mouth, vagina, anus, eyes, urethra).

Bleach is the preferred cleaning agent. A bleach and water solution should be prepared daily, and any leftover solution disposed of at the end of the day. If blood or bodily seepage is excessive, a stronger mixture of bleach should be used.

Hot soapy water kills HIV. If dishes are visibly soiled with blood or other bodily substances, they should be soaked in 10% bleach solution before being cleaned with soapy water.

Bathroom surfaces are only hazardous if they are visibly soiled with tainted bodily waste or substances. Any contaminated substance would have to encounter a mucous membrane surface or an open wound in order to contaminate another person. Bathrooms should always be cleaned as if they were contaminated.

Human immunodeficiency virus is not the only virus of concern. Other diseases such as herpes, human papillomavirus (venereal warts), and HBV are also spread from body fluids, including during sexual contact. Massage professionals must be concerned about the spread of all types of disease and should conscientiously follow sanitation techniques and universal precautions.

The CDC has recognized the following three levels of solutions and products that destroy HIV, hepatitis, and other viral organisms. These recommendations should be used in every practice.

1. High level: These products will be labeled as "sterigent/disinfectant glutaraldehyde - air dry." Massage therapists do not need to practice high-level sanitation techniques
2. Medium level: Bleach solutions—one cup bleach to one gallon water made up daily (10% solution) or hospital disinfectants that indicates they are a tuberculocidal.
3. Low level: Hot soapy water (that is allowed to air dry) or a hospital disinfectant that is effective against viruses and bacteria. Hands are to be washed in hot soapy water or surgical soap.

Medium- and low-level procedures are adequate for therapeutic massage. Massage professionals should update their information on recommended sanitary practices at least every six months. The CDC can provide the most current information. The number for the National Centers for Disease Control and Prevention voice information system is (404) 332–4555.

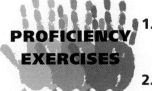

PROFICIENCY EXERCISES

1. Contact the local hospital, police, fire department, and emergency rescue team and investigate their procedures concerning universal precautions.
2. Practice putting on and taking off gloves.

UNDERSTANDING AND PREVENTING AIDS AND HEPATITIS

SECTION OBJECTIVES

Using the information presented in this section, the student will be able to do the following:

❶ Define AIDS in detail.
❷ Identify behavior that is suspected to transmit HIV and hepatitis virus.

A "syndrome" is a group of clinical symptoms that comprise a disease or abnormal condition. ("Clinical" means reported or observed symptoms not discovered by laboratory tests.) In a syndrome, all symptoms do not have to appear in any one patient. Syndromes may be caused by many different things, but in AIDS the cause is a dysfunction in the body's immune system, which defends the body against disease.

The diseases of the AIDS syndrome are caused by germs we encounter every day. In fact, some of these germs live permanently in small numbers inside the human body. When the immune system weakens, these germs have the opportunity to multiply freely, so the diseases they cause are called "opportunistic diseases."

The human immunodeficiency virus, which is responsible for AIDS, is a retrovirus. As a group, retroviruses can live in their hosts for a long period of time without causing any sign of illness. In most animals, retrovirus infections last for life. They are not very tough: these viruses die when exposed to heat; are killed by many common disinfectants; and usually do not survive well if the tissue or blood they are in dries up. However, retroviruses have high rates of mutation and, as a result, tend to evolve very quickly into new strains. HIV seems to share this and other traits with other known retroviruses. HIV replicates (lives) in the group of white blood cells called lymphocytes, or T cells. Among the T cells, HIV's favorite is the T4 cell. The T4 cell, also called the helper/inducer T cell, performs a vital job in the immune system. HIV infection of the T4 cell creates a defect in the body's immune system, which eventually causes AIDS.

Mechanics of Transmission

Human immunodeficiency virus must travel from the inside of one person to the inside of another person. Since viruses are unable to enter the body through intact skin, they must enter through an open wound or one of a number of possible body openings (most of which contain mucous membranes). *Mucous membranes* are thin tissues that protect most openings and passages in the human body. These membranes secrete mucus, which contains anti-germ chemicals and keeps the surrounding tissues moist. There are mucous membranes in the mouth, inside the eyelids, in the nose and air passages leading to the lungs, in the stomach, along the digestive tract, in the vagina, in the anus, and inside the eye of the penis. When placed on the surface of a mucous membrane, many viruses can travel through the membrane and enter the tiny blood vessels inside. The mucous membranes of the eyes and mouth are often doorways for such highly infectious viruses such as the flu. The danger with HIV is very different. With this virus, the major infection sites are the bloodstream and the central nervous system. HIV can be found in any body fluid or substance that contains lymphocytes (e.g., the T4 cell).

The presence of HIV within a substance does not necessarily indicate that the substance is capable of transmitting the infection. All of these body fluids are capable, in theory, of transmitting disease. In reality, however, the most dangerous substances seem to be blood, semen, and pre-ejaculate fluid, cervical and vaginal secretions, and perhaps feces. Despite much research, a clear-cut case of saliva causing transmission has not been found, although kissing theoretically could transmit the virus. The concentration (number of viruses per unit of volume) of HIV in these substances is very important when it comes to infectivity. If a substance contains a high concentration of HIV then it is more likely that the virus will be transmitted. The concentration of HIV in mother's milk, saliva, urine, and tears is low, but theoretically they are infectious substances and can transmit HIV infection. No cases have been reported to be caused by contact with these secretions. Sweat cannot transmit HIV.

HIV Survival Outside the Host

If HIV is contained in any body substance that leaves the body, the viruses in the substances are capable of remaining infectious until these substances dry up. Depending on the circumstances, this period could be a matter of minutes or hours. If any of these substances stays moist, the viruses contained in them can survive much longer. For example, in water and blood solutions (10% blood, 90% saline), HIV can survive at room temperature for two weeks. In refrigerated blood, such as that used for transfusions, HIV can survive indefinitely.

No HIV Transmission Found

There is widespread fear of contracting AIDS through casual contact, such as shaking hands, being in the same room with an HIV-infected person, touching doorknobs, or sharing bathroom facilities. The fear is far, far greater than the risk. Diseases spread by casual contact invariably are spread via saliva or sputum, and exist in saliva or sputum in very high concentrations. HIV exists in saliva and sputum in very low concentrations if at all. After ten years of documenting the AIDS epidemic, there are no known cases of AIDS or HIV infection being transmitted by casual social contact, not even among people living in the same household. In some instances, household members have even shared toothbrushes with HIV-infected housemates without contracting HIV.

No medical or health care workers have contracted HIV from casual contact. The contact between the massage therapist and his or her client falls under this classification. We only touch the skin, which is not a transmission route.

Hepatitis

Hepatitis is an inflammatory process and infection of the liver caused by a virus. Hepatitis A is the less serious form and is usually transmitted by fecal contamination of food and water. Hepatitis B Virus (HBV) is a potentially fatal disease and is transmitted through similar routes as HIV. There are two types of vaccines available for the prevention of HBV. It is estimated that over one million people in the United States are carriers of HBV. HBV is one hundred times more contagious than HIV. Hepatitis C accounts for 85% of the new hepatitis cases each year. Hepatitis D only infects those who have HBV and its symptoms are more severe than other forms of hepatitis. Vaccines do not appear to be effective for this virus. Hepatitis E is transmitted through feces-contaminated food and water.

Universal precautions prevent the spread of hepatitis. It is important to avoid all behaviors that are potential transmission routes for HIV and HBV.

PROFICIENCY EXERCISES

1. **Call the National AIDS hotline (800) 342-AIDS and ask a representative to send you information (open 24 hours).**
2. **Contact the information center at the CDC in Atlanta, Georgia. Ask them to send you information about communicable disease.**

FIRE AND PREMISE SAFETY

SECTION OBJECTIVES

Using the information presented in this section, the student will be able to do the following:

❶ Recognize and avoid fire and safety hazards.

❷ Complete an accident report.

The massage therapist's facility must be kept hazard-free. Some clients will need additional assistance to prevent falls or other injury. The following safety rules are guidelines for providing a hazard-free massage environment:

1. Infants and young children should not be left unattended. Parents or guardians should always be present during massage for minors.
2. Women in the last trimester of a pregnancy should not be left in the massage room alone and may need assistance getting on and off the massage table.
3. The elderly may be less steady on their feet and should not be left in the massage room unattended.
4. Anyone who is mobility-impaired, including the visually impaired, may need assistance getting on and off the massage table. Those with disabilities should be asked what assistance they need, and their instructions followed carefully.

Preventing falls is very important. To prevent falls:

• Provide good lighting. Never perform a massage in a dark room.
• Avoid loose rugs as they may slip or tangle in the feet.
• Avoid slippery tile floors.
• Keep floors and walkways uncluttered.

- Keep cords out of traffic areas.
- Regularly check all massage equipment to make sure that it is sturdy and in good repair.
- Make sure that all outside entrances are free from clutter and hazards from ice and rain.

Fire prevention is essential. To prevent fire:

- Provide for a nonsmoking environment. Where smoking is allowed, make sure proper ashtrays are used. Empty ashtrays only into a metal container that is partially filled with sand or water.
- Regularly check all electric cords and equipment to make sure that they are in good condition. Do not plug more that two plugs into an electrical outlet.
- Never use candles, incense, or any other open flame.
- Make sure the massage area is equipped with a smoke detector and fire extinguisher. Check them regularly to make sure they are functional.

If an accident does occur, all the information about the accident must be written down. An insurance company will need the following information:

- Where and when the accident occurred
- Detailed information about the accident
- Names and addresses of the person or people involved in the accident
- Names of any witnesses to the accident
- Names of manufacturers if equipment is involved

Most accidents can be prevented. Knowing the common safety hazards, recognizing which clients need extra assistance, and using common sense are all necessary to promote safety.

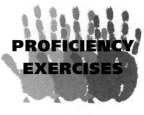

PROFICIENCY EXERCISES

1. **Contact your local fire marshal and learn more about fire prevention.**
2. **Develop a fire escape route and emergency plan for your massage business.**
3. **Contact the local building and safety inspector and find out more about accident prevention.**
4. **Contact a local insurance agent and find out about requirements for reporting accidents to the insurance company and what type of insurance is recommended for this type of protection.**
5. **Take a basic and advanced first aid class, and learn cardiopulmonary resuscitation (CPR).**

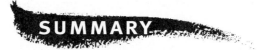

SUMMARY

The information in this chapter is primarily common sense, but it is a good idea to review these procedures regularly. We occasionally may become sloppy in the necessary attention to detail that is required to provide a safe and sanitary massage environment for our clients. It is our responsibility to be able to act reliably in emergencies. As professionals, understanding universal precautions, fire, and premise safety is necessary in order for us to touch our clients in a safe and hazard-free manner.

REVIEW QUESTIONS

1. Why is the hygiene of the massage therapist so important?
2. What odors may be offensive or a health risk to clients?
3. Why does the use of alcohol and certain drugs interfere with the ability to function as an effective and professional massage therapist?
4. Why should the massage professional study pathogenic organisms?
5. Why is the integrity of the skin so important?
6. What are the main ways diseases, caused by pathogenic organisms, are spread?
7. What are the aseptic methods?
8. What are the main concepts presented in the section on sanitation requirements?
9. What is the main goal of universal precautions?
10. Why should the massage professional understand hepatitis, HIV, and AIDS?
11. What one sanitation method is most effective in the control of the spread of disease?
12. What are the main precautions necessary for preventing falls and accidents?
13. What are the main ways to prevent fire?
14. Why should the massage therapist study emergency care and CPR?

REFERENCES

1. Ontario, Canada Therapeutic Massage Curriculum Guidelines, Toronto, Ontario, Board of Directors of Masseurs-Province of Ontario, 1992.
2. *Sanitation Requirements for the State of Oregon,* Oregon Board of Massage Technicians: Oregon Administrative Rules, July 1991.
3. Thibodeau GA and Patton K: *The Human Body in Health and Disease,* St. Louis, 1992, Mosby–Year Book.

CH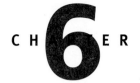ER

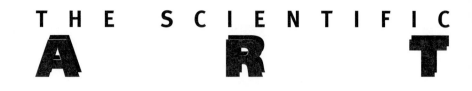

OBJECTIVES

After completing this chapter, the student will be able to:

1 Explain the effects of therapeutic massage in physiologic terms.
2 Classify massage methods into basic concepts.
3 Cite current research that validates therapeutic massage.

Student note: It will be helpful for the student to have a medical dictionary and an anatomy and physiology text book to use as references while reading this chapter. Many of the terms used are technical, and the student may need to do more in-depth reading to gain the best understanding of the information presented. See Appendix C for recommended texts.

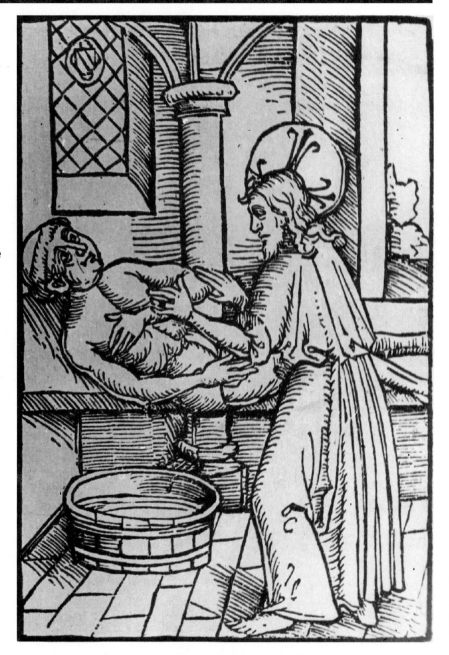

A medieval saint treats the sick by laying on of hands. Therapeutic massage was typically applied by medieval monks, many whom were canonized saints as part of their role as physicians. (Courtesy of Bettmann Archive)

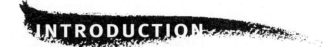

INTRODUCTION

According to the *American Heritage Dictionary,* **science** is defined as the intellectual process for using all of the mental and physical resources available in order to better understand, explain, and predict normal as well as unusual natural phenomena. The scientific approach to understanding anything involves observation, measurement of things that can be tested, the accumulation of data, and analysis of the findings. The scientific approach is classified differently than an intuitive approach.

Intuition is defined as knowing something without going through a conscious process of thinking. Other words for intuition include feelings, inspiration, instinct, revelation, impulse, and idea. The term *intuition* is not used in this textbook to mean a psychic or extrasensory experience. Intuition is the ability to purposefully act on subconsciously perceived information. Intuition is the ability to bring subconscious information into conscious awareness. This is the same principle on which biofeedback works. Through the use of equipment that detects heart rate, blood pressure, and skin temperature, a person can monitor and adjust the involuntary or subconscious responses. Centering is the ability to pay attention to, or focus on a specific area. Centering is the skill to screen sensation and the ability to concentrate.

Art is craft, skill, technique, and talent. Practice is needed to learn to pay attention to and focus on quiet, subtle information through all the loud and exaggerated stimulation that blasts our sensory receptors every day.

When the massage professional works with a client, it is important to trust his or her own intuition. It is important to maintain the art of the profession through recognizing that intuitional expression is valid. Massage professionals need to know that it is equally important to validate massage on a scientific basis to separate what science can know and what is speculated about massage and related bodywork methods. In a taped lecture called *Stress Without Distress: Evolution of the Concept,* the world renowned researcher Hans Selye talked about the importance of both. He said that if there is not an idea first (intuition), there is nothing to research. Without research (science), an idea does not develop form and usefulness. One does not function without the other. The scientific art of therapeutic massage depends upon development of the concept or idea, testing the idea through research to see if it works, and the skill and talent of application of the craft through its various techniques.

It is not difficult to scientifically validate the physiologic effects of massage. It is important to realize that the basis for the physiologic effectiveness of massage is simple. John Yates, Ph.D, in his book *A Physician's Guide to Therapeutic Massage, Its Physiological Effects and Their Application to Treatment* has done a wonderful job of compiling research. This book covers the existing body of knowledge and scientific validation in only thirty-four pages. Massage and its scientific basis is extraordinarily basic and simple.

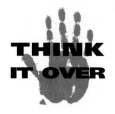

THINK IT OVER

1. What did Dr. Selye mean when he said that if there is not an idea first, there is nothing to research. Without research, an idea does not develop form and usefulness. One does not function without the other?
2. If Dr. Yates can explain the physiologic effects of massage in thirty-four pages, why does it seem so complicated?

FUNDAMENTAL CONCEPTS

Many effects of massage have been validated even though few studies that specifically focus on massage have been done. Massage is external sensory stimulation. Many studies have explained these effects. The manual techniques of massage are physiologically specific and well defined by the mode of application—rubbing, pulling, pressing, and touching; the speed and depth of pressure—sustained or slow, rhythmic, staccato, or fast; light touch, deep touch, and a combination of both; and the part of the therapist's body used to apply the techniques—fingers, hand, forearm, or knee. Massage is a form of organized, systematic, structured touch and movement.

The fundamental concepts of the effects of therapeutic massage can be broken into two categories: mechanical methods that directly affect the soft tissue through techniques that normalize the connective tissue or move body fluids and intestinal contents, and reflexive methods that stimulate the nervous system, chemical system, and endocrine system. The problem with this approach is that the mechanism by which the effect is produced cannot always be clearly identified. According to Dr. Philip E. Greenman, effects of the massage occur through the interrelationships of the peripheral and central nervous systems, their reflex patterns and multiple pathways, the autonomic nervous system, and neuroendocrine control.[8] Dr. John Yates says, "It appears far more reasonable just to recognize that massage produces effects that are due to a combination of mechanical, neural, chemical and psychological factors and to identify these wherever possible rather that to attempt to use them as a basis for classifying those effects."[20]

Because most stress patterns involve the nervous and endocrine systems, techniques that cause these systems to respond will influence the stress levels of the person. The nervous system responds to therapeutic massage methods that stimulate sensory receptors. An existing pattern in the central nervous system control center is disrupted by massage, resulting in a shift of motor impulses to reestablish homeostasis.

Massage methods that directly address the neuromuscular area stimulate reflexive responses. Benefits are achieved by substituting one set of sensory signals for another—hopefully resulting in a more efficient body pattern. Reflexology and acupressure are examples of reflexive techniques.

Methods that directly address the connective tissue do so by mechanically changing the consistency of the connective tissue, usually by softening it, and by creating physical space in the body. Mechanical dysfunctions call for more direct methods and depend on an actual physiologic change to the area. Cross-fiber frictioning and inhibitory (direct) pressure approaches are examples of mechanical massage methods. Methods that mechanically affect the circulation do so by causing changes in internal pressure of the vessels. Compression and long surface strokes accomplish these functions.

Either approach, mechanical or reflexive, changes the feedback loop response of the autonomic nervous and endocrine systems to affect responses of the body/mind and the circulatory systems. Both styles also influence the energy component of the body. The term *subtle energies* covers a wide range of techniques that affect the subtle electrical fields of the body. These electrical fields do exist. Animal behavior studies have shown that the platypus detects a living food source by sensing the weak electrical field around its prey.[1]

Massage is one of the best ways to reduce stress levels and to deal with the symptomatic relief of chronic pain. Stress and pain appear in the body through impingement of nerves by soft tissue, spinal reflex dysfunction, referred pain, problems in the motor control areas of the brain, responses of the autonomic nervous system, limbic system, and neurotransmitters. Most of these dysfunctions can be related to either "too much" or "not enough" of something such as too much energy or not enough muscle tone. Massage tends to even out the responses.

Some methods of massage, especially the more subtle approaches, are not as scientifically validated. However, research is being done in these areas. These methods, based on the subtle electrical energy of the body, have been around for eons. Most ancient healing practices are based on the interaction with these subtle energy fields. The massage profession would be wise to not discount these methods. Many of the methods will most likely show validity, or they would not have stood the test of time. It is possible that our technology is not advanced enough to verify what the human can perceive. These subtle weak energy fields do exist. Remember, the duck-billed platypus finds its living food by detecting these energy fields. It is possible that the effectiveness of the energy approaches is reflexive. Touch here and it causes something to happen there. Dr. Leon Chaitow cites Hans Selye's research that states that stress can either cure or aggravate a disease depending on whether the stress induced is of an adequate type, adequate intensity, and does not overload the system.[4] In homeopathy, minute quantities of a substance are given to provoke a healing response. It is a good comparison. Until our technology can prove the validity of energy techniques, it is important to remember the wisdom of Hippocrates, "Do no harm" and Bernie Siegal's, "There is no false hope." Represent subtle techniques simply, professionally, and free from false expectations and mysticism. Addititional training is required to learn to use the subtle energy approaches purposefully. It is also important not to discount the stimulation of the powerful placebo effect. If touch can activate it, why not use it?

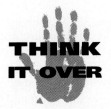

THINK IT OVER

1. **Is it not amazing that there are really only two types of massage styles—reflexive and mechanical?**
2. **What do you think will be the physiologic rationale for the effectiveness of energy or subtle types of bodywork?**

CURRENT RESEARCH

There are many exciting ongoing studies currently being conducted. Research is being conducted at the University of Miami School of Medicine Touch Research Institute. This program is funded by Johnson and Johnson and others and directed by Tiffany Field, Ph.D. Extensive research is also being done at the Menninger Clinic in Topeka, Kansas, by Dr. Elmer Green, who is credited with the validation of biofeedback, and the prestigious John E. Fetzer Institute in Kalamazoo, Michigan, that provided funding for the Public Television series *Healing and the Mind* with Bill Moyers. The International Society for the Study of Energies and Energy Medicine is located in Golden, Colorado, and sponsors and promotes research. Additional studies are being done by Dr. Krieger, developer of therapeutic touch, and Dr. Norman Shealy. Dr. Robert Becker has been researching the electrical component of the body for years. Dr.

Tiffany Field believes the clinical health care system will incorporate touch therapy in the same way it incorporated the approaches of relaxation therapy, exercise, and diet.[7]

Massage has shown promise in strengthening the immune system. Researchers have found that massage reduces stress, anxiety, and poor sleep patterns in hospitalized, depressed, and adjustment-disordered children. It improves caregiver–child relationships for abused and neglected children, decreases sensitivity to touch in autistic children, reduces arthritic pain, increases immune function in HIV-positive men, and enhances adult job performance. Massage appears to stimulate vagal activity, which slows the heart rate and stimulates the gastrointestinal system to produce glucose and insulin. Massage increases the production of serotonin, which in turn facilitates the production of natural killer cells in the immune system. Research has even shown that giving a massage is therapeutic. Administering massage actually reduces stress and improves sleep patterns in the massagers.[17]

Effective bodywork is achieved through massage methods interacting with the physiology. Studies of anatomy and physiology are fascinating because all humans share the same basic blueprint of their anatomy and physiology. Because this is true, the effects of massage can be studied through the scientific method. The scientific method is a way of objectively researching a concept to see if it is valid. Research begins with a hypothesis or "if this happens, then that will happen." In the next step the hypothesis needs to be tested. This is done with an experiment. The experiment needs to follow accepted design measures so that others can replicate or redo the experiment. Results of the experiment will either prove or disprove the hypothesis. Often the results of the research generate more questions that lead to more research. The subjective quality of massage complicates the research issue because of the complexity of human beings and the interaction of the client practitioner dynamics, which have effects on the results of massage. Only a growing body of research and data replication, establishing positive biochemical and behavioral reaction to touch, will convince the medical community that massage is therapeutic. Fortunately, this type of research is now being done. The National Institutes of Health Office of Alternative Medicine awarded grant money in 1994 for massage research.

Through the centuries, therapeutic massage has provided hands-on therapy for people. It is interesting to examine the historic literature and find that the benefits of massage were known in Hippocrates time and have resurfaced about every forty to sixty years. The last time massage was respected and popular was in the early 1940s. Today, an increasing amount of information about massage is being written. This textbook is an example. Because of technologic advances, the validation for massage can be more objective based on scientific methods instead of subjective observation from experiential evidence. With research, validation, and clinical usage of massage, two things will inevitably happen. Massage and bodywork systems will move from the arena of specialized and mystic knowledge into a solid, physiologic basis using a physiologically based terminology. The proliferation of styles and methods will decrease, and massage and bodywork will become more homogeneous. This progress is good as long as the profession does not forget the importance of the total body, mind, and spirit of ourselves and the people we touch, and as long as creativity is not stifled. Educational standards will increase for massage practitioners. This is also good as long as the profession does not educate the "heart" out of the profession, and the education stays focused on whole-person approaches as well as anatomy, physiology, and pathology. Massage is again proving itself important in many situations.

The beginning student of massage may find technical information intimidating. But without this understanding, the massage professional cannot intelligently use the simple methods of massage that are presented in this text. It is important to develop this knowledge at the beginning of the education because it is the foundation of the profession. This chapter's purpose is to build a strong physiologic basis for an understanding of the effectiveness of therapeutic massage. The student needs to build a firm foundation in the anatomy and physiology of why massage works, so that, trusting intuition, a massage can be designed according to the information received from the client during assessment procedures.

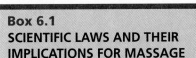

THINK IT OVER

• **What type of research study would you like to develop?**

THE NERVOUS SYSTEM

Responses and effects of massage on the nervous system are reflexive. A reflex is an involuntary response to a stimulus provided by massage. Reflexes are specific and predictable. They are also purposeful, adaptive, and explain most of the benefits of massage (see Chapter 4). Various neurologic laws come into play when exploring the effects of therapeutic massage. A **law** is a scientific statement that is true uniformly for a whole class of natural occurrences (Box 6.1).

Box 6.1
SCIENTIFIC LAWS AND THEIR IMPLICATIONS FOR MASSAGE

All-or-None or Bowditch's Law[13]
The weakest stimulus capable of producing a response produces the maximum response contraction in cardiac and skeletal muscle and nerves.

Implication for massage: Techniques do not have to be extremely intense to produce a response. All that needs to be done is enough sensory stimulation to begin the process.

Bell's Law[16]
Anterior spinal nerve roots are motor and posterior spinal nerve roots are sensory.

Implication for massage: Massage along the spine is a strong sensory stimulation.

Law of Facilitation[18]
When an impulse has passed through a certain set of neurons to the exclusion of others one time, it will tend to take the same course on a future occasion, and each time it traverses this path the resistance will be smaller.

Implication for massage: The body likes sameness, which produces habitual patterns. When a pattern is established, it does not take as much stimulation to activate the response.

Hooke's Law[16]
The stress used to stretch or compress a body is proportional to the strain experienced, as long as the elastic limits of the body have not been exceeded.

Implication for massage: Methods that lengthen the tissue need to be intense enough to match the existing shortening but not exceed it.

continued

Box 6.1
SCIENTIFIC LAWS AND THEIR
IMPLICATIONS FOR MASSAGE
(continued)

Law of Specificity of Nervous Energy[16]

Excitation of a receptor always gives rise to the same sensation regardless of the nature of the stimulus.

Implication for massage: Whatever the method used, if a sensory receptor is activated, it will respond in a specific way.

Weber's Law[16]

The increase in stimulus necessary to produce the smallest perceptible increase in sensation bears a constant ratio to the strength of the stimulus already acting.

Implication for massage: For a massage method to change a sensory perception, the intensity of the method must match and then just exceed the existing sensation.

Hilton's Law[16]

A nerve trunk that supplies a joint also supplies the muscles of the joint and the skin over the insertions of such muscles.

Implication for massage: It is difficult to figure out if a pain is from the joint itself, the muscles around a joint, or the skin over a joint. Stimulation of all areas in turn affects each part.

Pfluger's Laws:[18]

Law of Unilaterality[18]

If a mild irritation is applied to one or more sensory nerves, the movement will take place usually on one side only and on the side that has been irritated.

Implication for massage: Light stimulation remains fairly localized in response to massage.

Law of Symmetry[18]

If the stimulation is sufficiently increased, motor reaction is manifested not only by the irritated side, but also in similar muscles on the opposite side of the body.

Implication for massage: By using increasing levels of massage intensity, a bilateral effect can be created even if massaging only one side of the body. This is especially useful for massage applications to painful areas. By massaging the unaffected side, the painful areas can be addressed without direct massage work.

Law of Intensity[18]

Reflex movements are usually more intense on the side of irritation; at times the movements of the opposite side equal the movements in intensity, but they are usually less pronounced.

Implication for massage: (See Law of Symmetry)

Law of Radiation[18]

If the excitation continues to increase, it is propagated upward, and reactions take place through centrifugal nerves coming from the cord segments up higher.

Implication for massage: (See Law of Symmetry)

Law of Generalization[18]

When the irritation becomes very intense, it is propagated in the medulla oblongata, which becomes a focus from which stimuli radiate to all parts of the cord, causing a general contraction of all muscles to the body.

Implication for massage: This response needs to be avoided if possible. It is important to keep invasive massage measures, such as frictioning, below the intensity levels that cause a general body response.

Arndt-Schultz Law[18]

Weak stimuli activate physiologic processes; very strong stimuli inhibit them.

Implication for massage: To encourage a specific response use gentler methods. To shut off a response use deeper methods.

Cannon's Law of Denervation[5]

When autonomic effectors are partially or completely separated from their normal nerve connections, they become more sensitive to the action of chemical substances.

This "denervation supersensitivity" involves injured nerves responding to all sensory stimulation regardless if the stimulation is specific to that nerve or not. Denervation supersensitivity is a universal phenomenon affecting muscles, nerves, salivary glands, sudorific glands, autonomic ganglion cells, spinal neurons, and even neurons in the cortex. There are also changes in muscle structure and biochemistry and progressive destruction of fiber's contractile elements. Furthermore, unlike normal muscle fibers that resist innervation from foreign nerves, degenerated muscle fibers accept contacts from other motor nerves, preganglionic autonomic fibers, and even sensory nerves.

Implication for massage: If a client has had an area injured, that area will hyperreact to all sensory stimulation. Therefore, if the person has a cold or is stressed at work or cannot sleep, the injured area will flare up.

The nervous system is divided into the central nervous system, consisting of the brain, spinal cord, and coverings, and the peripheral nervous system, which consists of nerves and ganglions. The peripheral nervous system is further divided into the autonomic and somatic divisions. The autonomic division is subdivided into the sympathetic and parasympathetic systems. The sympathetic autonomic nervous system is responsive for functions that expend energy to respond to emergency situations of "fight or flight." The parasympathetic division is more restorative and normalizing and returns the body to a nonalarm state (Fig. 6.1).

The influence of the nervous system regulates the endocrine system and neurochemicals. The endocrine system influences the nervous system. It is a big feedback loop similar to the thermostat of a furnace. The feedback system and autoregulation (maintaining of internal homeostasis) is interlinked with all body functions. The control for initiation of a reaction comes through the nervous system and the endocrine system.

The stimulation of the body by massage influences the autonomic nervous system and the limbic system response. The limbic system is a group

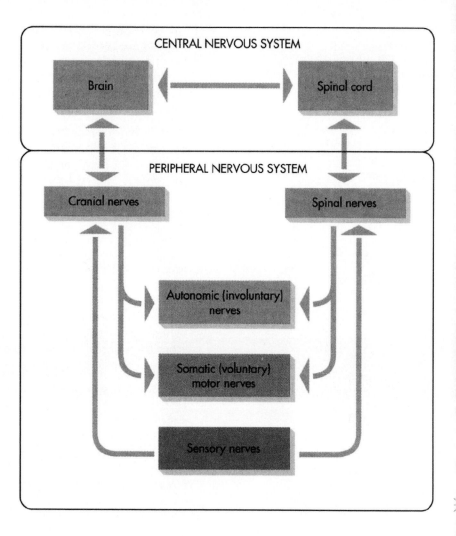

CENTRAL NERVOUS SYSTEM

Brain ↔ Spinal cord

PERIPHERAL NERVOUS SYSTEM

Cranial nerves   Spinal nerves

Autonomic (involuntary) nerves

Somatic (voluntary) motor nerves

Sensory nerves

Figure 6.1
Divisions of the nervous system. (From Thibodeau/Patton: The human body in health & disease, St. Louis, 1992, Mosby–Year Book, Inc.)

of brain structures, activated by emotional behavior and arousal, that influences the endocrine and autonomic systems. The responses activated are more general and are reflected in an alteration of mood and feelings of well being or distress. A property of limbic neural circuits is their prolonged after-discharge following stimulation. This may explain why emotional responses are generally extended and outlast the stimuli that initiate them. Studies done using slow-stroke back massage suggest a complex interaction between the autonomic, somatic, emotional, and cognitive elements in response to massage.[12] These findings agree with the mechanical, neural, chemical, and psychologic effects described by Dr. Yates. The results suggest that slow, long stroking of the back causes reflex inhibition of the muscle spindle. If massage is continued for a least six minutes, slow-stroke back massage lowers the autonomic arousal. The long-term effects of slow-stroke back massage show decreased psychoemotional and somatic arousal.[12] In simple language, slow-stroke back massage calms people.

The autonomic nervous system is part of the central nervous system. It is regulated by centers in the brain, particularly the cerebral cortex, the hypothalamus, and medulla oblongata. The hypothalamus largely controls the autonomic nervous system and receives impulses from the visceral (organ) sensory fibers and from some somatic (muscles and joints) sensory fibers. The hypothalamus plays an important role in the body/mind connection.[10] The hypothalamus is a main component of the limbic system. The cerebellum controls subconscious movements of skeletal muscle, input from proprioceptors, feedback loops, posture, future positioning, and regulates sensations of anger and pleasure. Research indicates that the cerebellum, the limbic pain and pleasure centers, and the various relay centers are all part of one circuit.[10]

Therapeutic massage techniques that stimulate the cerebellum have a wide-spread influence on the person receiving the massage. The strongest of these techniques is rhythmic rocking produced during the application of massage. Rocking produces movement at the neck and head that influences the sense of equilibrium. Rocking stimulates the inner ear balance mechanisms, including the vestibular nuclear complex and the labyrinthine righting reflexes, to keep the head level. This is a bodywide effect stimulating muscle contraction patterns that pass throughout the body. Pressure on the side of the body may stimulate the body-righting reflex. There is a close interrelationship between the vestibular nerves and the cerebellum. Massage alters body positional sense and initiates specific movement patterns that change sensory input from muscles, tendons, joints, and the skin. This feedback information, which adjusts and coordinates movement, is relayed directly to the motor cortex and to the cerebellum. The output from the cerebellum goes to the motor cortex and brain stem. Stimulation of the cerebellum by altering muscle tone, position, and vestibular balance also stimulates the hypothalamus to adjust autonomic nervous system functions to restore homeostasis.

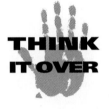

THINK IT OVER

- **Why do you think the functions interplay with each other and become one large neuroendocrine circuit?**

HYPERSTIMULATION ANALGESIA AND COUNTERIRRITATION

In 1965 the **Gate Control Theory** was proposed by Melzack and Wall. It explained the relationship between pain and emotion. According to this theory, there is a hypothetical gating mechanism occurring at the level of the spinal cord—a "gate" through which pain impulses reach the lateral spinothalamic system. Painful impulses are transmitted by large-diameter and small-diameter nerve fibers. Stimulation of large-diameter fibers prevents the small-diameter fibers from transmitting signals. Stimulating (rubbing, massaging) these fibers helps to suppress the sensation of pain, especially sharp pain. Many parents and small children seem to know this instinctively. They rub the injured spot, thus activating large-diameter fibers. Tactile stimulation produced by massage travels through the large-diameter fibers. These fibers also carry a faster signal. In essence, massage sensations win the race to the brain, and the pain sensations are blocked out because the gate is closed.

It is well known that soldiers wounded in the heat of battle may feel no pain until the battle is over (stress analgesia). Many people have learned from practical experience that touching or shaking an injured area decreases the pain of the injury. This is another practical application of therapeutic massage. Acupuncture has been used for four thousand years to prevent or relieve pain. Using this technique, it is possible in some instances to perform major surgery without any other type of anesthesia. These observations make it clear that pain transmission and perceptions are subject to inhibition or modification.

All methods of massage can be used to produce counterirritation. *Taber's Cyclopedic Medical Dictionary* defines **counterirritation** as the superficial irritation that relieves some irritation of deeper structures.[16] Counterirritation may be explained by Melzack and Wall's Gate Control Theory. Inhibition in central sensory pathways through rubbing or shaking an area may explain counterirritation. This theory is another of the

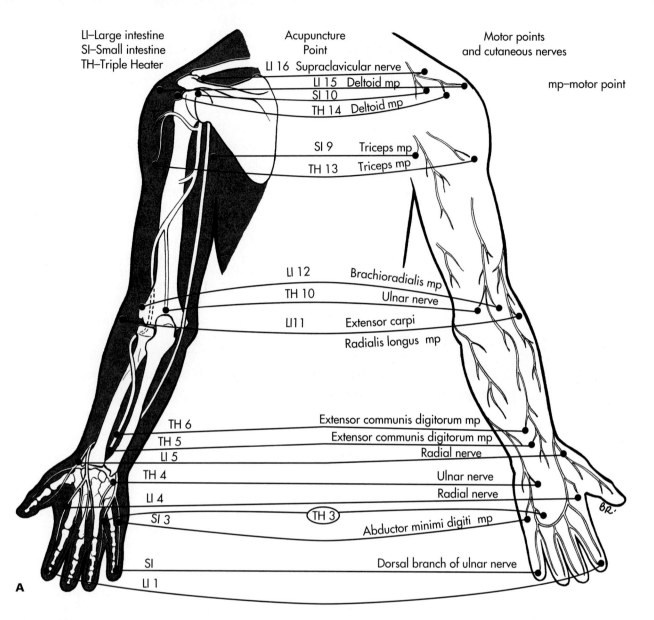

LI–Large intestine
SI–Small intestine
TH–Triple Heater

Acupuncture
Point

Motor points
and cutaneous nerves

mp–motor point

LI 16 Supraclavicular nerve
LI 15 Deltoid mp
SI 10
TH 14 Deltoid mp

SI 9 Triceps mp
TH 13 Triceps mp

LI 12 Brachioradialis mp
TH 10 Ulnar nerve
LI 11 Extensor carpi
Radialis longus mp

TH 6 Extensor communis digitorum mp
TH 5 Extensor communis digitorum mp
LI 5 Radial nerve
TH 4 Ulnar nerve
LI 4 Radial nerve
SI 3 TH 3 Abductor minimi digiti mp
SI Dorsal branch of ulnar nerve
A LI 1

Figure 6.2
A & B, Comparison of traditional acupuncture points, motor points, and cutaneous nerves of the arm and leg.

proposed explanations for the action of acupuncture. Studies done on effects of acupressure can be generalized to effects of certain styles of massage especially compression, percussion, and frictioning methods.[9]

The skin over the entire body is supplied by spinal nerves that carry somatic sensory nerve impulses to the spinal cord. Each spinal nerve serves a specific, constant segment of the skin called a dermatome. These dermatomes can be affected by massage techniques that stimulate the skin and may account for **hyperstimulation analgesia.** Reduction of pain by stimulation (hyperstimulation analgesia), using massage and acupuncture, has been used for many years.[9] Noxious stimuli suppress nociceptive (pain) impulses. Changes in the perception of pain by introducing a different pain signal is akin to the old adage of stepping on someone's foot to give relief from the pain in the thumb just hit by a hammer. Inhibition in central sensory pathways may explain the effect of counterirritants. Stimulation of the skin over an area of pain or dysfunction produces some relief from the pain. The old fashioned mustard plaster works on this principle. So do therapeutic massage and various rubs and creams on the market.

Stimulating techniques (massage) that produce analgesia have long been recognized. In recent years, transcutaneous neurostimulation has

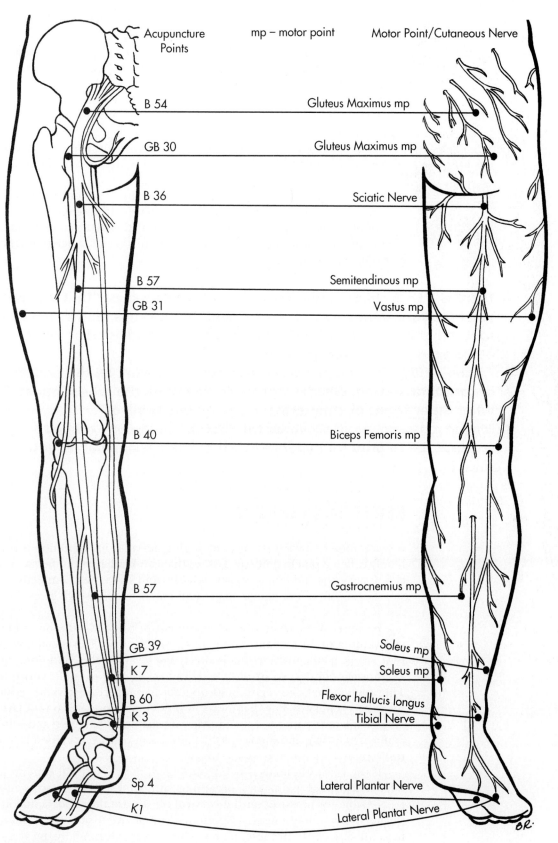

Acupuncture Points	mp – motor point	Motor Point/Cutaneous Nerve

B 54 — Gluteus Maximus mp

GB 30 — Gluteus Maximus mp

B 36 — Sciatic Nerve

B 57 — Semitendinous mp

GB 31 — Vastus mp

B 40 — Biceps Femoris mp

B 57 — Gastrocnemius mp

GB 39 — Soleus mp

K 7 — Soleus mp

B 60 — Flexor hallucis longus

K 3 — Tibial Nerve

Sp 4 — Lateral Plantar Nerve

K 1 — Lateral Plantar Nerve

BR.

B – Bladder
GB – Gallbladder
K – Kidney
B Sp – Spleen

Figure 6.2 *continued*
For legend see opposite page.

become very popular. Dry needling by acupuncture may also be considered another form of "stimulation-produced analgesia." Stimulating techniques, such as percussion of painful areas to produce "stimulation-produced analgesia" or hyperstimulation analgesia, have been used for a long time. It has only been within recent years that the mechanism has been studied. Stimulation of the peripheral nervous system may produce analgesia by neurophysiologic and neurohumoral inhibitory effects at the spinal gating mechanism. Evidence suggests that the development of analgesia depends on the stimulation of specific points in the muscle that corresponds to certain types of muscle receptors. It is now accepted that most acupuncture points correspond to muscle innervation points or motor points. The transmission of painful stimulus may be blocked by other afferent inputs at the spinal and thalamic levels. If massage stimulates these motor points at a sufficient intensity, stimulation of the large-diameter fibers can be produced and the gating mechanisms and hyperstimulation analgesia may be activated (Fig. 6.2).

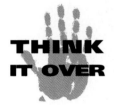

THINK IT OVER

1. **There is a trick children play with each other. One says, "Oh I see that you hurt your thumb. Let me fix it," and then stomps on the other's foot. What is the physiologic basis for why this trick works? What other examples can you think of?**
2. **All the ointments that promise relief from pain work on the principle of counterirritation. What receptors do you think the rubs stimulate? What other forms of counterirritation can you think of?**
3. **Maybe massage was discovered the first time someone rubbed a stubbed toe to produce hyperstimulation analgesia. What do you think?**

NERVE IMPINGEMENT

It is common to have soft tissue impinging nerves. This condition is commonly called a pinched nerve. Tissues that can bind are skin, fascia, muscles, ligaments, and joints. Spastic muscles and shortened connective tissue (fascia) often impinge on major and minor nerves, which gives rise to discomfort.

Because of the structural arrangement of the body, these impingements often occur at major nerve plexuses (Fig. 6.3). The specific nerve root, trunk, or the division that is affected determines the condition, such as thoracic outlet syndrome, sciatica, or carpal tunnel syndrome. Therapeutic massage techniques operate in numerous ways to reduce pressure on nerves. The main ways to reduce pressure are to reflexively change the tone pattern of the muscles, mechanically lengthen and soften connective tissue, and interrupt the pain-spasm-pain cycle caused by protective muscle spasm in response to pain.

If the cervical plexus is being impinged, the person will experience headaches, neck pain, and breathing difficulties. The muscles most responsible for pressure on the cervical plexus are the suboccipital and sternocleidomastoid muscles. Shortened connective tissues at the cranial base will also press on these nerves. This plexus is formed by the ventral rami of the upper four cervical nerves. The phrenic nerve is part of this plexus. It innervates the diaphragm. Any disruption to this nerve will affect breathing. Many cutaneous (skin) branches of the cervical plexus transmit sensory impulses from the skin of the neck, ear, and the shoulder. The motor branches innervate muscles of the anterior neck.

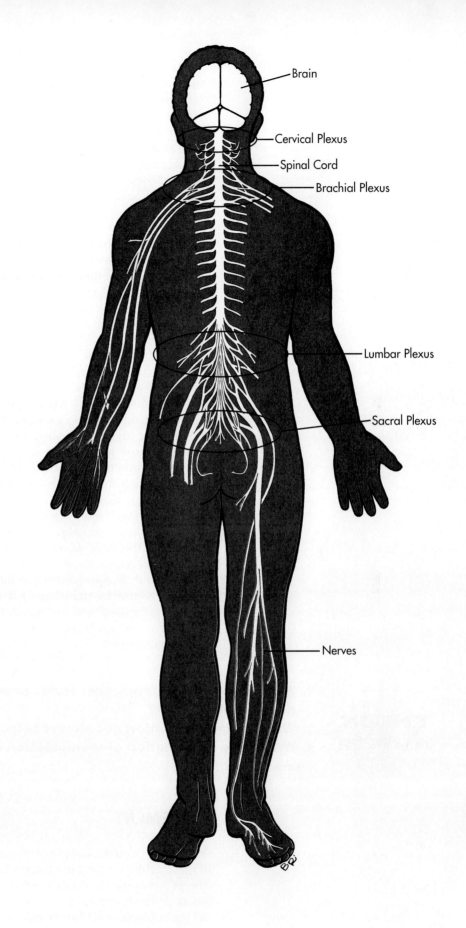

Figure 6.3
Major nerve plexuses.

The brachial plexus is situated partly in the neck and partly in the axilla and provides virtually all the nerves that innervate the upper limb. Any imbalance that brings pressure on this complex of nerves will result in shoulder pain, chest pain, arm pain, wrist pain, and hand pain. The muscles most often responsible for impingement of the brachial plexus are the scalenes, pectoralis minor, and subclavius. Muscles of the arm occasionally will impinge branches of the brachial plexus. Brachial plexus impingement is responsible for thoracic outlet symptoms, which are often misdiagnosed as carpal tunnel syndrome. Whiplash injury involves the brachial plexus. Massage is listed as one of the treatment modalities for whiplash in the text *Correlative Neuroanatomy* by deGroot.

Lumbar plexus nerve impingement may give rise to low-back discomfort with a belt distribution of pain, lower abdominal pain, genital pain, thigh pain, and medial lower leg pain. The main muscles that impinge the lumbar plexus are the quadratus lumborum and the psoas. Shortening of the lumbar dorsal fascia will exaggerate a lordosis and cause vertebral impingement of the lumbar plexus.

The sacral plexus has about a dozen named branches. About half of these serve the buttock and lower limb; the others innervate pelvic structures. The main branch is the sciatic nerve. Impingement of this nerve by the piriformis muscle gives rise to sciatica. Ligaments that stabilize the sacroiliac joint can affect the sacral plexus. Pressure on the sacral plexus can cause gluteal pain, leg pain, genital pain, and foot pain.

Input from the sensory systems plays a role in the control of motor functions by stimulating spinal reflex mechanisms. All forms of therapeutic massage use some aspect of touch. These tactile sensations stimulate the various touch receptors found in the skin. Methods of massage that use light touch stimulate root hair plexus, free nerve endings, Merkel's discs (tactile), Meissner's corpuscles (touch), and end organs of Ruffini (cutaneous mechanoreceptor). Techniques such as compression, deep gliding strokes, and joint movement stimulate the pressure receptors known as Pacinian corpuscles (lamellated) and type II cutaneous mechanoreceptors. Rapid and repetitive sensory signals of vibration and percussion techniques directly influence the corpuscles of touch and the Pacinian corpuscles (lamellated). Therapeutic massage introduces touch, pressure, vibration, and positional stimuli, which causes sensory receptor neurons to respond, changing tone patterns of muscles and reducing pressure on nerves.

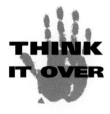

THINK IT OVER

1. **Why do chiropractic and other forms of skeletal manipulation help nerve impingement?**
2. **Why does manipulation not always help a nerve impingement?**
3. **Why is the combination of manipulation and massage such a good one?**

MOVEMENT

Movement, stretch, and pressure methods of massage focus the effects of these activities on the muscles, tendons, joints, and ligaments to stimulate the proprioceptors. Proprioceptors provide the body with information about position, movement, muscle tension, joint activity, and equilibrium. As the massage practitioner moves, stretches, and applies tension to the muscles and joints the following receptors are stimulated:

• Muscles spindles located primarily in the belly of the muscle respond to both sudden and prolonged stretches.

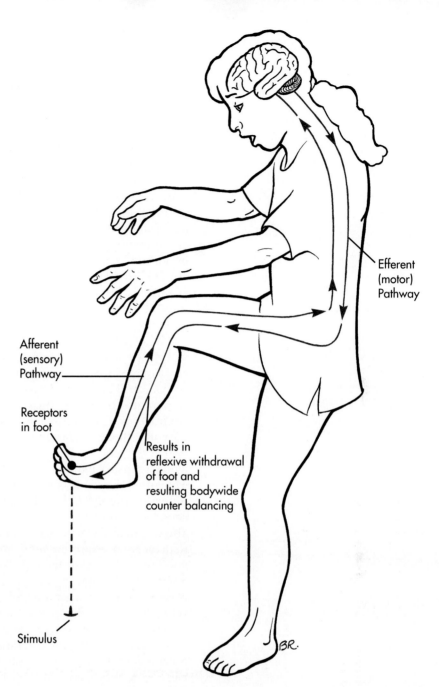

Efferent
(motor)
Pathway

Afferent
(sensory)
Pathway

Receptors
in foot

Results in
reflexive withdrawal
of foot and
resulting bodywide
counter balancing

Stimulus

Figure 6.4
Reflex response. The localized stimulation of a few specific receptors leads to a large number of outgoing impulses to effect a large number of muscles.

- Tendon organs found in the tendon and musculotendinous junction respond to tension at the tendon. Articular (joint) ligaments contain receptors similar to tendon organs that adjust reflex inhibition of the adjacent muscle when excessive strain is placed on the joints.
- Joint kinesthetic receptors in the capsules of joints respond to pressure, acceleration, and deceleration of joint movement. There are two main types of joint kinesthetic receptors: type II cutaneous mechanoreceptor and Pacinian (lamellated) corpuscles. Stimulation of nervous system receptors will be interpreted and processed through the somatic reflex arcs.

Reflexes are fast, predictable, automatic responses to a change in the environment and help to maintain homeostasis (Fig. 6.4). Therapeutic massage stimulation constitutes a change in the environment. When the body is called on to restore homeostasis, nonproductive nerve transmission pathways often can be overridden.[4] The reflexes most often stimulated are the stretch reflex, tendon reflex, flexor reflex, and crossed extensor reflex.

The stretch reflex is activated by the muscle spindles, which sense muscle stretching. In response to therapeutic massage methods that stretch muscles, a muscle spindle produces nerve impulses stimulating a somatic sensory neuron in the posterior root of the spinal nerve. When the motor nerve impulse reaches the stretched muscle, a muscle action potential is generated, which causes the muscle to contract. Muscle contraction stops spindle cell discharge. The effect of the muscle stretch stimulates the stretch reflex, resulting in shortening of the muscle. The sensitivity of the muscle spindle in response to stretching sets the level of muscle tone throughout the body. Therapeutic massage methods can make use of this reflex to tone weak muscle patterns by stretching the muscles and initiating the stretch reflex. An awareness of this reflex response is important in all stretches that are intended to lengthen and relax the muscles. In these instances, the reflex must be avoided. Often this system of reflexes becomes hyperactive, which results in an increase of muscle tone. Massage techniques that use isometric and isotonic muscle contraction to relax and lengthen muscles are helpful in resetting muscle tone.

Whereas the stretch reflex operates as a feedback mechanism to control muscle length by causing muscle contraction, the tendon reflex operates as a feedback mechanism to control muscle tension by causing muscle relaxation. This reflex is mediated by the tendon organs that detect and respond to changes in muscle tension caused by the stretch of muscular contraction. The most common massage technique used to stimulate the tendon reflex is post-isometric relaxation. This technique increases tension at the tendon. The tendon organ is stimulated, which sends a signal along a sensory neuron. In the spinal cord, the sensory neuron synapses with an inhibitory association neuron, which inhibits motor neurons that innervate the muscle associated with the tendon organ. This inhibition causes the muscle to relax. The sensory neuron from the tendon organ also stimulates an association neuron in the spinal cord. The association neuron synapses with a motor neuron, controlling antagonistic muscles and causing them to contract. To simplify, when one muscle contracts, its antagonist or opposing muscle group must relax. This is called *reciprocal innervation* and is often used by the massage therapist to avoid the stretch reflex response and to prepare a muscle for lengthening and stretching.

The flexor (withdrawal) and crossed extensor reflexes are polysynaptic reflex arcs. When these reflexes are stimulated, both sides of the body are affected through intersegmental reflex arcs. A single sensory neuron can activate several motor neurons. The flexor reflex is involved in moving away from a stimuli, and the crossed extensor reflex is involved in maintaining balance. Synchronized control over the muscles that are contracting and those that are being inhibited (allowing for relaxation) is conducted though contralateral reflex arcs. By creating a noxious (unpleasant) signal, therapeutic massage can stimulate a withdrawal response in order to stimulate opposite side patterns of tension or weakness. This is a powerful response because withdrawal reflexes take priority over all other reflex activity occurring at the moment. These reflex patterns also explain why tension patterns are seldom on only one side of the body. Massage therapy can reset reflex patterns that are unproductive and lead to discomfort and postural distortion from uneven contraction and relaxation patterns of muscles.

Therapeutic massage effects heavily depend on the reflex mechanism. The effectiveness of the techniques is dependent on how efficiently the receptors for these reflexes are stimulated. It is important that the receptor being targeted is accessed with the appropriate technique and intensity, so that the reflex stimulated is allowed to function in the appropriate manner.

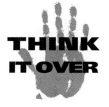

THINK IT OVER

1. **What do movement systems such as the Alexander technique, tai chi, or dance and stretching systems like yoga have in common with massage?**
2. **How could combining a movement and stretching system with massage be beneficial?**

BODY/MIND EFFECT

Much of the body/mind connection takes place through autonomic nervous system activity. As mentioned, the autonomic nervous system consists of two divisions. The parasympathetic division is the energy conservation and restorative system associated with what is commonly called the *relaxation response*. The sympathetic division is associated with the "fight or flight" response of arousal that expends energy and dominates in stressful situations. Excessive sympathetic output is what causes a majority of the stress-related diseases that physicians encounter. Problems with headaches, gastrointestinal difficulties, high blood pressure, anxiety, muscle tension and aches, and sexual dysfunction can all be related to excessive sympathetic stimulation (Table 6.1).

Massage works to initially stimulate sympathetic functions. This really surprises students who think that they are giving a relaxation massage. The increase in autonomic function resulting from massage is followed by a decrease when the massage is slowed or terminated. Hans Selye's general adaptation syndrome responses are commonly sympathetic activation. When the "fight or flight" response occurs, blood pressure increases, muscles tense, digestion and elimination shut down, circulation patterns shift, and glycogen is mobilized.

Activation of the sympathetic nervous system usually results in sensations that people call *stress*. Excessive stress can cause bodywide distress. Intense emotion, such as fear, rage, or anxiety, plays a part in activating the "fight or flight" response. Which comes first, the emotion or the release of the hormones? Science has discovered that it is rather like the chicken and the egg problem.

The release of the hormones adrenaline, epinephrine, and norepinephrine occurs within the "fight or flight" response too. In cases of long-term stress, cortisol may also be released. Cortisol is a cortisone manufactured by the body. Long-term high blood levels of cortisol cause similar side effects as the drug cortisone, such as fluid retention, hypertension, muscle weakness, osteoporosis, breakdown of connective tissue, peptic ulcer, impaired wound healing, vertigo, headache, reduced ability to deal with stress, hypersensitivity, weight gain, nausea, fatigue, and psychic disturbances. When the body can no longer tolerate the effects, the exhaustion phase begins. In long-term sympathetic stress, tension builds until the body basically wears out. Cardiovascular problems, upper respiratory, and gastrointestinal problems tend to develop. The body begins to break down.

In our society, we do not physically fight (most of us anyway) or "flight" (run away), although the chemical reactions may be activated several times a day. So what happens to the chemicals? We each find our own way to dissipate them, for example, yelling at our family. Hopefully we can find more appropriate ways to release the chemicals. Moderate exercise is one of the best ways to burn up "fight or flight" chemicals.

When we become fatigued, parasympathetic functions signal for rest. Chronic fatigue syndrome is a good example of a parasympathetic reaction to stress. Parasympathetic patterns are restorative, therefore, physical activity is curtailed and digestion and elimination increase. Peace, calm-

Table 6.1
AUTONOMIC FUNCTIONS

Visceral	Sympathetic Control	Parasympathetic Control
Heart Muscle	Accelerates heartbeat	Slows heartbeat
Smooth muscle		
Of most blood vessels	Constricts blood vessels	None
Of blood vessels in skeletal muscles	Dilates blood vessels	None
Of the digestive tract	Decreases peristalsis; inhibits defecation	Increases peristalsis
Of the anal sphincter	Stimulates—closes sphincter	Inhibits—opens sphincter for defecation
Of the uninary bladder	Inhibits—relaxes bladder	Stimulates—contracts bladder
Of the urinary sphincters	Stimulates—closes sphincter	Inhibits—opens sphincter for urination
Of the eye		
Iris	Stimulates radial fibers—dilation of pupil	Stimulates circular fibers—constriction of pupil
Ciliary	Inhibits—accommodation for far vision (flattening of lens)	Stimulates—accommodation for near vision (bulging of lens)
Of hairs (pilomotor muscles)	Stimulates "goose pimples"	No parasympathetic fibers
Glands		
Adrenal medulla	Increases epinephrine secretion	None
Sweat glands	Increases sweat secretion	None
Digestive glands	Decrease secretion of digestion juices	Increases secretion of digestive juices

ness, or more drastically, depression can manifest with parasympathetic dysfunction.

Hyperstimulation analgesia can be used to move the body from a sympathetic pattern. Repetitive stroking, noise, or movement initiates these responses. It is the old "follow the watch" hypnosis induction trick. Rhythmic bodywork creates a trance-like effect. (People are very open to suggestions at this time, therefore be very attentive to any type of leading discussion or suggestions.)

There is exciting, ongoing research concerning state-dependent learning in the areas of sympathetic and parasympathetic patterns of function. Triggering a pattern of movement or particular pressure sensation resulting from a trauma is sometimes enough to access a particular state, which results in a second release of the chemical codes of the emotions involved.

Simple active muscle energy techniques can replace exercise and dissipate sympathetic stress and help to alleviate depression. Point holding, such as acupressure, reflexology, or dry needling of acupuncture, will release the body's own painkillers and mood-altering chemicals from the entire endorphin class. These chemicals stimulate the parasympathetic responses of relaxation and contentment. Acupressure is a specific pinpoint compression over motor points of the body, the focal meeting of superficial nerves in the sagittal plane, superficial nerves or plexuses, and muscle tendon junction at the golgi tendons.[9] These areas where nerves are close to the surface of the body correspond with the traditional acupuncture points. Acupressure produces sympathetic inhibition.[6]

It is much more difficult to deal with a parasympathetic depression pattern. Encouraging participation in muscle energy techniques is helpful. Compression and a fast-paced massage style, similar to pre-event sports massage, stimulates sympathetic responses and may lift the depression temporarily.

Whenever there is emotional involvement, it is important to refer clients to a competent counselor. Once the client is seeing a counselor, it is important for the massage professional to work in conjunction with the counselor.

Breathing is a powerful way to interact with the autonomic nervous system. Chest breathing and hyperventilation are common components of increased sympathetic stimulation. The muscular patterns of breath must be normalized in order to deal with stress. Most meditation breathing patterns, singing, and chanting are a way to do this. The heart rate tends to follow a base rhythm beat. A heart rate of below sixty beats per minute will induce a parasympathetic state, whereas sixty beats or more per minute induce a sympathetic state. Just by altering the muscles to be more toned or less toned or by changing the consistency of the connective tissue will affect the autonomic nervous system through the feedback loop, which will have an effect on our own powerful body/mind phenomenon. See Chapter 14 for additional breathing information.

This autonomic reaction to massage may be explained by a concept known as *toughening* or *hardening*. Toughening/hardening is the repeated exposure to stimuli that elicit arousal responses. The planned presentation of stimuli teaches the body to manage more efficiently with sympathetic stress responses. Forms of passive toughening/hardening, such as repeated exposure to cold shock, have been found to increase an individual's tolerance to stress. During cold exposure, two hormones of the adrenal medulla, epinephrine and norepinephrine, are released into the bloodstream. Although massage is not as severe as cold shock, the increase in autonomic functioning and its passive nature may indeed characterize massage as a form of passive toughening/hardening.[11] Like exercise, massage methods that use active participation of the client help to dissipate (burn off) sympathetic stress hormones (sympathoadrenal response), which allows the system to reestablish homeostasis.

In 1969, Reynolds observed that stimulating the periaqueductal gray matter in the brainstem eliminated pain in rats without any anesthesia.[2] Soon after, other important discoveries confirmed this. The dedicated work of Dr. Candice Pert and others led to the discovery of the endogenous (made in the body) endorphin and nonendorphin pain-inhibiting systems of the central nervous system. There are several endogenous opiate-like compounds within the body, including enkephalin and beta-endorphins (β-endorphin is a fragment of the pituitary hormone β-liptropin). These peptides attach to opiate receptors, as does morphine, and relieves pain and produces euphoria. In most cases, pain, especially chronic pain, is relieved.

It takes a larger pain or stress stimulus to generate the endorphin response than the perception of the existing pain. Some methods of massage depend on the creation of a moderate, controlled pain to relieve pain. A negative feedback system activates the release of serotonin and opiates, which inhibit pain.[2] When pain is triggered with the release of substance P, enkephalins are released and suppress the pain signal through presynaptic inhibition. Serotonin is a hormone that affects relaxation and sleep, among its other functions. Massage has been shown to increase serotonin levels. Therapeutic massage methods can be used to create a controlled, noxious stimulation that would trigger this mechanism. Clients will refer often to this noxious stimulation as "good pain."

There is some evidence that acupuncture exerts its analgesic effect by causing the release of enkephalins, and the analgesia is said to be blocked by the morphine antagonist, naloxone. In addition, there appears to be a component of stress analgesia that is mediated by endogenous opiates because in experimental animals, some forms of stress analgesia are prevented by naloxone. Acupuncture probably works by taking advantage of the body's natural inhibitory influences that can normally block pain pathways. For example, it has been established that sensory pain fibers release a neurotransmitter called substance P. Substance P increases the transmission of pain impulses. Enkephalin blocks the release of substance P, which inhibits pain transmission to the brain. The effects of these and other neurotransmitters released during massage may explain and validate the use of sensory stimulation methods for treating chronic pain, anxiety, and depression.[15]

The onset of the effect of acupuncture is delayed until the enkephalin level rises to inhibitory levels. It usually takes fifteen minutes for blood levels to begin to rise. The implications for massage are that the pain inhibiting effects are not immediate. Massage therapists should keep this in mind in regard to the intensity and duration as they work. Similarly, the effect of acupuncture lingers after the twirling or vibration of the needles stop. Again, the implication for massage is that the client should experience a prolonged effect from the massage, typically lasting about forty-eight hours.

People have known throughout history that treatment itself influences the course of a disease, even if the treatment is not specific. The placebo effect is probably caused by several mechanisms, most of which are not yet clearly understood. The environment, suggestions from and attitude of the person giving the placebo, and the patient's confidence in its effectiveness act together to produce a placebo effect. Some studies have reported a success rate of 70% to 90% with the use of placebos. It is possible that the gentle, caring attention focused on the client during therapeutic massage interacts with this powerful and important placebo effect. Dumbo was an elephant with big ears. He believed that if he held a magic feather, he could fly. But the magic was not in the feather; the magic was in the belief.

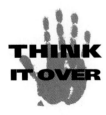

THINK IT OVER

1. **How are the day-to-day activities listed below dependent on the autonomic nervous system?**
   - **Eating when tired, not hungry.**
   - **The driver of the car does not have to stop to use the restroom and the children in the backseat do.**
   - **When the driver of the car tells the children in the backseat that they are not going to stop to use the restroom and they have to wait, the children start fighting.**
   - **Stomach growling a half an hour after a lecture begins.**
   - **Watching a scary movie makes you feel like doing something exciting and active.**
2. **What other daily experiences are influenced by the autonomic nervous system?**

3. **How does music set or change a mood?**
4. **How is exercise a form of "hardening?"**
5. **What are some behaviors that will stimulate the opiate peptides?**

CONNECTIVE TISSUE

Connective tissue massage was formalized in 1929 by Elizabeth Dicke, a German physiotherapist. Dr. James Cyriax contributed extensively to the research of deep transverse friction massage. Studies indicate that massage may reduce the adhesions and the scarring that often result from soft tissue injury. Fibrotic tissue responds well to the specific approaches of connective tissue massage (see Chapter 13).

Other approaches to the fascial or connective tissue component of muscles are called myofascial techniques. Connective tissue is mostly thought of as ligaments and tendons. Few anatomy texts show fascia other than as a structure to be removed to expose the important organ system. Cailliet lists fascia as a type of connective tissue along with tendons, ligaments, cartilage, muscle, and bone.[3] The fascia is actually divided into three layers. The first is a superficial layer that contains fat, nerve endings, and blood vessels. The second layer is called a *potential space*. This space may enlarge with the escape of fluids into the surrounding tissue or edema, which suggests that the fascia can be disrupted and stretched by any injury no matter how minor. The third layer is the deep, investing layer, and below that lies layers of other tissues such as pleura, peritoneum, and pericardium. Individual muscle groups are enveloped by fascia, which separates one muscle group from the next. Fluid between the fibers of the fascia act as a lubricant and allow free movement of one muscle past another. Bursae are formed between muscles, between muscles and tendon or bone, or beneath the skin over bony prominences. Septa extend from the outer fascial layers into the muscle. These septa divide the muscle into progressively smaller units, ultimately surrounding each myofibril. The connective tissue fibers that form the fascia also form membranes. The fibers run in various directions so that they appear interwoven with no one prevalent direction. This is in contrast to tendons, in which fibers run roughly parallel to each other. Because the fibers in fascia run in all directions, they allow the fascia to be stretched to accommodate changes in muscle bulk. All the fascia in the body is directly linked together like a three-dimensional body stocking. There is a lot of fascia in the body. Fascia tends to shrink when it is inflamed. It is a focus of pain because of its rich nerve supply.

Massage that provides for a gentle, sustained pull on the fascial component will affect this type of connective tissue. The specific "pull" on the connective tissue can stimulate cutaneovisceral (skin to organ) reflex, and together with autonomic reflex pathways and endocrine response, produce the body-wide reactions to connective tissue massage. Connective tissue massage helps to harmonize the relationship between the sympathetic and parasympathetic parts of the autonomic nervous system. It helps to normalize the circulation between organs and organ systems and other tissues. Locally, it improves the blood supply of the surface tissues in the area being treated, especially in the particular connective tissue element.

Dr. Janet Travell has spent much of her professional career researching and developing treatment for myofascial trigger points. A plethora of terms, including myalgia, myositis, fibrositis, fibromyalgia, myofibrositis, fibromyositis, fascitis, myofascitis, rheumatism, fibrositic nodule, and myogelosis all seem to be describing the myofascial trigger point.[3] Travell and Simons and others suggest that the effects of massage on the myofascial trigger points are from the stimulation of proprioceptive nerve endings, the release of enkephlin, the stretch of musculotendinous structures that initiate reflex muscle relaxation through the Golgi tendon organ and spindle receptors, and increased circulation.[2,3,18]

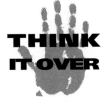

THINK IT OVER

1. **If the fascia is like a body stocking and there is a knot in the toe, how will the rest of the body feel?**
2. **If the fascia is like a body stocking that connects all the inside and outside body parts, what will happen if one part of it is pulled on?**

CIRCULATION

Increases in the blood and lymph circulation are the most widely recognized physiologic effects of massage therapy. According to Dr. Yates' information, many studies validate the increase in lymphatic movement produced by massage. He quotes a study done by Yamazaki and others in 1979. This study seemed to confirm that edema was reduced, lymphatic movement from the tissues to the blood increased, and blood circulation improved by the application of a mechanical device producing a rhythmic massage in a proximal direction.[19]

Increased blood flow on a local level is achieved by compression of tissues, which empties venous beds, and lowers venous pressure and increases capillary blood flow that is quickly counteracted by autoregulation. Massage stimulates the release of vasodilators, especially histamine. Blood flow changes may also be induced through the autonomic vascular reflexes. This increase in blood flow will have a body-wide effect. Compression against arteries will mechanically influence the internal pressure receptors in the arteries. It seems that there is no way to not affect the blood and lymph circulation when giving a massage.

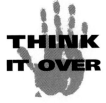

THINK IT OVER

- **Is there really any way to separate the various effects of massage? Can you only massage connective tissue, or affect the circulation, or the autonomic nervous system?**

SUMMARY

Therapeutic massage methods are simple and effective in producing responses mediated though the nervous system, the interaction with the endocrine system, the connective tissue, and the circulatory system. These techniques could be used to replace pharmaceuticals in mild manifestation of symptoms in some illnesses, and also as a supporting adjunct to drug therapy to reduce dosages and duration of treatment, thereby reducing the risk of side effects. The use of massage for anxiety, depression, and chronic pain would be beneficial in conjunction with other treatment protocols. Most forms of musculoskeletal pain and discomfort respond, at least temporarily, to massage. General daily stress responds well to massage. With an understanding of the physiologic effects of massage, it is hoped that individuals, in consultation with medical personnel, will consider the use of these very old and effective methods provided by trained massage professionals in the development of conservative treatment plans for chronic pain and stress-induced disease processes before resorting to more invasive measures. Therapeutic massage could play an important role in prevention programs by providing a natural mechanism to stimulate the body to adjust to the stress of daily life and restore the natural homeostatic balance.

As indicated at the beginning of this chapter, it is easy to validate massage. Additional information can be obtained by locating and studying the resources listed as references in this chapter as well as in Appendix C.

Professional experience shows that most clients get a massage because it feels good and helps them feel better. It will be difficult to scientifically research "good and better." The massage professional can provide the services of this art and be confident that there are scientific reasons for why massage works and feels good. Let us not forget, as professionals, the importance of the "feel good" part. Clients do care "how much you know," but they care more about "how much you care."

The massage profession needs research. Therefore, the massage profession needs to cooperate with researchers, and appreciate that research is tedious, painstaking work. The medical community and the public need the research to strengthen their beliefs in massage so that they can justify receiving or recommending massage. The massage profession needs the public and medical community to support massage. We all need touch because it is so beneficial and, most of all it, feels good.

REVIEW QUESTIONS

1. Why is it easy to validate massage?
2. What is meant by "Do no harm"?
3. Why is research and its replication to verify the positive biochemical and behavioral responses to touch important?
4. Why will educational standards increase with the scientific validation of massage?
5. Is it possible to separate the somatic, emotional, and cognitive elements in response to massage? Is it possible to separate the mechanical, neural, chemical, and psychologic effects of massage?
6. What is feedback?
7. How does the Gate Control Theory explain hyperstimulation analgesia and counterirritation?
8. What role does massage play in relief from nerve impingement?
9. Why are reflexes important to the understanding of why massage works?
10. How does massage interact with the powerful body/mind phenomenon?
11. How does massage stimulate the release of neurotransmitters, endorphins, and enkephalins?
12. What is the significance of the three layers of fascia?
13. What seems to be the effects of massage on myofascial trigger points?
14. In what ways does massage encourage circulation?
15. Why would the serious massage student want to obtain the references listed at the end of this chapter as well as in Appendix C and read them?
16. What does this statement mean, "Clients care what we know, but they care more about how much we care."

REFERENCES

1. Alcock J: Animal behavior: an evaluatory approach, Sunderland, Ma, 1989, Sinawer Assoc.
2. Baldry PE: Acupuncture, triggers points and musculoskeletal pain, New York, 1989, Churchill Livingstone.
3. Cailliet R: Soft tissue pain and disability, Philadelphia, 1977, FA Davis Company.
4. Chaitow LND: Soft-tissue manipulation, Rochester, Vermont, 1988, Healing Arts Press.
5. deGroot J and Chusid JG: Correlative neuroanatomy, ed 20, San Mateo, Ca, 1985, Appleton & Lange.
6. Ernest M and Lee MHM: Sympathetic effects of manual and electrical acupuncture of the tsusanli knee point: comparison with the huko hand point sympathetic effects Exp Neurol 1986.
7. Gewirtz D: Touchpoints, vol 1, no 1, Fall 1993.
8. Greenman PE: Principles of manual medicine, Baltimore, 1989, Williams & Wilkins.

9. Gunn CC: Reprints on pain, acupuncture and related subjects, 1992, University of Washington, Seattle, WA.

10. Hooper J and Teresi D: The three pound universe, New York, 1986, Dell Publishing.

11. Levin SR: Acute effects of massage on the stress response, Master's thesis, Greensboro, 1990, University of North Carolina.

12. Longworth JCD: Psychophysiological effects of slow stroke back massage in normotensive females, Nurs Sci, 4:44–61, 1982.

13. Anderson K, Anderson LE, and Glanze WD, editors: Mosby's medical, nursing, and allied health dictionary, ed 4, St. Louis, 1990, Mosby–Year Book.

14. Selye H: The Healing Brain: Understanding Stress, Stress Without Distress, Institute for the Study of Human Knowledge, Los Altos, Ca, 94022 ISHK Taperbacks.

15. Shealy NC: The neurochemical substrate of behavior. The psychology of health, immunity and disease, vol B, Mainsfield Center, CA, 1992, The National Institute for the Clinical Application of Behavioral Medicine, 434–455.

16. Thomas CL, editor: Taber's cyclopedic medical dictionary, ed 16, FA Davis Company, 1985, Philadelphia.

17. Research at TRI. In Touch Therapy Times, vol 5, no 5, 1994.

18. St. John Paul Workshop Notes Seminar I, St. John Neuromuscular Therapy Seminars, Largo, Florida, 1990.

19. Travell JG and Simons DG: Myofascial pain and dysfunction: the trigger point manual, Baltimore, 1984, Waverly Press, Williams and Wilkins.

20. Yates J: Physiological effects of therapeutic massage and their application to treatment, 1990, Massage Therapists Association of British Columbia, Vancouver.

CHAPTER **7**

BUSINESS AND PROFESSIONAL PRACTICE
MANAGEMENT

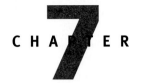

OBJECTIVES

After completing this chapter, the student will be able to do the following:

1. Determine his or her personal motivation for developing a massage business.
2. Develop a five-year business plan.
3. Design a marketing strategy and advertising materials for a massage business.
4. Negotiate rental and employment contracts.
5. Develop a business management and record-keeping system.
6. Write a comprehensive client/practitioner agreement and policy statement booklet.

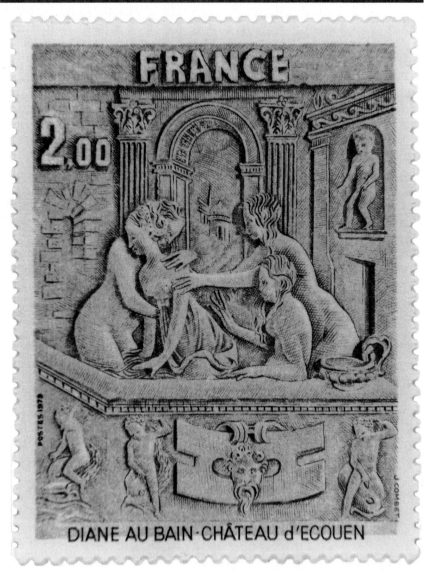

This stamp depicts and celebrates the regimen of the spa, which is a traditional resource for treatment and prevention of disease in France since Roman times. The routine represented includes drinking the waters, enjoying the climate, and receiving massage under the influence of heat and sunlight. (Courtesy of France)

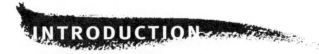

INTRODUCTION

Many massage practitioners are currently self-employed. Being self-employed successfully requires an entrepreneurial spirit. According to *The American Heritage Dictionary,* an entrepreneur is one who organizes, operates, and assumes the risk of a business venture. Many people believe that there will be a steady increase in available jobs in the more traditional employee market, where the massage practitioner will go to work for an individual or company at an hourly wage or salary. Regardless of whether you are self-employed or an employee, an understanding of business practices related to the massage profession is important.

Very technical business information often seems alien to the student of therapeutic massage. Those who seek to develop a career in massage are frequently gentle and intuitive people who may find the concepts of developing policy statements and fee structures difficult. Many people have difficulty with the discipline and organization required to manage a small business. This chapter shares information about business issues. It is important to be able to understand the steps required to set up and manage a small business. These issues are not contrary to the service orientation and the gentle caring attitude necessary for the practitioner of therapeutic massage. Instead, careful attention to these concerns is part of the responsibility of the massage professional.

MOTIVATION

SECTION OBJECTIVES

Using the information presented in this section, the student will be able to do the following:

1 Understand the commitment required to develop a massage therapy business.

2 Understand the importance of motivation for successful business development.

3 Determine a suitable market for an individual massage therapist.

4 Explore strengths and weaknesses in yourself that will add to or distract from the development of a successful business.

5 Develop a personal application of methods to prevent "burn-out."

To succeed at anything one must be motivated. There must be some sort of internal drive that provides the energy to do what is necessary to accomplish a goal. One of the biggest reasons businesses fail is the lack of drive and motivation. Without the *motivation* to stay with the commitment, people give up during the difficult times. This is especially true of small businesses with single owners. Most massage businesses fall into this category.

Therapeutic massage is the same as any other business. It is important to market the product—your skills as a massage practitioner—and to attend to the record-keeping and financial commitments required of the business person. Even if the practitioner chooses to be an employee rather than a self-employed professional, it is important to understand the obligations and time commitments required of the employer. This understanding helps a person be a better employee (Box 7.1).

Motivation begins with knowing what is wanted. Plans must be developed, but the massage professional must be willing to change when a strategy is not working. If success is the goal, then quitting cannot be an option.

When developing a business, it is important to know the market. Massage therapy is again beginning to prove itself as a wellness and health-enhancing system. There are many avenues open for the massage business, ranging from the service approaches of stress reduction massage to the allied health opportunities of working within clinical settings. The future for massage is bright. Research in the near future should provide

Consider your education in therapeutic massage as a pregnancy. It takes time for the baby to grow until it is developed enough to survive in an unprotected environment. So it is with going to school for therapeutic massage. The time will come for the baby to be born. This is a natural process, but not without its struggles and hard work. Graduation, the birth from school, comes for the student as well. Everyone is excited about the baby, but soon the parents realize that for about two years this new little life will require constant care, hard work, attention to detail, and very long, focused hours. The two-year-old child seeks independence, but constant supervision is necessary until the child is about five years old. At five, the child has learned many lessons and can begin self-care as the parents supervise from a little farther away. Each year after that, the child will become more independent. Attention from the parents continues to be necessary, just as it is with a new business.

A professional should plan to give a new business two years of constant attention for it to grow from strong roots and a solid foundation. It will be about five years before attention to the business can be relaxed and small portions of it entrusted to another supervising person for short periods of time. A business will always need attention and participation if it is to be successful. Building a business is hard work that in time reaps rewards.

the long-awaited verification for the benefits of massage. Educational standards will continue to increase and the profession will become standardized and formalized. These developments should provide a broader acceptance for therapeutic massage and bodywork methods. More people will consider using massage as part of health maintenance programs.

It is likely that massage will become a larger part of corporate stress reduction programs. Athletes will use the services of a massage therapist more frequently. Pain control clinics will see its value. Both the elderly and the young can benefit from the nurturing touch of the massage therapist. Opportunities for the development of the massage business will be even greater once people understand the benefits of massage. The need for consistently well-trained practitioners will increase.

Personal service wellness massage is a rewarding career. It has neither the demands nor the responsibilities involved with medical or rehabilitative massage. The focus of personal service massage is preventive stress reduction, relief from minor aches and pains, and the pleasure of safe nonsexual, nonjudgmental touch. The main marketing obstacle is convincing the public that regular massage is beneficial in a total lifestyle program focused on managing stress and striving for wellness. This type of business is built on those who obtain therapeutic massage regularly. Clients who get a massage on a weekly, bimonthly, or monthly basis are the mainstay of a personal service massage business. A successful business of this type depends on quality, consistent, individual personal attention to the client. A regular base clientele of about 100 is sufficient to support a thriving massage therapy business. Twenty clients and forty hours of business commitment per week will provide an average yearly gross income of approximately $40,000 and a yearly net income between $20,000 and $25,000. Personal service massage also lends itself well to a part time supplemental income (Fig. 7.1).

There is no typical massage business. Successful massage therapists are commonly found operating in many different formats. The massage therapist can be a full-time employee of a chiropractor, or may work part-time

Career Resource Directory

The variety of career opportunities available to a trained massage or bodywork practitioner is almost unlimited. Massage and bodywork practitioners work in a variety of atmospheres. Below is a list outlining some of the opportunities.

Airports
Athletic clubs
Beauty salons
Chiropractic clinics
Cruise ships
Corporate wellness programs
Dance studios
Dance touring companies

Golf & country clubs
Hospitals
Hotels
Medical clinics
Orthopedic clinics
Mall locations
Physical therapy clinics
Physicians offices
Plastic surgery rehabilitation clinics
Private establishments

Private employment by celebrities
Private out-call practice
Professional athletic teams
Resorts
Ski resorts
Spas
Sports medicine clinics
Truck stops

Hotels & Resorts

Most four- and five-star hotels and resorts include at least minimal spa facilities on their properties. The following chains are known for employing massage and bodywork practitioners. You should also contact privately-owned hotels and resorts in your area.

Clarion
Embassy Suites
Four Seasons Hotels
Hilton Hotels

Hyatt Regency Resorts
Intercontinental Resorts
Radisson Hotels
Registry Resorts

Sheraton
Ritz Carlton
Stouffer
Westin Resorts

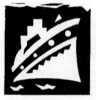

Cruise Lines

Cruise lines offer an exciting opportunity for both travel and employment. Hiring for several cruise lines is handled through the concessionaire, Coiffure Trans Ocean Inc. They hire for Princess, Crystal, Crown, Royal, Norwegian, Cunard, Commodore, Seaborne, Admiral, American Hawaii, and other cruise lines. *Coiffure Trans Ocean Job Line: 305/358-8739.*

Day & Destination Spas

Day and destination spas are very popular places to be hired as a massage or bodywork practitioner. Some destination spas such as the Golden Door, Canyon Ranch, and La Costa employ as many as sixty massage and bodywork practitioners. There is also an opportunity to be hired overseas as there are a tremendous number of spas in Europe, the Caribbean, and other exotic destinations. In these situations, practitioners will often be required to learn a variety of spa therapies, such as herbal wraps and paraffin baths, which can add to your skills and allow you more variety in your practice. For more information on approximately 250 spas in the United States, Canada, the Caribbean, the Bahamas, and Bermuda, get the book *Fodors Healthy Escapes,* available from any bookstore or your local library. Consult your local telephone book for information on day spas in your area.

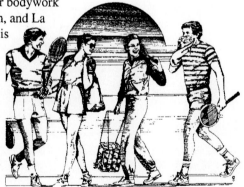

Figure 7.1
Career resource directory. (Reprinted with permission of Associated Bodywork & Massage Professionals (ABMP) . . . the source for massage and bodywork training, information, services, equipment, supplies and more. Telephone: 800/458-ABMP (2267), 303/674-8478; fax: 303/674-0859. Associated Bodywork & Massage Professionals, 28677 Buffalo Park Road, Evergreen, CO 80439-7347.)

out of the home. A business could be developed entirely at one location, or in three or four different locations. A therapist may do massage one day per week at a local manufacturing business for the employees. The next day, he or she may do home (on-site) visits for local business people. The following day could be spent teaching a self-help massage class for the local community education program. The therapist may see clients at a full-service cosmetology establishment in the morning of the next day, and then that evening might provide on-site massage for a local support group dealing with stress. With all the possibilities available to the massage practitioner, it will be necessary eventually to narrow the focus to one, two, or three specific markets so that advertising and promotional activities are manageable.

Answering the following questions begins the process for narrowing and developing a target market for a therapeutic massage business. Who are the people available within a half an hour drive of the location? What type of massage or bodywork does the therapist enjoy giving? Who are the people the practitioner wants to help most?

It is not only the massage skills that are brought to the massage therapy business. Each professional also brings personal strengths and weaknesses, successes and failures, experiences and learning. It is important to use our strengths. It is even more important to recognize those areas in which we are not as strong since it will be these limitations that influence our business activities. Other questions a therapist needs to ask are "How disciplined am I? Do I wait until the last minute to do a job? Am I on time or do I usually run late? Do I keep myself organized?" The very skills that make a wonderful massage therapist—intuition, sensitivity, responding to the moment—can be the source of difficulties in the business requirements of planning ahead, keeping bills paid on time, carefully planning business strategy, and staying in one place long enough to carry out the business plan.

The prospect of altering who we are at our core values is very difficult. A wise decision is to hire help to support those areas in which weakness is noticed. Each business person needs a diverse group of support people, including a lawyer, an accountant or skilled bookkeeper, an advertising-marketing consultant, and an adviser for business planning. Consultation with these resource people need not be expensive. The local Chamber of Commerce and Small Business Administration (SBA) offer services for free. The SBA supports an organization of retired business people called Service Corps of Retired Executives (SCORE). The people in this organization want to help others succeed.

It is essential that the massage professional talk to many people and listen to their experiences about successes and mistakes. This information can be extremely helpful with regard to inherent problems in business. This core information, like therapeutic massage fundamentals, is the underlying foundation for why businesses succeed.

Know thyself. No one should persist with something that goes against personal core values no matter how successful it may be for someone else.

Follow your dream. Success follows desire and motivation. Desire and motivation are the driving forces for those dreams that come from deep within us to bring us joy and healing. Hard times and hard work are part of the process of building a new business. If we are following our dreams, and living on purpose, the hard work provides for a rewarding intrinsic sense of satisfaction.

To succeed in any endeavor we need to realize what benefits will be gained from the process. "What's in it for me" is an important consideration in any decision, and is not a selfish attitude. Rather it is a smart approach. People will not give energy to something that does not provide satisfaction for them. This concept applies to money as well. Business is business, and making money is part of any successful business operation.

Experience is truly the best teacher, and we learn from our mistakes and successes. Implementing plans is the only way to know if they will work. It may become obvious that another approach is more advantageous, but being afraid to make mistakes will limit you as a professional.

There are many motivational tapes, books, and speakers that can be used to inspire us. The overlapping themes in all of them are the kernels of truth. No one person holds the entire answer or knows the whole truth. Each of us must find our own answers, especially when developing a business.

Whatever we believe—with emotion and feeling—becomes our reality. What we do with confidence can become our self-fulfilling prophecy. We attract into our lives that which harmonizes with our dominant thoughts. It is important to be aware of our self-concept. People have ideas about who they should be, and these often conflict with what we have been told and believe that we are. Self-esteem is very important to successful business practices. Trying to live up to others' expectations is a bad business practice. A successful business is built on who we are, not what others want us to be. Develop your ability to use all parts of yourself to the best advantage.

Believe in your product. Understand and be able to explain the benefits of therapeutic massage. It is most acceptable to explain the benefits of massage in terms of physiologic responses, which all people share. Explanations of this type are easy to understand.

Provide a quality product. It is important for the massage practitioner to be a skilled technician. Clients pay for the benefits they experience from massage. Repeat business is based on your ability to continue to produce those benefits. To be truly successful, the person (not his or her condition) must come first. People seek caring, nurturing, nonjudgmental touch as much as the technical skills.

Burnout

Burnout occurs when you use up your energy faster than you can restore it. For the massage therapist, this means taking care of others more than we take care of ourselves. You must take care of your physical needs. Get rest, eat well, and get regular massage. Pay attention to your emotional needs. Surround yourself with people who believe in you. Take care of your spiritual needs, which connect the value of what you wish to accomplish with a much higher purpose. Burnout can be a problem in most service professions. Taking care of others is a big job. If we do not take care of ourselves also, we will soon have nothing to give.

The actual practice of massage is simple, repetitive touch, which sometimes can get boring. It is important to keep yourself excited about the benefits of such simple applications of touch. One of the best ways to do this is with continuing education. Classes make you think and bring you together with other massage professionals. These are good opportunities to share and to learn together. State-licensed massage schools and professional organizations are the best sources for massage education. There are many classes available about business practices and motivation.

It is also important to get away from massage for a while. The massage therapist should occasionally take classes or vacations that have nothing to do with massage or muscles. If you commit to saving your earnings from one massage a week, you will have between $1000 and $2000 per year to spend for continuing education and vacations. You deserve it. Take care of yourself, and let others take care of you. Take a vacation and burnout will be less of a problem.

Once a person begins to live life—including business—**on purpose,** the energy to develop the business concept will be available. Living on purpose means drawing strength from knowing that what we have to offer is valuable. Massage therapy is a wonderful way to be "on purpose." When this is really believed, then the development of the business concept can begin.

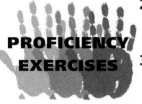

PROFICIENCY EXERCISES

1. With three other students, list strengths and weaknesses for yourself and each other. Compare what others see in you and what you see in yourself.
2. Talk with three small business owners. Make sure one is a massage therapist. Ask them about the first five years of business development. Find out what motivates them.
3. Look through current massage publications and choose three continuing education options you would like to explore. Write them down and keep for future reference.
4. Plan your dream vacation. Write it down and include an estimated cost. Figure out how many massages you will have to do to save enough money to give yourself this vacation.

BUSINESS DEVELOPMENT

SECTION OBJECTIVES

Using the information presented in this section, the student will be able to do the following:

❶ Write a resume.
❷ Develop a five-year business plan.
❸ Develop business goals.
❹ Develop a personal start-up cost worksheet.

The Resume

A resume is a professional and personal summary of a person. Before a business plan can be developed and goals set, it is important to find out who we are. Development of a good resume becomes a part of promotional materials when self-employed, and it is necessary when applying for a job in the massage field. Figure 7.2 illustrates a sample resume. Observe the self-awareness that developed as this massage therapist created her resume. Notice that not just the massage experience is included, but other work experience is listed as well. This is very important. We are a sum total of all our experiences, and we bring that knowledge base into all work and business situations.

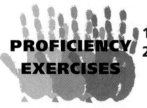

PROFICIENCY EXERCISES

1. Draft your resume.
2. Contact your local community college, library, or public service organization, and attend a class in resume writing.

The Business Plan

It is important to have a plan when setting up a business. To make the plan workable, the therapist needs to know where he or she is right now, where his or her path has been, and what was learned from the accumulated experiences. Once this information is available, future plans can be made. One option is to move gradually into a new business by working with massage part time for a while and letting the business grow slowly (while you keep your full-time job). Another option is to dive into the new massage business full time. If this is the choice taken, the therapist will need to have some money saved in order to support basic needs for about a year. Both paths are acceptable. You will need to decide what fits for you. This is the type of information that becomes formalized when developing a business plan. In all marketing it is important to find and

LAUREL D. FREDERICK

24 Disney Lane
Tyler, Michigan 00000
(000) 000-0000

PERSONAL PROFILE

Excellent sense of self-confidence, personal motivation, and self-discipline. Thorough knowledge of therapeutic massage skills. Adapts quickly to new responsibilities and challenging job requirements. Strong oral and written communication skills; extensive computer skills. Career plans include full-time therapeutic massage in a clinical setting, supported by advanced studies in clinical approaches and continuing education workshops.

THERAPEUTIC MASSAGE EDUCATION AND EXPERIENCE

1000-hour diploma. Tyler School of Therapeutic Massage. Tyler, Michigan. Curriculum included anatomy and physiology, applied kinesiology (Touch for Health), Swedish massage techniques, basic clinical evaluation and correction approaches, myofascial work, shiatsu and reflexology, hydrotherapy, sports massage, client-practitioner dynamics, professionalism, and relationship dynamics with other health professionals. Additional coursework in nutrition, muscle-skeletal anatomy, specific neck and shoulder applications, and advanced techniques.

Approximately 300 hours of therapeutic massage work experience (100 hours independent, non-supervised), with clients of all types, including infants, elderly persons, and pregnant women.

OTHER WORK EXPERIENCE

Senior Instructional Specialist, Performance Management, April 1990 - present. Designed and taught training courses for PC - based and mainframe computer systems. Wrote training and user manuals. Managed projects with companies such as Ford Motor Co., Chase Manhattan Bank, and Consumer's Power. Have trained approximately 2500 persons with varying levels of computer experience.

Editor, *Tournaments Illuminated*, Society for Creative Anachronism, Inc., February 1990 - January 1992. Responsible for 48-page quarterly, circulation 14,200. Supervised Art Director and Advertising Manager.

Editorial Assistant, *The Hanover Review*, July 1987 - January 1989. Worked closely with Editor-in-Chief, edited manuscripts, wrote ad copy and correspondence, implemented marketing proposals.

OTHER EDUCATION

B.A., English Literature, 1987, University of Virginia Dean's List, Intermediate Honors. Supporting coursework in French language, studio art, and theater arts

Figure 7.2
Sample resume.

fill a need. What is the massage demand that you, as a practitioner, are willing to fill?

The business plan begins with exploration of the possible educational options and the development of a financial plan to support the educational process and the first year of business when income is low. Development of the business plan begins in school. This is a great time to use the expertise of the instructing staff and other students to explore career options. Many markets and options are available. It will become important to begin to narrow the target market. By the fifth year, a solid focus, a narrow target market, and a consistent clientele is usually established.

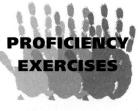
PROFICIENCY EXERCISES

1. **Pretend that you are a successful massage practitioner five years from now. You have been asked to return to your massage school and speak to the business class about how you succeeded in your business. Talk into a tape recorder for thirty minutes as if you were addressing the class. Play back the tape and write down the points used to develop a business plan.**
2. **Meet with ten other students and share your business plans with each other.**

The Goal-Setting Plan

Goals are important because they provide direction and landmarks for achievement (see Box 7.2). Goals may change over time. Goal-setting can be compared to taking a trip. To stay fresh and alert during a trip, it is important to stop and rest. If these stops are planned ahead of time, the journey seems shorter. The journey to a successful business is the same when attainable goals are placed along the way.

When planning for a trip, it is important to identify any obstacles that may be encountered. So it is with a business. Review the support available from others. It is important to realize that most of the learning will happen along the way. What are your financial and personal resources? Basic survival skills aid in providing self-sufficiency. Again, development of a business is the same. A good question to ask is, "What is the worst possible thing that could happen from this decision?" Think ahead to possible

---

Box 7.2
HINTS FOR SETTING GOALS

1. State goals in the present tense. Act as if your goal has already been achieved. Make sure you are the main character. Use the pronouns I, me, and my.
2. Make sure your goals are realistic and attainable. Can you achieve these goals from your own resources with little help from others? If the activity of a specific person is necessary for the achievement of your goal, re-think it. What other people may be able to be part of the goal? Avoid depending on only one other person.
3. Speak in the positive. Avoid words like should, would, could, try, and never.
4. Set target deadlines for yourself. They will give you something to work toward.
5. Make sure your goals are small steps toward your ultimate plan. For example, graduating from school is too big to be a goal, while completing all the exercises in this chapter within four weeks is realistic.

solutions should the worst happen, and to whether or not survival of this experience is a probability. What would be gained? It is important to take calculated risks. If these risks are small and entered into slowly, you can get out easily if need be.

PROFICIENCY EXERCISES

1. **Picture yourself five years from now enjoying a successful massage therapy business. A new student comes to you and asks you how you achieved your success. You begin to tell the story about the last five years and all the steps it took toward achieving your success. All the steps you list are the goals. When you begin with the whole picture, all you have to do is decide how you got there.**
2. **Using the hints listed in Box 7.2, write down three goals pertaining to one of the proficiency exercises in this chapter that can be achieved within two days.**

Start-Up Costs

Start-up costs are the initial expenses of beginning a business. When giving a massage, the student is taught to keep it simple and to go slowly. The same ideas apply to business. In the beginning of a massage business, it is not necessary to have a suite of offices. Beginning small with the bare essentials will incur start-up fees less than $1000. A basic portable table should not cost more than $350. Business cards and a simple brochure are needed as well as client/practitioner statements and policy and procedure booklets, receipt books, and client information forms. Total cost for these is about $200. It is a good idea to have a separate phone line and answering machine. Total cost for these is about $150. Membership in one of the professional organizations will also provide liability insurance; the membership and insurance usually cost under $300. Development of an on-site massage business for homes or offices is the least expensive way to do business, and often the most lucrative. Renting office space often requires the first and last months' rent up front, which may add an additional $1000 to the start-up costs.

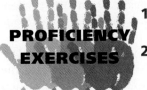

PROFICIENCY EXERCISES

1. **Talk with three massage practitioners and ask them what it cost to start their massage businesses.**
2. **Use professional massage publications and other resources to complete a start-up cost worksheet.**

MARKETING

SECTION OBJECTIVES

Using the information presented in this section, the student will be able to do the following:

❶ **Develop a word-of-mouth marketing plan.**

❷ **Develop an informational brochure, business card, and media story.**

❸ **Design a fee structure for therapeutic massage services.**

Marketing is the advertising and other promotional activities required to sell a product or service. Advertising of some type is a must when starting a new business, many forms of which are very costly. For massage, some types work better than others. Word-of-mouth is the best advertising. Meeting people and talking with them is far more effective than placing an ad in a newspaper. Satisfied clients telling other potential clients about you is even better. In the beginning, the therapist will have to talk with many people to find clients. It takes time to build a business. It is important not to become discouraged, because if you want to succeed, quitting is not an option.

Not everyone supports massage, so negative responses should not be taken personally. The massage practitioner should keep handing out business cards and brochures, and giving demonstrations until the clients are found. Placing an ad and then sitting in an office waiting for clients to call

4 Determine if third-party insurance reimbursement is available or appropriate for the practice of therapeutic massage.

does not work. Better success will come by arranging to speak at service clubs and churches in the area or volunteering to work at races and local events. Businesses may want to offer a stress management class. Local school districts will have adult education classes, and a short class teaching simple massage routine is popular. Charitable organizations often have auctions, which provide wonderful opportunities to give away gift certificates for massage (Fig. 7.3). Being visible in the community will help to generate business.

Experience has shown that the client base for a successful massage practice, developed around repeat business, is about 100 clients. Some will have weekly appointments, others biweekly, and the rest will visit monthly or occasionally. It may be necessary to talk to two thousand people to find 100 clients. Clients who are happy with the work will be the best source of word-of-mouth advertising.

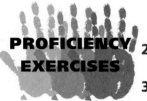

PROFICIENCY EXERCISES

1. **Locate the phone numbers of all the service clubs, e.g., Rotary International, in your community. (The local phone book often lists these organizations.) Write a short letter of introduction and offer to do a thirty-minute presentation about massage therapy.**
2. **Send the letter to three of the organizations and follow-up with phone calls. Arrange to do a presentation (as a student) for the group.**
3. **Find a company, organization, or church where you can volunteer to do mini-massage with the neck and shoulders or feet. Commit to at least eight hours of volunteer time.**

The Brochure

The brochure is the primary tool to educate the public and potential clients concerning the services being offered. It should be specific regarding the following items:

1. *The nature of the services offered.* The brochure should explain clearly that therapeutic massage is a general health service. It should state that no specific treatment of any kind is given for pre-existing physical or mental problems. All specific problems of a medical, structural, psychological, or dietary nature should be referred to the appropriate licensed professional. Written permission and supervision by the medical or other licensed health professional will be required in order for the massage therapist to work with any conditions that fall within their scope of practice.
2. *Description of the services offered.* The brochure should simply explain the process of a massage. It should include a full description of the types of services offered and the procedures followed in rendering those services. It should explain that the client may remain dressed and will always be properly draped. It should be clearly stated that the client may stop the session at any time and may choose to not have any area of the body touched or particular techniques used.
3. *Qualifications of the practitioner.* Verifiable credentials documenting education, training, and experience should be outlined to allow potential clients to verify the accuracy and competency of the practitioner. A valid organization issuing the credentials, such as a school or continuing education provider, must have a record of completion of the course.
4. *Client financial and time investment.* Include a realistic statement of costs and fees in the brochure. Emphasize that the effects of massage are temporary and that massage is best used as a maintenance system. Indicate that the effects of the massage session can be increased with

sample coupons:

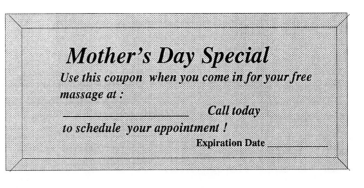

> ## Mother's Day Special
> *Use this coupon when you come in for your free massage at :*
>
> _____ **Call today**
>
> *to schedule your appointment !*
>
> **Expiration Date** _____

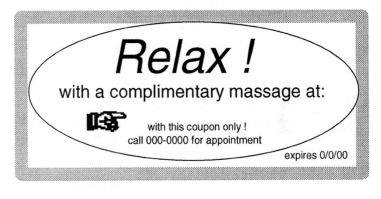

> # Relax !
> ## with a complimentary massage at:
>
> ☛ with this coupon only !
>
> call 000-0000 for appointment
>
> expires 0/0/00

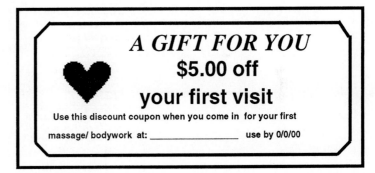

> ## A GIFT FOR YOU
> ## $5.00 off
> ## your first visit
> ♥
> Use this discount coupon when you come in for your first
>
> massage/ bodywork at: _____ use by 0/0/00

Figure 7.3
Sample coupons and gift certificates.

simple exercises. The massage practitioner will teach self-help to the client if requested. The best results from massage are maintained when implemented on a weekly or biweekly basis. Therapeutic massage, when used occasionally, will provide only temporary effects.

5. *Role of the client in health care.* Include the importance of the client's responsibility in his or her personal health care. It is important for the client to realize that the role of the massage therapist is as a facilitator in the wellness process.

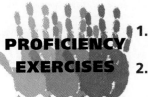

PROFICIENCY EXERCISES

1. **Locate three different professional brochures. Evaluate them against the criteria listed.**
2. **Develop a professional brochure for your future business.**

The Media

The local paper will often run a story about a new and unusual business. A word of caution about newspapers: the therapist should write the story in order to eliminate embarrassing mistakes. Including a black and white photo of the therapist giving a massage is a great idea. Also beneficial are copies of other good news stories about therapeutic massage.

Media advertising (newspaper, radio, and television) is very expensive and not the best idea initially. The clientele developed most likely will be located within a thirty-mile radius of the business location. A direct mailing to a specific area is more effective than newspaper advertising. Before advertising in the yellow pages of the phone book, which is also very expensive, the therapist must be sure that his or her business location will not change for at least a year. The phone number will be locked in for a

Ad Samples

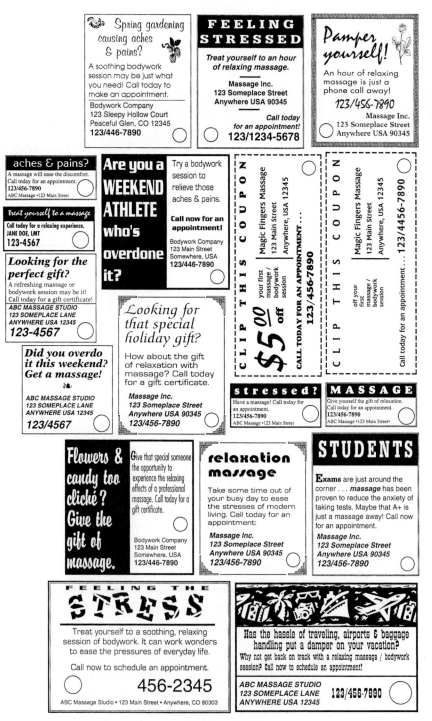

Figure 7.4
Sample advertisements. (Reprinted with permission of Associated Bodywork & Massage Professionals (ABMP) . . . the source for massage and bodywork training, information, services, equipment, supplies and more. Telephone: 800/458-ABMP (2267), 303/674-8478; fax: 303/674-0859. Associated Bodywork & Massage Professionals, 28677 Buffalo Park Road, Evergreen, CO 80439-7347.)

year once the phone book is distributed, and the contract must be paid even if the business moves. It is much more cost-effective to advertise the way automotive companies do: a group of massage professionals in the area can advertise together. By splitting the costs, newspaper, radio, and television advertising (difficult to pay for alone) would be affordable. Whenever a cooperative venture such as group advertising is formed, the therapists *must get the agreement in writing with the help of an attorney.* Verbal contracts or agreements must never be made (see Fig. 7.4 for sample advertisements).

As mentioned, it is important to target your market. This can be accomplished by answering the following: with whom would you want to work? What type of massage do you want to do? Where do you plan on working? When do you want to be available to do massage? How are you going to reach those potential clients?

Potential clients need to know the answers to these basic questions. Who? (You.) What? (Therapeutic massage.) Where? (Address and phone number.) When? (Appointment times.) How? (They can reach you by phone.) This is the information that should be on a business card. The card should be simple and direct, and should not list all of the therapist's credentials. It is convenient to put the next appointment date information on the back (Fig. 7.5).

PROFICIENCY EXERCISES

1. **Collect three newspaper stories about new businesses in your area.**
2. **Write a newspaper story about yourself. Include a picture of yourself.**
3. **Collect three current supportive magazine or newspaper articles about therapeutic massage.**
4. **Design a small ad suitable for the yellow pages. Call an ad representative from your local phone company and find out how much it will cost to run the ad.**
5. **Design a business card.**
6. **Develop an incentive plan. Include how you will track the discounts.**
7. **Locate a direct mail advertising source and develop a direct mail piece. Find out how much it will cost and what is the expected rate of return on this type of advertising investment.**
8. **Contact your local paper and ask an ad representative to help you design a display ad. Find out how much it will cost to run the ad.**

SAMPLE BUSINESS CARD

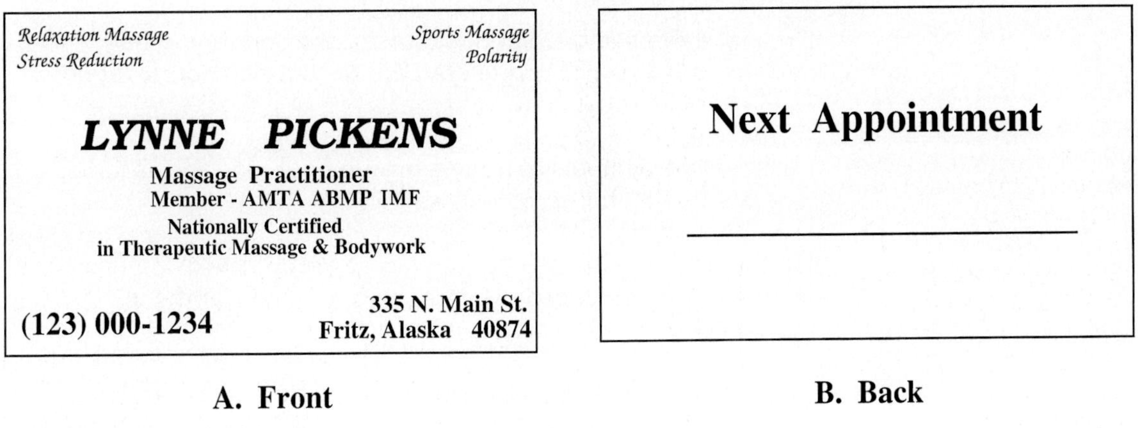

Relaxation Massage Stress Reduction	Sports Massage Polarity
LYNNE PICKENS **Massage Practitioner** Member - AMTA ABMP IMF **Nationally Certified** **in Therapeutic Massage & Bodywork**	
(123) 000-1234	**335 N. Main St.** **Fritz, Alaska 40874**

A. Front

Next Appointment

_____

B. Back

Figure 7.5
Sample business card.

SETTING FEES

Another concern for the client is how much the massage will cost. Setting fees and using incentives are great marketing tools. When trying to decide how much to charge for massage services, it is helpful to investigate what others located within a one-hour radius of the business location are charging. Consider setting your fees at the mid-range of current fees in the area. It is possible to offer incentives and coupon offers to generate business interest, but it is usually unwise to attempt to undercut the competition by charging very low fees (Box 7.3). There is much to be gained by massage therapists working together to educate the public about the advantages of massage. The national average for massage fees based on a recent job analysis is as follows: thirty minutes, $23.12 and a full hour, $38.74.

The half-hour massage is the most expensive per minute for the client because of the linen usage and necessary paper costs. It costs the therapist

---

Box 7.3
MASSAGE PRICING AVERAGES

Half-hour	$25.00
Full hour	$40.00
1.5 hour	$55.00

On-site one-hour massage $80.00 (Special circumstances may reduce this fee.)
The pricing structure for rural areas will be somewhat lower than for urban areas. It is essential to consider "real time" when planning the business. There is always time between massage sessions. It will take:

Forty-five minutes to do a half-hour massage.
An hour and fifteen minutes to do an hour massage.
An hour and forty-five minutes to do an hour-and-a-half massage.
Three hours to do an hour on-site massage.

Now consider the actual amount of money generated per hour:

Two half-hour massages can be done in an hour and a half. Income generated is $50 or $33 per hour.

It will take three hours to do two one-hour massages. Income generated is $80 or about $27 per hour.

It will take three and a half hours to do two hour-and-a-half massage sessions. Income generated is $110 for an hourly rate of $33.

It will take three hours to do one on-site hour massage. Income generated is $80 for an hourly rate of $27.

You should always remember to plan on half of the gross income being spent on overhead expenses, and one third of the net income being set aside to pay income taxes.

Always remember that each hour spent doing massage requires at least one hour of business management time. Giving twenty one-hour massage sessions is at least forty hours of work.

as much to do a half-hour as it does an hour massage. The hour massage and the hour-and-a-half massage are more cost effective. With an on-site massage session, where the practitioner travels to the home or business of a client, travel and set-up time must be figured into the cost. Since the therapist is already organized to do massage, other sessions at the same location can be provided at the regular rate. If someone is house-bound for health reasons, it is common for the massage therapist to take this into consideration when setting fees. The massage therapist who has only an on-site business is saving on rental and utility costs, which may influence the on-site fee structure. Remember that time is money and it takes longer to do an on-site massage than an office visit.

Many therapists give a discount to clients who schedule regular visits. This can be done in a variety of ways. One suggestion is a package of massages that the client pays for in advance. For example, a client will pay for ten massage sessions in advance with a $5 discount for each massage. The package deal would include ten massages for $350 as opposed to $400. Another option is to give a $5 discount to anyone who books a weekly appointment.

Many massage therapists underestimate the value of their service, while others overestimate themselves. When considering money and how much to charge for a service, it is important to realize that people usually live based on an equal exchange for services rendered or for goods received. This is called the *equity hypothesis*. It is important to charge what a massage is worth in time value. If the fee is too high, the therapist does not support those stable weekly and biweekly clients who are the mainstays of a massage practitioner's business. However, if fees are too low, the clients may begin to feel as if they are taking advantage of the therapist, and the therapist may begin to resent the time spent with the clients. This situation does not foster a gentle, caring, nonjudgmental touch. It is important to review fees yearly. A good time is at the end of the year when taxes are filed (this usually happens in April, so May is a good time to raise rates). Clients should be notified at least thirty days in advance of any price changes. Also, a full schedule of clients for three months is an indicator that a rate increase might be considered.

PROFICIENCY EXERCISES

1. Investigate the fee structure for massage therapy in your area.
2. Budget in your personal financial plan how many massages you could receive per month at the going rate in your area.

INSURANCE OR THIRD-PARTY REIMBURSEMENT

It is not common for insurance companies to pay for wellness-oriented, personal-service therapeutic massage. Paperwork requirements to collect insurance are extensive. Most massage therapists are unable to bill the insurance company directly for reimbursement. Payment by the client for services rendered is a more dependable income base. If the therapist is an employee of a licensed medical professional who has access to insurance billing codes, and is working under direct supervision, the massage services may be available for billing. In this situation, the massage therapist is receiving an hourly wage or salary. The burden for collection from the insurance company falls to the doctor, chiropractor, physical therapist, dentist, or psychiatrist.

Occasionally, a client can collect from an insurance company by providing a prescription for massage, and a receipt showing payment. It is important to have the insurance company pre-approve payment for therapeutic massage. This is done by having the client contact the insurance company before any massage begins. Documentation on the benefits of massage, the doctor's prescription, and any other necessary information required by the insurance company is presented for review. This is the responsibility of the client. A decision is made and written notification is given to the client.

There is a good deal of controversy about the advisability of dealing with insurance companies. There are some massage therapists who seem to be doing well with insurance reimbursement. Workers' compensation and smaller insurance companies are more apt to pay. Should a therapist choose to deal with insurance, however, he or she is cautioned to be very careful. Many massage practitioners have been unable to collect insurance payments due and have lost a considerable amount of money.

It is not likely that personal service massage will fall under the acceptable coverage of current or future health care plans. There is a possibility that future insurance coverage will be available for preventive heath care. Massage is a wonderful addition to any wellness program. If insurance coverage becomes available in this realm, it is likely that it will still fall under the medical umbrella and not be accessible to the independent personal service massage practitioner. This should not discourage the new massage professional seeking to begin business. It is beneficial for both the client and the therapist to have options. As the future unfolds, both business opportunities will continue to develop. Jobs will become available for those who wish to work within the medical system and have access to insurance reimbursement, and for those who wish to be independent business people providing the personal service massage outside the medical establishment on a cash for services rendered basis.

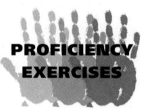

PROFICIENCY EXERCISES

1. **Contact a local chiropractor, physical therapist, or doctor and talk with the billing clerk about insurance reimbursement paperwork requirements. Ask how much the insurance company will cover for various treatments.**
2. **Call your personal health insurance company and ask if they cover massage therapy, what requirements are in place to receive coverage, and how much they will reimburse for a massage session.**

BUSINESS STRUCTURE

SECTION OBJECTIVES

Using the information presented in this section, the student will be able to do the following:

❶ **Choose to be self-employed or an employee.**

❷ **Negotiate lease agreements based on either a percentage of gross receipts or a flat fee.**

❸ **Determine average overhead expenses and yearly income.**

The most common type of massage practitioner is the self-employed massage therapist. A typical practice is to become affiliated with an established business such as a health club, chiropractor, or full-service cosmetology business by renting a room in the business establishment. It is important to make sure that any agreement of this type is written in contract form and reviewed by an attorney (Fig. 7.6).

One of the pitfalls of this type of an arrangement happens when the owner or manager of the business wants the massage practitioner to function as an employee, but for payment purposes be classified as self-employed. If the massage therapist is self-employed, the business owner does not have to pay matching payroll taxes or benefits.

If a self-employed status is desired, then it is important to realize that the therapist is essentially renting space from the owner. The massage business is totally independent as far as how business is conducted. The business owner cannot tell the therapist what hours to work, what kind of work to do, or what to wear.

SAMPLE CONTRACT:

FACILITIES AND SERVICES AGREEMENT

Agreement, made this ____ day of _____ , 19 _____,

by and between _____Therapist, DBA, Catonsville, Maryland,

and _____.

Whereas, _____ Massage Therapist, DBA, is a massage therapist and an independent contractor wishing to use the facilities and services of _____ at _____ for the express purpose of the rendition of therapeutic massage services or activities related to massage therapy.

TERMS OF AGREEMENT

1. Fee for a one hour therapeutic massage is $35.00 - Massage Therapist receives 75%, of Massage Fees and _____ receives 25%. The same percentage applies regardless of the cost of the massage.

2. Fees may be adjusted only upon agreement by both parties.

3. This contract is in effect through March 31. At that time either party may cancel or modify the agreement. A new contract will be issued from April 1.

The following *facilities* and *services* will be provided by the chiropractor for massage therapist:

A. Storage for all massage supplies.
B. Use of the facility and its services, i.e. telephone, bathroom, microwave, refrigerator.
C. Booking and confirmation of all massage therapy appointments.
D. All collection of money, whether cash or insurance.
E. Furnish a room for massage therapist use in the rendition of theraputic massage services or activities related to massage therapy, and _____also furnishes electricity, heat, cleaning for this room.
F. Promote therapeutic massage as an enhancement to chiropractic care.

Massage Therapist will:

A. Bring all necessary supplies associated with therapy.
B. Launder all sheets.
C. Pay any and all own costs associated with being an independent contractor, i.e., liability insurance and professional membership.
D. Control own hours and schedule.
E. Not be held accountable for any expenses incurred by facilities or services not included in this agreement.
F. Keep all tips.
G. Keep all client information confidential.
H. Work at facility by appontment only.
I. Reconcile all accounts & pay proper percentage to chiropractor at the end of each month.

Cancellation of use of facilities and services is to be in writing, giving at least 30 days notice, thereafter releasing each party from all financial and legal obligations with the other.

Having read the terms of this agreement does hereby agree to terms and by signing does agree to use _____facilities and services to begin on _____.

Figure 7.6
Example of a facilities and services agreement written in the form of a contract.

_____   _____

Date:_____   Date:_____

There are two basic ways to pay the owner of the existing business. One is to give the owner a percentage of every massage performed. The rate varies from 10% to 50% (average, 30%). With this arrangement, the business owner profits from every massage done, and may be more likely to support your business with word-of-mouth advertising and referrals. It is also common to advertise together.

Another common agreement is for the person to pay the owner a monthly rent. Rental fees vary depending on location and area of the country. It is difficult to provide a range, but most rooms in established businesses can be rented for $100 to $500 per month. One formula is to calculate the percentage of the total square footage of the space. For example: The room you wish to rent is $12' \times 12'$. This is 144 square feet. The business occupies two thousand square feet. The $12' \times 12'$ room is about 7% of the total available space. The owner pays $2800 per month for rent ($14 per square foot). Seven percent of $2800 is $196. The business owner needs to make some money in order to apply the good business principle of making a reasonable profit. A 50% return is normal; 50% of $196 is $98. The rent for the space would be $196 plus $98 for a total of $294.

It may be a better choice at first to pay a percentage for each massage. If there is a slow week or very few massages, the therapist is not obligated to pay a monthly bill. It is common to end up paying more per month on a percentage agreement than a flat fee. If a mutually beneficial relationship is desired, then a compromise can be negotiated. This is the type of information that needs to be in a written legal agreement (contract).

It is becoming more common to hire massage technicians at an hourly wage. The average yearly net income for a full-time technician is about $20,000. This would be about $10 per hour based on a forty-hour work week. Remember that income taxes must be paid on this amount. A beginning wage is between $7 and $10 per hour. When working for an hourly wage, the therapist can be paid for the time spent at the job, whether or not a massage is given. To earn $20,000 of net income, the self-employed massage therapist would have to generate about $40,000 gross income. Based on 50 weeks of work per year, and twenty massage clients per week at $40 per client, the gross receipts would be $40,000 per year. Fifty percent will be spent on overhead costs (including rent, advertising, linens, supplies, phone, mailings, and postage). It is also important to remember that the self-employed massage therapist must figure real time, which is the amount actually put into the business. At a minimum, for every hour spent giving a massage, at least an hour will be spent with business work such as records, clean up, advertising, and marketing. Self-employed persons never really leave their business. Remember that.

When all the pros and cons are considered, the salary ends up being about the same whether the practitioner is an employee of someone at an hourly wage, or owns his or her business. The advantages of being self-employed are to be considered. It is possible to increase the business income by subletting the space (make sure any rental agreement allows for this). Likewise, after the first few years, the advertising and marketing expenses decrease because you have established a repeat business with clients returning regularly for massage.

The Massage Employee

If the information in this chapter seems like too much to handle, if the therapist is not especially self-disciplined and driven, or if he or she prefers to go home and get away from it all, then finding a job working for someone else may be the best business option. If this is the best choice, the therapist must take care to not let those with their own businesses imply that he or she is inferior. Being employed is an excellent career choice for massage therapy. More and more opportunities are becoming available within the personal service or medical establishment for massage professionals. The biggest opportunity for employment is within the health system. Working as technicians for doctors, physical therapists, and other professionals is a growing opportunity. This type of career may require some additional training. If advanced training for massage is not available locally, then combining massage training with a community college or private school-based program for a medical assistant, receptionist, or physical therapy assistant program is an option. Cross-training or the ability to do more than one job increases employment opportunities.

More massage clinics are opening in which one person, the owner or manager, provides for all the business responsibilities and hires massage practitioners to do the work. Hotels, cruise ships, full-service cosmetology businesses, health spas, retreats, and resorts are active employers of massage practitioners. Understanding business operations will make someone a better employee.

To apply for a job, a resume and expectations for the job will be needed. An interview may include a massage session to test skills. An hourly wage may seem like less than if the applicant were self-employed, but overall the actual money in the therapist's pocket is about the same. It is important to understand the job description, the hours that will be spent on the job, and obligations to the employer; and it is vital to get all this in writing along with any special arrangement that may be made. This document should be signed and dated by all parties involved, so everyone has an original copy.

Not everyone is cut out to be self-employed. The hours are long, and the commitment is 100%. Self-employed people must be self-starters with a broad range of professional and business skills. Some people mistakenly think that self-employed persons get to run their own shows. Instead of having one or two bosses, every client becomes the boss. It takes the entrepreneurial spirit and a deep internal commitment to do it. The key is "know thyself."

PROFICIENCY EXERCISE

- Provide two sample facility agreements for rental space. Base one on a percentage and the other on a flat fee. Be very specific about details.

MANAGEMENT

SECTION OBJECTIVES

Using the information presented in this section, the student will be able to do the following:

1. Use a step by step procedure to set up business management practices.
2. Set up business files.
3. Develop the paper trail required for business records.

Management is all the activities that are required to maintain a business, particularly record-keeping and financial dispersement. The KISS principle (Keep It Simple and Specific) is an excellent concept to help organize the details of business practices. Of course, there are many ways to set up a business operation. A business consultant and attorney are usually the best advisers. The simplest business arrangement, the sole proprietorship, is detailed in this textbook.

Here are the steps to follow:

Licenses

Massage therapists usually deal with two distinct types of licenses: professional and business. Professional licensing shows that you have achieved the skills to practice your profession, and can be state- or local-issued (see Chapter 2). With massage, difficulties occasionally arise with local licensing in the form of massage parlor ordinances. If this problem is encountered, it is important to organize a group of therapists in the local community and change the ordinances.

If a state licenses massage, the therapist usually must show proof of a certain level of education and pass some sort of licensing test. To find out about licensing in any state, it is best to contact the Department of Licensing and Regulation at the state capital. Usually the licensing department for massage is in the occupational license department. This agency can provide the necessary information.

A business license is obtained from the local government, and allows the local government to regulate the types and location of business operations. If a profession is licensed, the professional may need to show a copy of the license to obtain a business license. Any required forms should be filled out carefully.

Location of Business

When deciding where to locate your business, remember that each community has specific zoning regulations. These regulations protect the investment of those who own property. Without zoning, someone could put a junkyard next to a home. Usually the zoning that a massage business will require is general office or commercial zoning. Because of difficulties with local ordinance control of massage establishments, it is possible that there will be restrictions on locations for massage business. To obtain this information, the practitioner should visit local government offices and ask to see the zoning ordinances. A permit or business license may be needed. It is important that the relationship developed between the business owner and the government officials is a good working relationship. These officials usually have a sincere concern for their community, and the therapist must be respectful. Often, they will need to be educated about therapeutic massage. As with a massage, go slow and be gentle and understanding.

Business Legal Structure

Sole proprietorships are the simplest way to set up a business. A meeting with an attorney will allow for careful discussions regarding these more complicated forms of business structures to serve business needs. (This chapter is structured around the sole proprietorship business structure.)

Obtaining a DBA

A DBA is a registration of the business name, i.e., Doing Business As _____. When choosing a business name, the public's interpretation must be considered. One person chose "BODY-WORKS" and received calls about automotive body repair. The fee to register your business name is about $20, and it is usually done at the county clerk's office. The clerk will check to see if anyone else in the county is using the name and will then issue the DBA. This document may be needed to open a business checking account.

Arranging for Registration of Taxes

Federal, state, and local taxes must be paid. A sales tax number may also be needed. Information about federal taxes can be provided by the Internal Revenue Service (IRS) at 1-800-829-1040. State tax information can be obtained from the Department of the Treasury in any state. Information about local taxes can be obtained from both the county and local government offices. The IRS has many helpful publications and counseling services.

One third of a gross business income is usually needed to cover various taxes. This money must be set aside every month and not spent. One of the biggest problems new business owners have is nonpayment of taxes because they spent the tax money on overhead expenses. The best protection is to pay the government first since penalties are high and tax laws are difficult. A professional tax preparer can help a great deal with your taxes.

Arranging for Insurance

The massage practitioner will need professional liability insurance (often called *malpractice insurance*). Malpractice refers to professional negligence. Negligence is an unintentional wrong. A negligent person fails to act in a reasonable and careful manner and consequently causes harm. Clients expect a certain level of professional education, standards of practice, and responsibility for conduct. Unfortunately, in the highly litigious climate of today's world, the best protection against a lawsuit is insurance. Insurance will reduce the risk of having a liability claim filed against you. To advertise this, however, only invites a lawsuit. Accurate and comprehensive records are the next protection; anything that seems even slightly important must be documented. The massage practitioner must stay within the scope of his or her practice and refer clients when in doubt.

The best place to obtain liability insurance is through the professional organizations. Those in existence for five years or longer are the Associated Massage and Bodywork Professionals (AMBP), the American Massage Therapy Association (AMTA), and the International Myomassetics Federation (IMF). Addresses and phone numbers are located in Appendix B. There are other fine professional organizations for the massage and bodywork community, but at this time these are the only ones that offer comprehensive malpractice insurance programs. The insurance costs are usually part of the dues structure of these organizations. It is very expensive to obtain insurance from other companies.

Premise liability insurance is also needed. This is often called "trip-and-fall" insurance. It can be obtained from professional organizations or a local insurance agent. Home business offices are not covered under a homeowner's policy, so additional coverage in the form of a rider is needed. The insurance agent can also discuss fire and damage insurance on equipment.

The more complicated a business, the more comprehensive the insurance coverage will need to be. Sale of products will require product liability insurance. Independent contractor liability protects the contractor against third-party claims from hired independent contractors and so on. The insurance agent and insurance representative from the professional organization can provide additional information.

Business Banking Accounts

A business checking account can be started at a local bank. The DBA is usually needed to use a business name. Self-carbon checks make records easier to keep. All income from the business must be deposited into the checking account which will serve as a record of gross income. All expenses must be written out of this checking account, which provides a record of business deductions. What is left over is called the *net income*. Taxes are paid quarterly on the net income. It is wise for the therapist to contact a good bookkeeper or accountant to help set up the payment schedule for taxes. After all business expenses and taxes are covered, the therapist may then write a paycheck. This check should be deposited into a personal checking account. Personal and business money must not be mixed. If the therapist is disciplined enough to pay off a charge card every month, then a business credit card is a good idea. The monthly statement is a good record of business expenses.

Because many massage therapists are self-employed, it is a good idea to set up a retirement plan. After paying the government taxes, 10% of income could be invested in a long-term growth investment. A local bank or insurance company may have access to stable mutual funds. Individual retirement accounts (IRAs) are also available. There are many ways to invest money in compound interest-bearing accounts. This takes discipline, but we will inevitably get older. It is important to plan for that time now.

Another investment to consider is giving one massage away per week to someone who really needs it. What is given out does truly come back tenfold. Remember the equity hypothesis. There is something that this person can return to the therapist. Maybe it is only a smile of appreciation; which can be worth more than gold.

Records

All receipts must be saved. Copies of all important documents should be stored in a different location than the originals. Everything must be dated, and no verbal contracts should be made. Information should be organized monthly on a spreadsheet so that when it is time for the tax preparer to do the business and personal taxes everything can be verified. This so-called "paper trail" is very important for a properly run business and it must be made.

Comprehensive client files must be in order. Information on each client should include a client information form (Fig. 7.7) and an ongoing record of each visit, including the date, a summary of what was done, notation of any special or unusual circumstances, and payment records. Note whether the payment was cash, credit, or check. If given a check, provide the check number. If cash, note the receipt number. If a monthly billing system is used, post the date the bill was sent and the date the check was received along with the check number. Any credit card information should be taken and recorded. Records must be kept current. If it is necessary to use professional liability insurance, or if billed by a client's insurance company, the first thing the insurance company will ask for are client records.

Any business person is advised to take some small business management classes at a community college or workshops offered by the local Chamber of Commerce. There is no way to avoid accurate record-keeping when self-employed. There are many commercial record-keeping systems available. One should be chosen and consistently used. Accurate and comprehensive client files must be maintained by all massage professionals whether self-employed or an employee. The success of your professional life will depend on it.

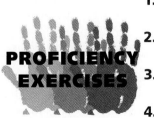

PROFICIENCY EXERCISES

1. **Provide a budget for the first year of running a business. Include your program for setting up payment schedules for the required taxes.**
2. **Provide a list of your advisers, including your tax adviser, attorney, and advertising consultant.**
3. **Collect three different client information forms from practicing massage therapists. Compare them with the samples given in this text.**
4. **Design a client information form. Include questions that would help to determine client expectations and outcome for the massage.**

CLIENT INFORMATION FORM

Name_____

Address_____

City_____ State_____ Zip_____

Telephone(Home)_____(Work)_____

Occupation_____ Employer_____

Medications_____ Physician_____

Age_____ Birth Date_____ Referred by_____

Primary Reason for Appointment:_____

Please answer the following questions by circling the appropriate answer. Please explain any YES answers below.

Have you had a professional massage before?	YES	NO
Have you ever had surgery?	YES	NO
Do you have any spinal problems?	YES	NO
Are you pregnant? Do you have an IUD?	YES	NO
Do you wear contact lenses or dentures?	YES	NO
Do you take any prescribed medication?	YES	NO
Do you have chronic back pain?	YES	NO
Do you have frequent headaches?	YES	NO
Are you constantly tired?	YES	NO
Do you have any heart problems?	YES	NO
Do you have high blood pressure?	YES	NO
Do you have varicose veins?	YES	NO
Do you have any blood clots?	YES	NO
Have you ever had cancer?	YES	NO
Do you have arthritis?	YES	NO
Have you suffered any acute injury?	YES	NO
Do you have pain which radiates down legs or arms?	YES	NO
Do you suffer from tension?	YES	NO
Do you have chronic diarrhea?	YES	NO
Do you have chronic constipation?	YES	NO

Please explain YES answers. _____

_____

_____

Do you have any other medical condition of which I should be aware?

If so, please specify._____

I, _____, understand that the massage therapy given here is for the purpose of stress reduction, relief from muscular tension or spasm, or for increasing circulation.

I understand that the massage therapist does not diagnose illness, disease, or any other physical or mental disorder. As such, the massage therapist prescribes neither medical treatment nor pharmaceuticals, nor performs any spinal manipulations. It has been made very clear to me that this massage therapy is not a substitute for medical examinations and/or diagnosis and that it is recommended that I see a physician for any physical ailment that I might have.

Because a massage therapist must be aware of existing physical conditions, I have stated all my known medical conditions and take it upon myself to keep the massage therapist updated on my physical health.

Signature: _____ Date: _____

Figure 7.7
Sample client information form.

CLIENT-PRACTITIONER AGREEMENT AND POLICY STATEMENT

Using the information presented in this section, the student will be able to do the following:

1 Develop a comprehensive client practitioner agreement and policy statement booklet.

It is essential to have the client read a *client-practitioner agreement and policy statement*. This booklet is more comprehensive than the brochure. It is appropriate for the client to sign a statement that the material has been read, that the therapist has explained the document, and that the client understands and agrees with all the points listed. This becomes part of the informed consent process, but is not protection against a lawsuit. It does have value in that it can do the following:

1. Develop clarity for the client as to the nature of the service being rendered.
2. Help in protecting against unwarranted and unrealistic expectations by the client.
3. Act as a constant reinforcement to the practitioner of the scope and limits of his or her practice within acceptable legal parameters.
4. Serve as a valuable factual tool in potential court actions.

   The agreement or policy statement should be in simple, easily understood language. It provides the practitioner with an opportunity to define his or her practice. The practitioner-client agreement will be of little value if it does not accurately describe the type of service being offered to the public (Box 7.4).

Box 7.4
POINTS TO CONSIDER WHEN DEVELOPING A CLIENT AGREEMENT AND POLICY STATEMENT

Type of Service:
- Explain what type of work you provide.
- Explain what this particular style of bodywork is good for and what are its limitations.
- Specify whether you specialize in working with any particular group, such as the elderly, athletes, or persons with specific problems like headaches and back pain.
- Indicate if there are certain situations or conditions that you do not care to work with, such as pregnancy or certain medical conditions.
- Have a referral network of related professionals that you use.

Training and Experience:
- Does your state require licensing? If so, have available the facts confirming that you are licensed.
- State how long you have been in practice, what school you attended, if the school was approved by any professional organization, and how many classroom hours were required for graduation.
- Provide information regarding continuing education.
- Provide additional education, if pertinent, such as that you are also an athletic trainer.
- Include the names of any professional affiliations of which you are an active member.

Appointment Policies:
- Define the length of an average session.
- Inform clients which days you work, your hours, and whether you do on-site residential or business work.

**Box 7.4
POINTS TO CONSIDER WHEN
DEVELOPING A CLIENT AGREEMENT
AND POLICY STATEMENT**
(continued)

- Tell the client to expect that the first appointment will be longer than subsequent appointments, whether or not you take emergency appointments, and how often you suggest clients come for a massage session.
- Be clear with the cancellation policy and your policy for late appointments.
- Explain to the client whether to eat before an appointment, or if physical activity should be altered or restricted before or after the session.

Client/Practitioner Expectations and Informed Consent:
- Explain in detail what happens at the first bodywork session (i.e., paperwork, medical history, and other preliminaries).
- Clients should know that they can get partially undressed, or undressed down to their underclothes, and that clients are always covered and draped during the session.
- Explain the order in which you massage: face up or face down to begin, what parts of the body you work on and in what order, if you use oils or creams, if a shower is available before or after the massage or if bathing at home before the massage appointment is expected.
- Make sure the client understands whether talking is appropriate during the session and that you should be informed if anything feels uncomfortable.
- If you have low lighting and if music is provided, the client should be comfortable with that atmosphere of the massage.
- Make clear to the client the possibility of any reactions that may be expected such as tenderness over any trigger point where direct pressure methods were used. Indicate that the goals for the massage session and proposed styles and massage methods will be discussed with the client prior to the massage and that consent will need to be provided for all massage procedures.
- Inform the client that your profession has a code of ethics and indicate your policy on confidentiality.
- If the client is in any way uncomfortable, he or she can be accompanied by a friend or relative.

Fees:
Make sure your fee structure is clearly defined regarding the following:
- how often you raise your fees
- if you have a sliding fee scale
- if you take only cash or will accept money orders, checks, or credit cards
- if you bill
- if you take insurance
- how often insurance covers your services
- different fees for various lengths of sessions
- if a series of sessions can be purchased for a discount price
- if you pay any referral fees for new clients

continued

Sexual Appropriateness:
- Sexual behavior by the therapist toward the client or by the client toward the therapist is always unethical and inappropriate. It is always the responsibility of the therapist or health professional to see that sexual misconduct does not occur.

Recourse Policy:
- If a client is unhappy or dissatisfied, do you offer a refund or a free session? Let the client know that if the matter is not handled satisfactorily, there is a professional organization or licensing board where complaints can be registered.
- Send the client policy and procedure booklets before the scheduled appointment. Include a personalized cover letter asking the client to read the booklet carefully and stating that you will discuss it with him or her at the first appointment.

Important Note: If you do go to homes, you need to be extra cautious about entering a home alone. It is important to screen your clients carefully. The initial intake interview is a good opportunity to do this. Have the client come to your location where you have more professional control for the screening process. Individual circumstances will dictate when the following recommendations are necessary, but remember, it is better to be safe than sorry. An on-site massage session for a bedridden elderly person will have a different level of concern than a female massage therapist providing on-site massage to a single male client. At the very least, make sure someone always knows where you are and check in with someone periodically throughout the day. If you are anxious about doing an on-site massage session, then consider referring the client to someone else.

- Hire someone to go with you to the client's home. This person does not need to be a massage professional, but he or she should be able-bodied in case there is a need to leave the home in a hurry. This person remains within hearing distance of where the massage is being given, and will act as a witness should the client claim inappropriate behavior by the massage professional. This person will also provide protection from any type of entrapment or illicit advances against the massage practitioner. It is appropriate to charge for this protection, and it is reflected in the fee structure.

- It is also important to use the phone when entering a home or other location where less control is available to the massage practitioner. Call a prearranged number and give an associate the name, address, and phone number of the client, the time of arrival, and the expected time of departure. Tell this person that you will call just before you leave. Leave instructions to call the authorities should you not call at the agreed upon time. Make sure that your client hears this conversation.

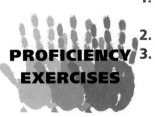

**PROFICIENCY
EXERCISES**

1. **Contact three practicing massage therapists in your area. Ask if you may have a copy of their client policy statements.**
2. **Write a comprehensive client policy and procedure booklet.**
3. **Combine all of the proficiency exercise material from this chapter and generate a business resource manual. In the front of this notebook include a mission statement. A mission statement is a one- or two-sentence statement of your purpose. On the next page write a one-page statement about why you want to be a massage professional**

and what motiviates you toward success in this career. On the following page define for yourself what a successful massage therapy
career means to you.

4. Refer to this notebook often. Continue to add resources, plans, and
goals. Be persistent in recording all your business successes and disap-
pointments. This notebook will become a history as well as providing
a tool to assist you in making future projections for your career.

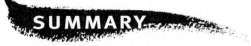

SUMMARY

This chapter is full of details, regulations, requirements, obligations, paperwork, and responsibility. Someone once said that the job is not complete until the paperwork is done. Be sure to do the paperwork, and use professional help where necessary. Success takes time and does not usually happen overnight. Persistence, flexibility, and determination are your keys to a successful business practice. Keep goals realistic and your professional dreams before you to fuel the motivation to strive for success. Define success not only by the money made, but by the value obtained from providing professional services. Take care of yourself to avoid professional burnout so you are able to continue to serve your clients in this wonderful and needed profession.

REVIEW QUESTIONS

1. Why is motivation so important in building a massage business?
2. Why is it important for a massage professional to explore individual strengths and weaknesses when developing a business?
3. What is "burnout" and how can it be prevented?
4. Why is it important to develop a good resume?
5. What is a business plan?
6. What are start-up costs?
7. What are the most effective marketing and advertising strategies?
8. What is the importance of a brochure?
9. How do you set fees?
10. What is real time?
11. What are the prospects for obtaining medical insurance reimbursement for personal service massage?
12. What are the three main types of business opportunities available for the massage professional?
13. What is the KISS principle and why is it important?
14. What types of insurance does the massage professional need?
15. What is the importance of the paper trail?
16. Why is the client-practitioner agreement and policy statement so important?
17. Why does everyone, including employees, need to understand business operations?

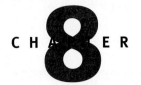

CHAPTER 8

BODY MECHANICS

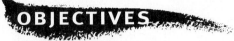

OBJECTIVES

After completing this chapter, the student will be able to:

1 Use the body, especially the hands and forearms, in an efficient and biomechanically correct manner when giving a massage.

2 Alter position of both the client and the therapist to maximize body mechanics.

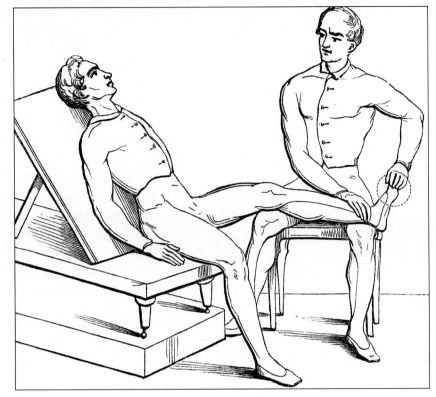

Passive mobilizations of soft tissues and joints as part of Per Henrik Ling's Swedish Movement Cure as depicted in the first English language textbook. (Courtesy of Brown University Library)

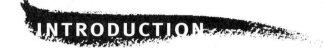

INTRODUCTION

Body mechanics allow the practitioner's body to be used in a careful, efficient, and deliberate way. They involve good posture, balance, and the use of the strongest and largest muscles to perform the work. Fatigue, muscle strain, and injury, including overuse syndromes, can result from improper use and positioning of the massage practitioner's body while giving a massage. In this chapter, the student will learn methods of working more efficiently so that giving eight hours of massage a day does not cause any dysfunction or pain. To make a full-time living doing bodywork, the practitioner must be able to give fifteen to thirty sessions per week. Efficient use of the body will help to prevent burnout.

The information in this chapter has been taken from standard recommendations for service professions, personal observation, and the author's professional and teaching experience. The principles of body mechanics presented rely on leverage, balance, and biomechanics. Static and dynamic postures assumed at work and during recreational activities may have adverse effects on the body. These problems usually manifest in the musculoskeletal system. Massage therapy has unique posture and physical demands. Injury will result if the massage professional is not careful. The massage practitioner makes extensive use of the forearms, wrists, hands, fingers, and thumbs. The massage professional will need to consider his or her own body type and musculoskeletal limitations. The suggestions in this chapter will help most students to individually develop the best personal body mechanics style.

A NOTE TO THE READER:
Most models in this chapter are pictured in leotards or sportswear in order to enhance and clarify the various body positions. The properly groomed massage professional would wear a uniform as shown in Figure 5.1 on page 108.

DYSFUNCTIONS RESULTING FROM IMPROPER BODY MECHANICS

Areas of the body commonly affected in the massage professional who is not attentive to body mechanics include the neck and shoulder, the wrist and thumb, lower back, knee, ankle, and foot. The most common reason for neck and shoulder problems results from the massage therapist using upper body strength to exert the pressure for massage. Tense wrists and hands will also contribute to shoulder problems. These problems can be avoided if the student learns to use leverage, leans with the body weight to provide pressure, avoids pushing and the use of upper body strength, and maintains a relaxed hand and wrist while giving a massage.

The massage professional will need to protect his or her wrists by avoiding excessive compressive forces developing from delivery of massage methods. Using a proper wrist angle and staying behind the massage stroke will protect the wrist. Some reasons for lower back problems include inappropriate bending, bent static positions, twisting, and reaching while giving a massage. The massage therapist must learn to keep the lower back straight and avoid bending or curling at the waist while working. The maintenance of a stable spinal line will help to avoid this problem. Frequent posture shifting of the massage therapist's body will also help protect the lower back as will learning to lift by leaning back during stretching. An asymmetrical stance, along with variations using a short and tall stool will provide methods of protection. The lower back is further aided by avoiding twisting

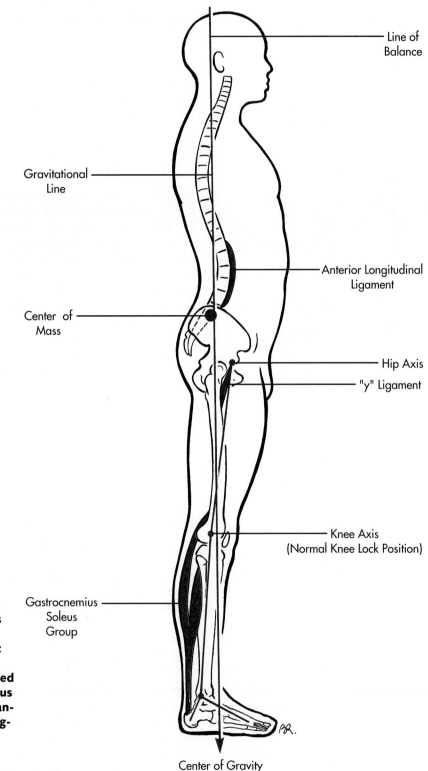

Line of Balance

Gravitational Line

Anterior Longitudinal Ligament

Center of Mass

Hip Axis

"y" Ligament

Knee Axis (Normal Knee Lock Position)

Gastrocnemius Soleus Group

Center of Gravity

Figure 8.1
Relaxed standing posture supporting gravitational line with normal knee locked position in the last 15 degrees of extension. The gravitational force line falls behind the hip joint, in front of the knee joint and in front of the ankle joint. The only muscle group used for balance is the gastrocnemius-soleus muscles. The relax stance involves leaning on the y ligament or iliofemoral ligament, the anterior longitudinal ligament, and the posterior knee ligaments.

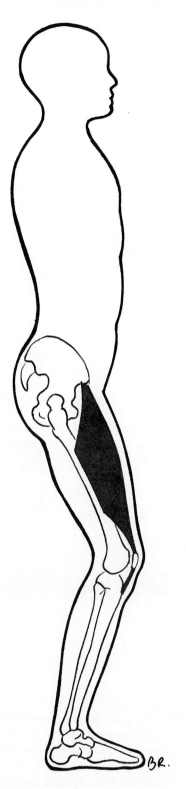

Figure 8.2
Improper leg position putting excessive strain on joints and requiring muscle activity to maintain balance. The gravitation line improperly falls behind the knees.

and reaching while working and keeping the point of contact with the client below the therapist's waist[1] (Fig. 8.1).

Knee problems can be avoided by respecting the basic stability design of the knee and by frequently shifting the weight from foot to foot. The most efficient standing position involves the normal screw home or knee lock position in the last fifteen degrees of extension. This position provides the least compressive force on the knee capsule and the least muscular action for stability. As the knee is flexed, compressive forces increase in the joint capsule, and muscular action for stability increases (Fig. 8.2). Full hyperextension must be avoided. The body mechanics presented in this chapter are developed to support the knee.[3,4]

Asymmetrical standing is the most efficient standing position. The weight is shifted from one foot to the other in an energy conservation mechanism. Symmetrical standing with the weight equal on both feet is fatiguing, interferes with circulation, and should be avoided.[3] The body mechanics presented are based on the asymmetrical stance to best use the massage professional's energy and avoid fatigue. Methods to support this stance, such as using a stool on which to place one foot, using a high stool to sit on, or putting a knee on the table, further protect the lower back and conserve energy (Fig. 8.3). The ankle and foot are protected by the asymmetrical stance, frequent position change, and sitting when possible to do massage.

The human body is designed for movement and range of motion and not the applied compressive forces required when giving a massage. Because of this, it is vital to use body weight and not muscle strength to provide the pressure required during a massage.[2] This is accomplished by shifting the body weight so that the balance point is at the contact point between the massage professional's hand or forearm and the client's body. It is important to redistribute the body mass and change the location of the body's center of gravity (Fig. 8.4).

Massage primarily uses a force generated forward and downward. Therefore, it is necessary to redistribute the center of gravity and the weight force by keeping the weight on the back leg and the balance point at the object-contact point. The body's stance increases to enlarge the base of support. The arm generating the pressure is opposite of the weight-bearing leg, which allows proper counterbalance and prevents twisting of the body.[2]

There is no one way to use the human body efficiently. Each body is different. The important thing is that the massage practitioner must learn to remain relaxed, comfortable, and not to strain when doing massage. If a person feels and looks like he or she is "working hard" while giving a massage, then something is wrong with the body mechanics. If the proper body mechanics are used, the therapist will look and feel relaxed and graceful while giving a massage. Massage is physical work, but it is more like dance or gymnastics than construction work. Shifts in balance apply the various degrees of pressure, not harder pushes. In fact, using body mechanics effectively eliminates the need for pushing to create compressive pressure when giving a massage (Fig. 8.5).

BASIC PRINCIPLES

The basic concept of this style of body mechanics is the use of leverage by "leaning" on the client just as someone would comfortably lean against a wall or on a table. The therapist seldom "pushes" against the client. Pushing requires a locked and stabilized body using muscle contraction to exert pressure. By leaning, muscle tension in the therapist's shoulders, neck, wrist, thumbs, elbows, and lower back is substantially reduced.

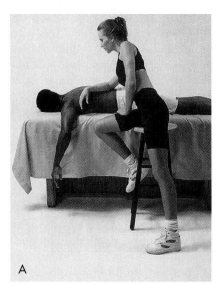

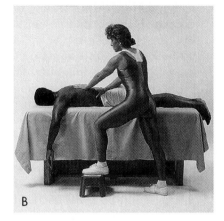

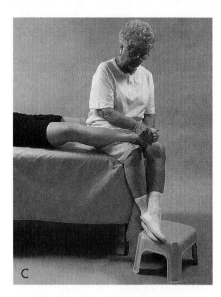

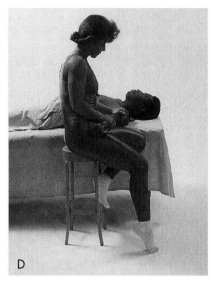

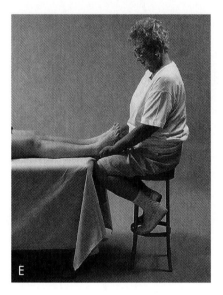

Figure 8.3
A, Use of high stool. B, Use of stool for massage therapists's foot. C, Massage therapist sits on table to protect the lower back. D & E, Massage therapists using low stools to protect the lower back.

The practitioner's body is balanced and relaxed, which allows body weight to do the work. The point of contact between the therapist and client is the balance point. With the balance point located at the point of contact with the client's body, the therapist can be moved or swayed by the subtle movements of the client's body. This prevents the use of too much pressure and allows the client to direct the movement and pressure intensity of the massage without feeling pressed and pinned against the table. The client should never feel trapped or constrained by the massage therapist (Fig. 8.6).

If the pressure levels are too intense or a sensitive area is touched, the client's body will automatically respond with a protective movement by either pushing or moving away. These subtle evaluation cues are easily missed if the massage practitioner is pushing on the client and stabilizing the movement. This style of body mechanics provides the essential component necessary to enable the therapist to receive feedback by body signals. The practitioner becomes extremely sensitive to subtle body changes in the client, which supports the ongoing assessment process during massage (see Chapter 11).

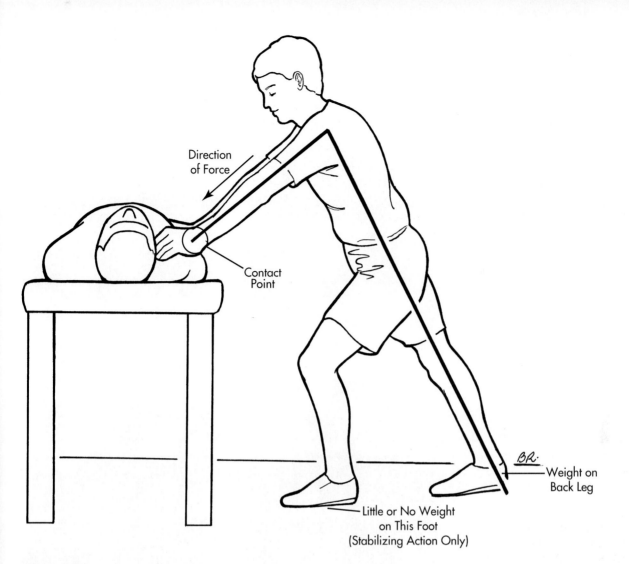

Direction of Force

Contact Point

Weight on Back Leg

Little or No Weight on This Foot (Stabilizing Action Only)

Figure 8.4
Correct body mechanics for compressive force required for massage.

ADDITIONAL BODY MECHANICS CONSIDERATIONS

Attention to body mechanics begins before the massage even takes place. The therapist's body should be warmed up with general aerobic activity and stretching. The massage professional needs to be comfortable and dressed in loose nonrestrictive clothing that does not interfere with movement. Throughout the massage day, breaks should be taken between each massage, and all of the muscles used to give a massage should be stretched. Besides getting a professional massage weekly, the therapist should massage his or her own hands, arms, and shoulders during the day (Fig. 8.7).

The massage table must be at a comfortable height, which depends on the body size and style of the therapist. Those with a long torso and long arms may need a shorter table than a person with short arms. A person with a short torso, short arms, and long legs will need a taller table. A general rule is that the table height should reach the finger tips or the first knuckle when the arms are hanging at his or her sides. This is only a place to begin, and each therapist must experiment to find what height is most comfortable.

It is helpful to have a short stool to put a foot on during the massage.

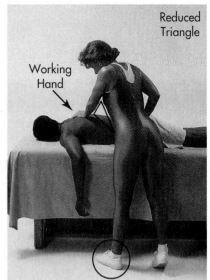

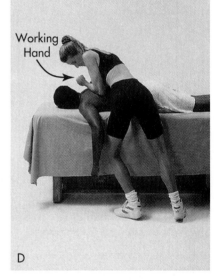

Working
Hand

Weight on Back Foot Opposite
Working Hand

A

Reduced
Triangle

Working
Hand

Weight Front Foot Same Side
Working Hand

B

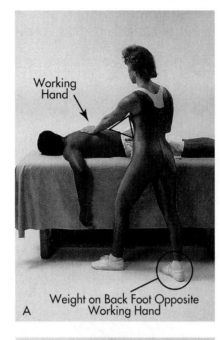

Working
Arm

Weight on Back Foot Opposite
Working Arm

C

Working
Hand

D

Figure 8.5
Comparison between correct and incorrect body mechanics in two positions. A, Correct position using hand. B, Incorrect position using hand. C, Correct position using forearm. D, Incorrect position using forearm. Notice the equilateral triangle that is formed between hip, axilla, and client contact point in correct positions.

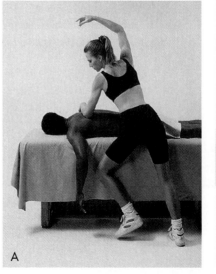

A

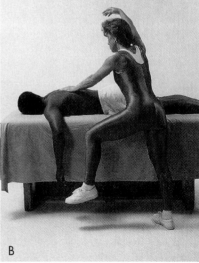

B

Figure 8.6
Comparison of correct leaning position to apply compressive force and pushing. Exaggerated leaning position for emphasis in two positions (A, Forearm & B, Hand). When leaning correctly, the massage practitioner should be able to lift the front supportive leg from the floor and raise the opposite arm.

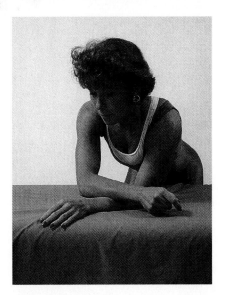

Figure 8.7
Self massage.

A low stool or chair is helpful when working on the face, neck, and feet. It is appropriate to sit while doing massage as long as the therapist is comfortable, relaxed, and can obtain the appropriate leverage for the pressure the client needs. It is permissible to sit on the edge of the table to work on the feet or put the knee on the edge of the table while working on the client's back. However, some professionals feel that sitting on the table is inappropriate. Both options will be offered because this decision is a personal choice. The various illustrations included in this chapter offer some ideas. Should a mat on the floor be chosen for the work, the same principles will apply. The balance points will then be from the knees instead of the feet (Fig. 8.8).

If the massage professional is carrying a portable table, attention should be paid to the body mechanics used to lift and move the table. Lifting the table is done with the knees and hips and not from the waist. A table that is twenty-eight inches wide will be easier to transport than a table thirty inches wide. The extra two inches of lift required to clear the ground require additional effort, especially if the practitioner is short. Some manufacturers of tables have developed shoulder straps, wheel bases, and other aids to help with the transport of tables. These aids help to redistribute the weight load. If a table is carried into the location using the left arm, then it should be carried out with the right arm. It could be harmful to repeatedly carry the table on one side of the body.

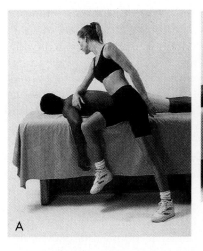

Figure 8.8
Various positions for use of tall tables, short tables, or massage mats. A, Tall table. B, Tall table with therapist sitting on end of table. C, Short table with stool. D, Short table with therapist using a chair. E, Massage mat.

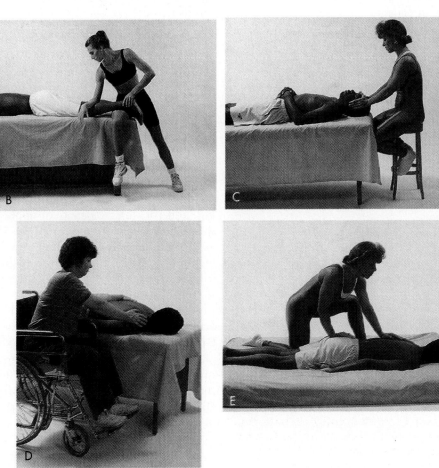

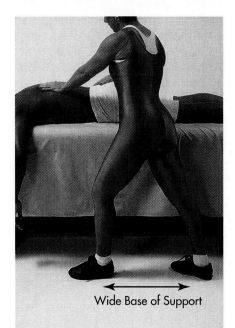

Figure 8.9
Therapist's feet positioned to provide a wide base of support.

BODY MECHANICS WHILE GIVING A MASSAGE

The following general rules apply to body mechanics:

1. The therapist's body must be in good alignment, with the feet placed apart for support. The arm generating the downward pressure is opposite the back weight-bearing leg (Fig. 8.9).
2. The body weight is kept on the back leg and foot and the client's body is in front of the practitioner. This position will provide adequate leverage. If the weight is put on the front leg and the client's body is directly under the pressure, there is no leverage, and all pressure will result from pushing with the upper body muscles instead of using body weight. The front non-weight-bearing leg is used to modulate pressure levels and provide some stability. The massage practitioner should be able to lift the front leg off the floor and still maintain a stable balance point at the client–practitioner contact point. It is important that the student uses body weight. While muscle strength is not a big factor, leverage is essential (Fig. 8.10).
3. It is important to stay behind the stroke. The student should be able to sight down the arm at a 45° to 60° angle and see the hand at the point of contact with the client. If the angle is 90°, the student is on top of the stroke, and muscle tension in the arm will result. If the student is pushing, a good practice technique is to lift the nonworking arm over the head and keep the head up to prevent pushing and promote leaning (Fig. 8.11).
4. The wrists and hands must always be relaxed. Tension in this area transfers to the shoulder and may develop into shoulder and neck problems. When applying a manipulation, the deltoid and shoulder muscles should remain soft, and the wrist and hand relaxed (Fig. 8.12).
5. Avoid the use of the fingers and thumbs. These joints are not built for compressive forces. An eloquent description is provided by Emily Cowall of Ontario, Canada. "The thumb is a unique, versatile, and efficient aspect in relation to hand function. The ability of the thumb to perform the movement of opposition assists the massage therapist in maximizing optimum performance during manipulations. Repetitive compressive force and incorrect use of the thumb and fingers, rigid positioning of the wrist, and excessive tension placed into the hand can give rise to biomechanical dysfunctions."

Cowall states, "The combined activity of proper body mechanics is communicated down through the arms into the hands. Some massage manipulations and techniques can be accomplished by using leaning, lifting, and rocking. A variety of approaches can include use of the arm, specifically the forearm and elbow. Use of the arm reduces stress at the wrist and hand. However, the therapist must accomplish biomechanical techniques to maximize the use of the hands during manipulation of the soft tissues. The hands deliver the resulting advantages of leverage and strength."

Most massage methods can be done by using the whole hand or forearm. Creative use of the forearms and palm of the hand is important. Grasping manipulations, such as *petrissage,* are stressful on the hands. Massage is not applied with the fingers. Instead, the fingers are used as a unit and closed against the pad of the thumb. The position is similar to that of a lobster claw. Massage is provided with the palm of the hands. Direct pressure is best applied with the forearm and not the thumb, except in small areas when using the forearm. The other hand is placed near the contact point to assess the tissue and the client's response when using the elbow or the forearm (Fig. 8.13). The ulnar nerve can be damaged by the use of the tricep portion of the arm.

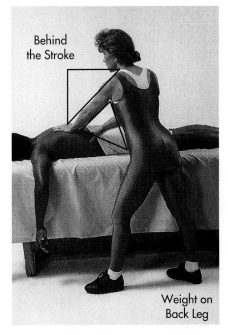

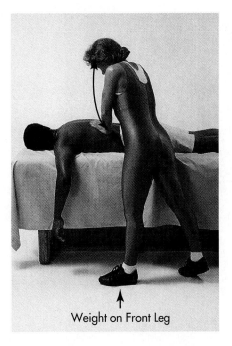

Figure 8.10
Correct position—weight on back leg. Wide base of support in asymmetrical stance; equilateral triangles are maintained so that therapist stays behind the stroke.

Figure 8.11
Incorrect position—weight is on front foot, moving the therapist on top of the stroke losing the triangles.

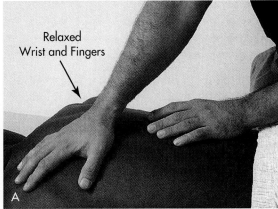

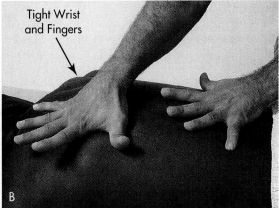

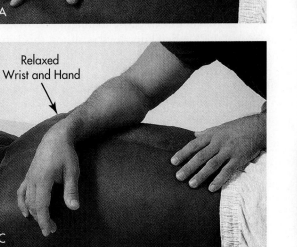

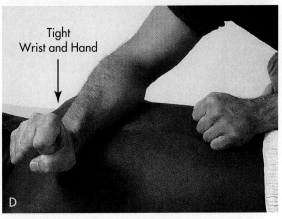

Figure 8.12
Comparison of correct and incorrect wrist and hand positions. A, Correct hand positions. B, Incorrect hand positions. C, Correct forearm position. D, Incorrect forearm position.

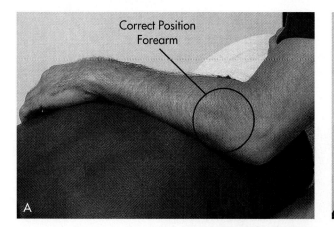

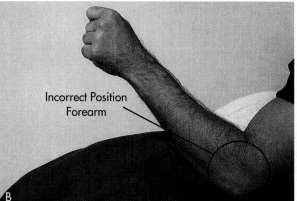

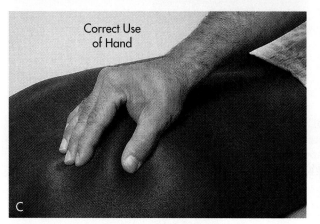

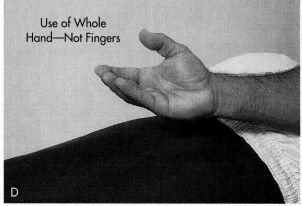

Figure 8.13
A & B, Comparison of correct and incorrect forearm positions. C & D, Demonstration of effective use of the whole hand to apply massage.

6. Positioning the client's body will allow the therapist to lean "uphill," or conversely, to slide "downhill" while protecting the shoulders. Leaning keeps the lower back relaxed (Fig. 8.14).

7. The stroke should be kept at a 45° to 60° angle in front of the therapist. Reaching further may cause lower back strain and a shift of the weight to the front foot, which pins the client to the table. An equilateral triangle is formed by the hip, shoulder, and client contact point (Fig. 8.15).

8. Hyperextension of the wrist or knees can cause damage. The weight-bearing knee will move into the normal knee-lock position; this is not hyperextension. The wrist angle must never be less than 110° to avoid compression of the nerves in the wrist (Fig. 8.16).

9. To avoid twisting, the student should face the area being worked on, with his or her navel pointed at the area being massaged. When the direction of movement is changed, the whole body must be turned, and the weight shifted to the back foot (Fig. 8.17).

10. If using *petrissage*, grasp and rock back to lift the tissue. A rhythm of rocking should be developed, moving forward as the tissue is grasped, and back as the tissue is kneaded and pulled (Fig. 8.18).

11. Pushing must not be used, even if intense pressure is required. Instead, lean and lift into the therapist's body. By shifting the weight on the feet as the client's body is grasped, the client is automatically lifted into the therapist. There is no set pattern or particular point to grasp. Anything available and comfortable for the client can be used. The original contact arm pressure will increase as the body area is

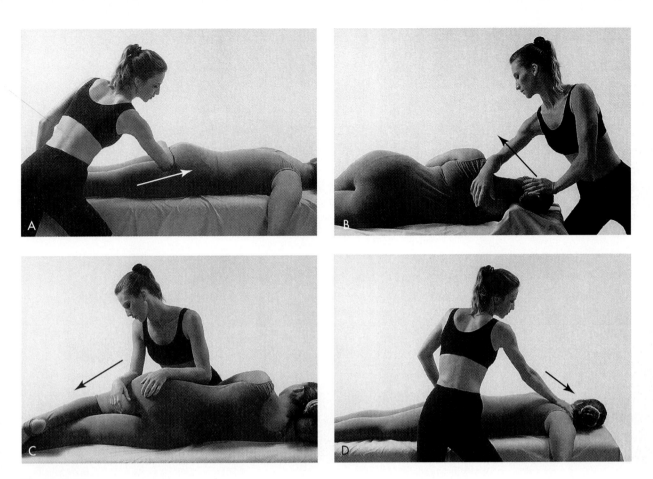

Figure 8.14
Examples of leaning up hill and sliding down hill. A & B, Correct leaning up hill. C & D, Correct sliding down hill.

pulled into it. As the pulling arm leans back, the contact arm moves forward into the client. This technique needs to be monitored by the client for pressure levels (Fig. 8.19).

Allowing the therapist's body to rock and sway with the massage movements is important. Slow rocking keeps the massage manipulations slow. This is critical for efficient adaptation or change in the client's muscle tissue or in the consistency of the connective tissue. The resulting rhythmic movement keeps the therapist's body relaxed and is comforting to the client. Remember to work with smooth and even movements, shifting position often.

The same principles apply to stretching methods used during massage. Range of motion is most often restricted by faulty physiologic signals rather than an anatomic barrier. The protective proprioceptive mechanism sets up this physiologic barrier. If a massage therapist is pushing or pulling the stretches or range- of-motion movements, this physiologic barrier can be bypassed, which fully activates the protective neuromuscular mechanism. Spasms may result. Leaning and going slow with the stretches automatically accesses the physiologic barrier. The therapist can then feel the subtle push back as the stretch reflex response signals that the muscles have been stretched enough (Fig. 8.20 and Fig. 8.21).

The "lean" pressure can also be used to evaluate the client. Evaluation means gathering information but making no changes. If a change in soft tissue is desired, the signal to the tissues must be carefully overridden and intensified slightly to substitute a different pattern. In order for the client's body to accept this change, it is vital that the new signal be presented in a nonthreatening manner and applied slowly. As soon as the client feels trapped, pressed, or pushed on, he will tense up to protect

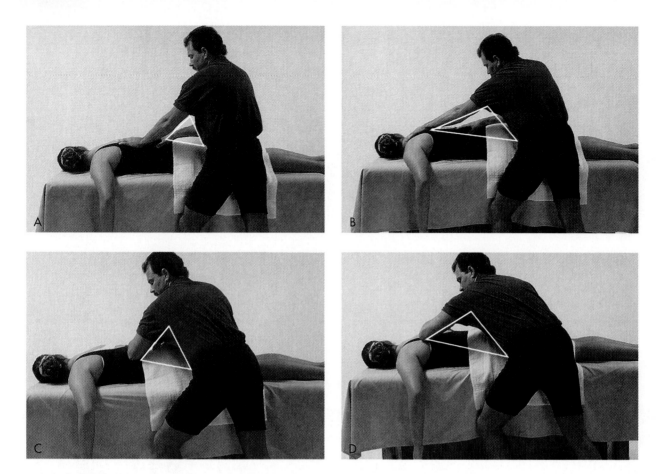

Figure 8.15
Comparison of correct position (45° to 60° angle of the stroke) and incorrect position (reaching for the stroke) in two positions—hand and forearm.
A, Correct hand position. B, Incorrect hand position (reaching). C, Correct forearm position. D, Incorrect forearm position (reaching).

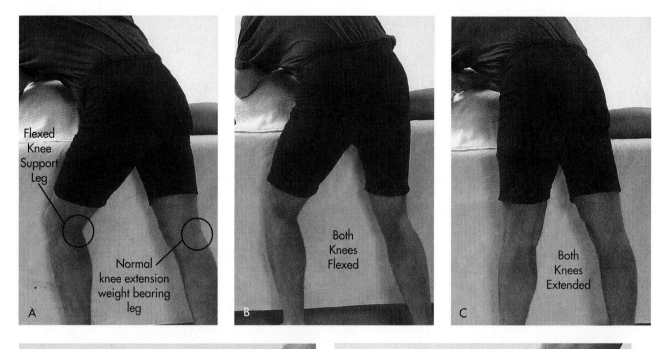

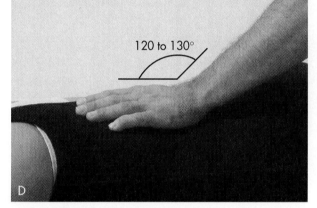

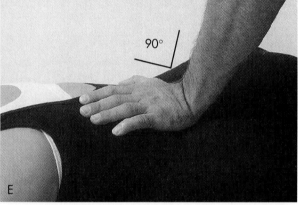

Figure 8.16
Comparison of correct and incorrect knee and wrist positions. A, Correct knee position. B, Incorrect knee position, both knees flexed. C, Incorrect knee position, both knees extended. D, Correct wrist position. E, Incorrect wrist position.

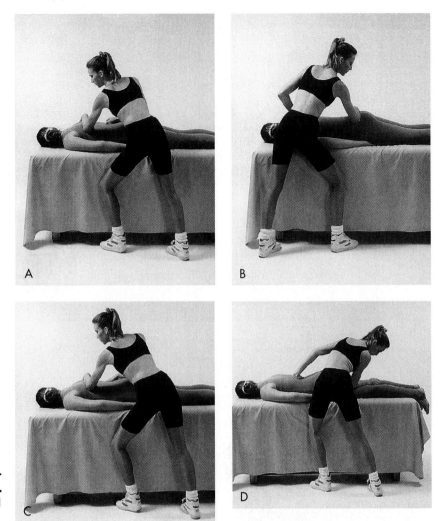

Figure 8.17
Comparison of facing the area to be massaged to avoid twisting and the incorrect twisted position. A, Correct starting position. B, Correct shifted position. Turn entire body; shift weight-bearing leg. C, Correct starting position. D, Incorrect (twisted) position. Feet did not move; torso becomes twisted.

himself. The old pattern will be reenforced, and little or no change will occur.

General transverse friction (Chapter 10) can be an energy consuming and fatiguing massage manipulation. Adapting the frictioning process to use body mechanics principles can reduce fatigue. Using compression on an area to be frictioned and simultaneously moving the joint or bone under the compression, creates cross fiber friction from the inside out, using the client's bone as the mechanism moving the tissue. The tissue can be felt moving. It is important that the compression does not slip so that tissue under the hand or forearm is effectively moved. The movement also acts as a distraction, which allows more pressure to be used. This is very important if the client is uncomfortable (Fig. 8.22).

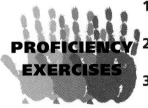

PROFICIENCY EXERCISES

1. **Practice leaning on a wall the correct way and the incorrect way. Feel the difference.**
2. **Videotape yourself giving a massage. Do you look graceful and relaxed, or are you working too hard?**
3. **Experiment with different positions with the client so that you can effectively "lean."**

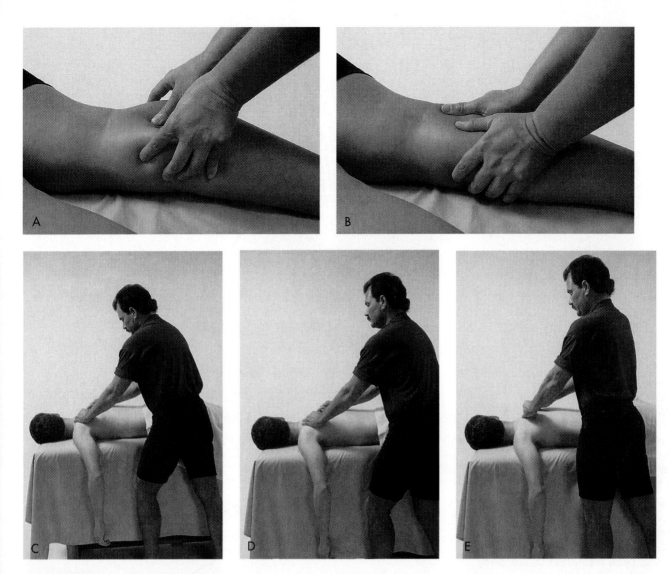

Figure 8.18
Comparison of correct grasp and rock back position for petrissage and incorrect position of grasp and lift up.
A, Correct finger position, petrissage.
B, Correct whole hand position, petrissage. C, Correct position to begin petrissage. D, Lean back and allow tissue to roll from grasp. E, Incorrect position. Instead of leaning back, massage therapist is lifting up with his shoulders and pulling the tissue.

4. Tie one end of a short rope around your waist and the other end around your wrist. The length of the rope should allow you to reach out at a 45°–60° angle, as in Figure 8.18C. Do a massage. The rope will prevent you from reaching too far with the stroke and will tug at the waist when it is time to shift the body.

5. Practice with a standing partner. Lean on your partner as you would lean on a wall. Pay attention to how you feel as your "wall" slightly changes position by moving forward, backward, or twisting. If your partner cannot easily move you with subtle body shifts, you are stabilizing your body and pushing.

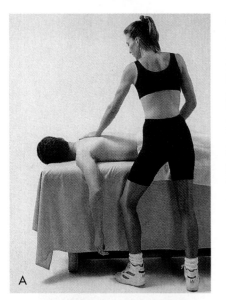
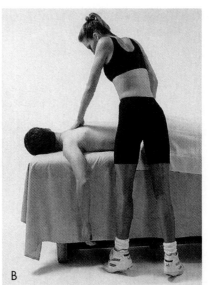
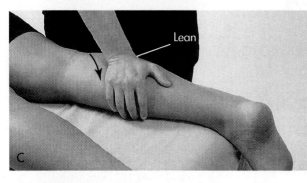
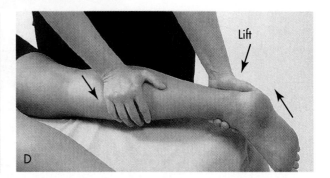

Figure 8.19
Lean and lift into the compression to increase pressure instead of pushing. A, Correct position. B, Incorrect position. C, Lean into area. D, Lift body area while maintaining compression to increase pressure.

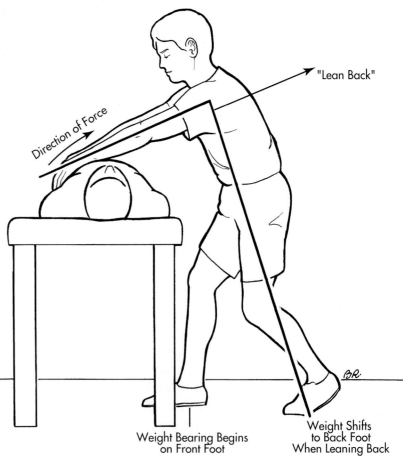

Figure 8.20
Proper position for lift and lean back for petrissage and stretching.

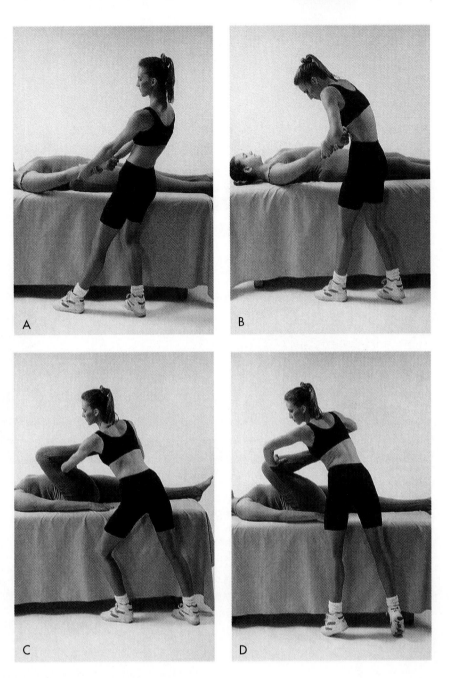

Figure 8.21
Comparison of correct and incorrect position for stretching using leaning for correct position and pushing or pulling in incorrect position. A, Correct—lean back to stretch. B, Incorrect—pull to stretch. C, Correct—lean to stretch. D, Incorrect—push to stretch.

6. Have your partner lie on the table and repeat exercise number five.
7. Practice using the hand as a unit and grasping objects with the palm of the hand.
8. Practice a massage using all of the positions illustrated and explained in this chapter.

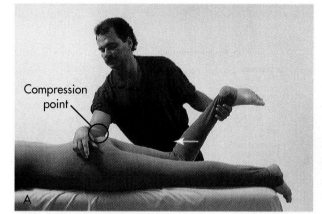
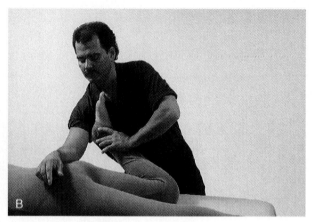
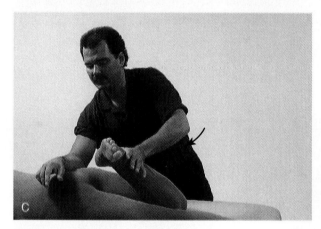
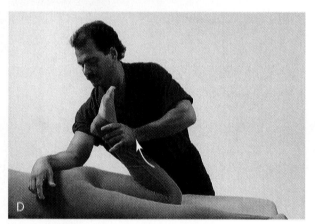

Figure 8.22
Friction using compression and movement. A–D, Move client's hip to various positions. Tissue moves under compression to create a friction movement.

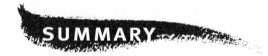

SUMMARY

The massage professional's body is a very important tool that is not replaceable. It is critical to take care of ourselves while giving a massage. If the professional is uncomfortable, the client will become uncomfortable. If the massage therapist can give a massage in a relaxed, efficient, and energy-conserving manner, the client will be able to relax and more easily accept the touch. Practice, practice, practice until your body mechanics are graceful and efficient.

REVIEW QUESTIONS

1. How does a practitioner maintain good body mechanics?
2. How can the massage professional protect his or her neck and shoulders?
3. How can the massage professional protect his or her wrists?
4. How can the massage professional protect the thumbs and fingers?
5. How can the massage professional protect his or her lower back?
6. How can the massage professional protect his or her knees?
7. How can the massage professional protect the ankles and the feet while giving a massage?
8. What is asymmetrical standing, and why should it be used instead of symmetrical standing?
9. What are the basic principles of body mechanics?
10. Where is the balance point during a massage?
11. What pre-massage preparations are important to support good body mechanics?
12. What are the general rules for body mechanics?
13. How do the general principles of body mechanics apply to stretching?
14. How is general transverse friction adapted to this style of body mechanics?

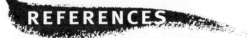

REFERENCES

1. Birnbaum JS: The musculoskeletal manual, ed 2, Philadelphia, 1986, WB Saunders Co.
2. Kreighbaum E and Barthels KM: Biomechanics: a qualitative approach for studying human movement, ed 2, New York, 1985, Macmillan Inc.
3. Lehmkuhl LD and Smith LK: Brunnstrom's clinical kinesiology, ed 4, Philadelphia 1983, FA Davis Co.
4. Norkin CC and Levangie PK: Joint structure and function: a comprehensive analysis, ed 2, Philadelphia, 1992, FA Davis Co.

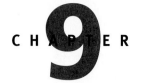

CHAPTER 9

GETTING READY TO
TOUCH

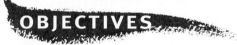

OBJECTIVES

After completing this chapter, the
student will be able to:

1 Develop a massage setting in different
types of environments.

2 List equipment, supplies, and set-up of
location needed to begin a massage
practice.

3 Perform a basic history taking and
informed consent process, which determines client expectations and outcome
for the massage.

4 Explain massage procedures to clients.

5 Effectively drape and position the client.

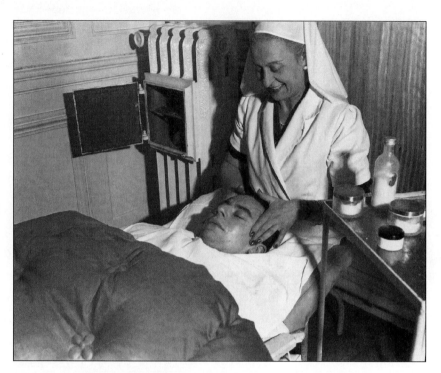

Facial massage as part of hygienic care. (Bettmann Archive)

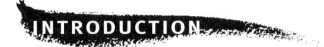

Certain preparations need to be done before the massage begins. The room is to be set up, and all necessary supplies need to be acquired. Consider the type of lubricant to be used and how it will be properly dispensed, the temperature of the massage room, as well as the warmth of the practitioner's hands. The massage professional needs to develop a method, referred to as *centering*, to help focus on the client and the session. Client positioning and modest, appropriate draping procedures must be considered. Finally, the approach for the massage is formed by using history taking and assessment procedures. Informed consent is obtained by discussing the plan with the client before the massage.

EQUIPMENT

SECTION OBJECTIVES

Using the information presented in this section, the student will be able to:

❶ Care for and protect the hands and his or her general health.

❷ Make informed decisions about the purchase of a massage table, chair, mat, body supports, draping materials, and lubricants.

❸ Be able to effectively use massage equipment.

The most important pieces of massage equipment are the massage therapist's hands. Make sure that they are protected from abrasion and damage by wearing gloves when doing outdoor work. Using the forearms will protect and limit use of the hands. In some circumstances, knees and feet are used to deliver certain techniques. It is the massage practitioner's professional responsibility to always be attentive to efficient and proper body mechanics and body health maintenance.

The next piece of equipment to consider is a surface for the client to sit or lie on while receiving the massage. The first choice of most practitioners is a massage table. It must be sturdy and properly assembled so there is no chance it could collapse when a client is lying on it. Two basic types include the portable table, which folds into a smaller unit and is easily moved from place to place, and the stationary table, which remains in one location.

Most manufacturers offer a basic model, and many have more detailed tables with all sorts of features, including those with automatic height and tilt adjustments, arm supports, and face cradles. The more features, the more expensive the table (Box 9.1).

Almost all portable tables are built with a hinge that allows them to fold in half and become more compact. This hinged area is a weak spot in

Box 9.1	A portable massage table is the most versatile and should have the following:
	• Sturdy construction using cable support on the legs
	• Manual height adjustment
	• A face cradle
	• A washable and disinfectant covering, usually vinyl
	• Padding adequate for comfort and firm support
	• It should be twenty-eight inches wide (most tables are about six feet long). Tables less than twenty-eight inches wide are too narrow for client comfort; if wider, they become difficult to carry.

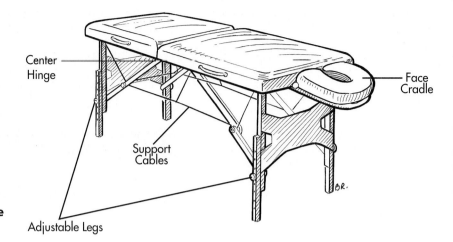

Figure 9.1
Generic portable massage table with center hinge, support cables, and face cradle.

Center Hinge

Face Cradle

Support Cables

Adjustable Legs

the table; cable supports on the legs counterbalance this weakness. Most tables are strong and will hold about three hundred pounds if the weight is evenly distributed over the entire surface of the table. Problems occur when the client sits in the middle of the table when lying down or sitting up, which focuses all the weight in one spot. It is important to consistently check the cable tension to ensure there is no sag. Otherwise, the table may buckle, which may damage the table and harm the client (Fig. 9.1).

Stationary tables avoid this problem because the table is heavier and more stable. Cross bracing and leg supports will make the table even safer. The lack of portability is a major drawback if the massage practice involves any on-site work (Fig. 9.2).

Many people may be concerned about the sturdiness of the table. The lightweight portable tables may look weak, but they are sturdily built. Before the massage, demonstrate the stability of the table, or offer alternate settings such as a chair or massage mat. Adjustable legs allow the table to be lowered or raised to accommodate the various body builds of clients while permitting proper body mechanics of the practitioner.

Ideally, the massage therapist would have both types of tables. The stationary table can be easily built at home by an average carpenter for a reasonable cost. A portable table should be purchased from an experienced manufacturer. It is worth the investment to buy a product that has been tested for safety. All massage tables need to be checked daily for structural stability. It is important to do a complete maintenance check on all the connectors, bolts, cables, and hinges every week and repair any defects immediately.

An alternative to a massage table is equipment designed for seated massage. There are special massage chairs on the market today for this purpose and are a worthwhile investment. The sit-down massage usually takes place in a public setting, such as a business, is done over clothing, and referred to as an on-site or corporate massage. Massage chairs are also excellent for working with anyone who is more comfortable sitting upright, such as a woman in the last trimester of a pregnancy or a person who has difficulty getting on and off a massage table (Box 9.2). Clients with certain respiratory, vascular, and cardiac conditions are best given massage in a seated position (Fig. 9.3). A straight-back chair with no arms can also be used. The client sits facing the back of the chair while leaning on the chair back, supported by pillows. Another option is to use a stool or chair pushed up to a table or desk. The client leans forward on a supporting pillow placed on the top of the table. Special triangular or block-shaped foam forms can be purchased and used to provide an effective support. Also available is a professionally manufactured desk-top support, which could replace the pillows (Fig. 9.4).

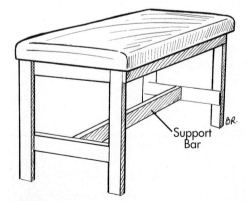

Support Bar

Figure 9.2
Generic stationary massage table.

Advantages of Using a Massage Chair:

1. The specially designed massage chairs are usually very comfortable and easy to use.
2. Professionally manufactured equipment adds to the atmosphere of the massage setting and provides safety through quality workmanship in the construction and design.
3. Professionally manufactured massage chairs are lightweight and portable.

Disadvantage of Using a Massage Chair:

1. Some people have difficulty getting in and out of the semi-kneeling position required to use the massage chair.

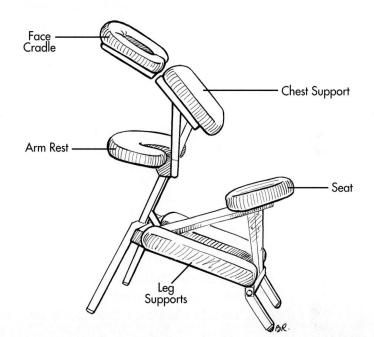

Face Cradle

Chest Support

Arm Rest

Seat

Leg Supports

Figure 9.3
Generic massage chair.

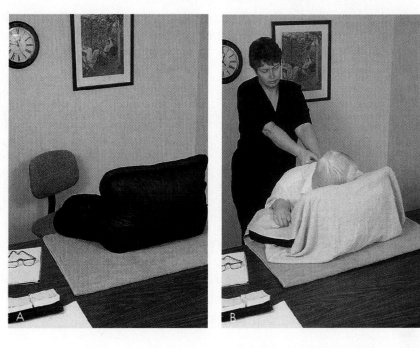

Figure 9.4
A, Use of support pillow to provide massage in office chair and desk. B, Positioning of client for massage.

The Key Elements of a Good Mat for Floor Work are:
- Provides sufficient softness and support for client comfort
- Large enough for the massage practitioner to move around the client's body while staying on the cushioned surface to protect his or her own knees and body
- Can be covered with a sanitary covering

The Advantages of a Mat are:

1. Often less expensive than a massage table
2. May be lighter to carry than a massage table
3. Safety—there is limited chance of a client falling off a mat
4. A popular choice when working with infants and children
5. Is portable
6. Mats may be desirable when working with clients with certain physical disabilities, especially because of the increase in comfort and safety. A transfer from a wheelchair to a mat may be more easily accomplished.

Disadvantages of a Mat are:

1. Proper training to work effectively on the floor is necessary; many massage therapists are not familiar with this kind of work.
2. May be drafty or colder on the floor for the client
3. Physically challenged or elderly clients may have difficulty getting up and down from the floor

Some methods of massage are done on a mat on the floor (Box 9.3). The mat can be a futon or exercise mat and must be protected by a sanitary covering (Fig. 9.5).

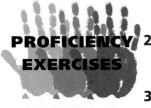

PROFICIENCY EXERCISES

1. **Collect information from at least three different massage table and massage chair manufacturers. Compare cost, quality, and construction of the equipment.**
2. **Locate massage therapists who work on a mat, a portable table, a stationary table, and a massage chair, and ask them questions about their equipment.**
3. **Using the resources in exercise 2, ask the massage therapists if you can sit or lie on their equipment to experience the feel of it.**

Body Supports

Body supports are used to bolster the body during the massage and to provide contour to the flat, working surface (Fig. 9.6). There are commercial body support products consisting of various shapes and sizes of pillows and foam supports. An alternative is to purchase hypoallergenic assorted shapes and densities of foam and to make covers for them. You will need the following shapes, each with a different depth and density: a wedge, round tube, and two or three square or oblong pieces. Additional supports are necessary when working with pregnant women.

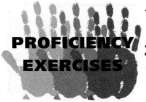

PROFICIENCY EXERCISES

1. **Research a variety of styles of body supports for clients with specific needs.**
2. **Locate a resource for foam; an upholstery or mattress company is a good start. See how many different body supports you can build from foam scraps.**

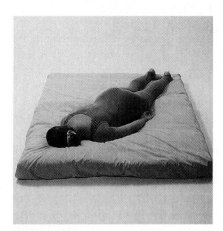

Figure 9.5
Generic massage mat covered with sheet

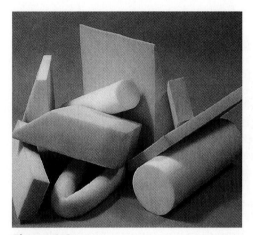

Figure 9.6
Various sizes and shapes of body supports.

Draping Materials

The purpose of using an opaque draping material is to provide the client with privacy and warmth. The most common coverings are standard bed linens because they are large enough to cover the entire body and are easily used for most draping procedures. Twin-sized sheets fit nicely on most tables. These can be purchased and laundered in a sanitary fashion by the massage therapist, or a linen service can be used. Sheets made out of cotton or cotton blends are the best choice because they do not slip on the client. Cotton flannel sheets are nice because they feel warm to the skin. Whatever linen is used, it needs to be able to withstand washing in bleach or other disinfecting solutions.

Large towels may be used for draping because they are both warm and opaque. They need to be at least beach towel size and have a soft texture. Be sensitive to the client's comfort and give a choice of towels or sheets. Because towels are smaller, a client may feel more exposed and prefer the security offered by a sheet. An alternative is to use sheets and towels in combination with a bath-size towel as a chest covering.

Disposable linen is also available. Some higher quality products may look and feel like a cotton fabric without having the warmth. They are convenient, but they cannot be washed or recycled.

The best recommendation is to use two twin-size flat cotton sheets, one for the bottom and one for the top. If fitted sheets are used, draping procedures may not make use of the bottom sheet. Some people are allergic to cotton blends, and skin irritation could result. Soft colors are nice and tend not to absorb lubricant stains. If working with someone who has sensitive skin, use white, pure cotton sheets to reduce the risk of a reaction. Drape face cradles with a hand towel, a pillow case, or an additional piece of fabric sewn just to fit the face cradle. Cover all body supports and pillows with pillow cases. Keep a flannel sheet or light blanket available should the client become chilled. Anytime linens come in contact with the client, they must be laundered in an approved fashion before being re-used.

At least ten full sets of draping material will be needed. This amount would be sufficient for two standard business days, with laundry done every other day. If using a laundry service, make sure that enough linen is ordered for ten days to assure that you do not run out of linens should delivery be late. Most linens need to be replaced every one to two years if used often. Lubricants build up and the bleach will wear the fabric.

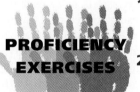

PROFICIENCY EXERCISES

1. **Obtain a set of sheets, some towels, and disposable linen, and then practice draping methods with them. See which type of material you prefer to use.**
2. **Working with another student or massage practitioner, receive a massage with the different draping materials, and see which type you prefer to have used on you.**

Lubricants

Lubricants serve only one purpose for the massage practitioner: they reduce friction on the skin during gliding-type massage strokes. Medicinal and cosmetic use of lubricants is out of the scope of practice for therapeutic massage.

Lubricants are classified as oils, creams, or powders (Fig. 9.7). Oils and creams can be vegetable-, mineral-, or petroleum-based, and powders can be talc- or cornstarch-based. If possible, use the most natural products available, and avoid petrochemicals and talc because many people are allergic to these substances. All lubricants must be dispensed from a contamination-free container.

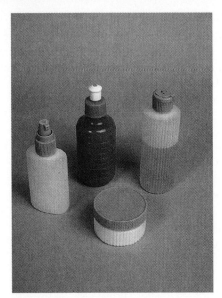

Figure 9.7
Massage lubricants.

The traditional lubricant for massage is oil. It is easy to dispense from a squeeze bottle and can be kept contamination-free. Natural vegetable oils can become rancid quickly. Some commercial products use additives that may cause allergic reactions in clients. The difficulty with oils is that they are messy, can spill and drip, and do stain linens. There are specialized laundry products available for the removal of oil stains.

Massage creams must be dispensed using a contamination-proof method. Some creams are thin enough and can be used in a squeeze bottle. Others are thick, and the amount to be used must be removed in a sanitary fashion before the massage. New processing methods have developed many natural vegetable oil-based massage creams and lotions that do not feel greasy. Some products are water-based and will wash out of linens without leaving stains.

Powders are used when creams and oils are undesirable, usually because of skin conditions like acne or excessive body hair. Do not inhale the dust from powders because it could cause respiratory problems. Powders with a cornstarch base are preferred in order to decrease the risk of respiratory irritation. If the client and the therapist are in agreement, disposable masks can be used to further decrease the risk of respiratory infection.

Headaches and other allergic responses to a lubricant are often from the volatile oils of scented products. Avoid the use of such scented lubricant products. This recommendation does not discount the therapeutic benefit of aromatherapy. The sense of smell is a very powerful sensory mechanism, and many emotional and physiologic processes can be triggered by deliberate use of aroma. This textbook does not cover all of these applications, and additional education is required to use aromas specifically, purposefully, and therapeutically. Until this training is received, avoid their use.

Very little lubricant needs to be used when giving a massage. Remember that the reason for using lubricant is to reduce friction on the skin from the massage movement. It does take more lubricant to work over hair. In some cases powder may be a better choice. Sometimes the use of all lubricants is contraindicated, so it is important to be able to do massage without the use of lubricants.

In Chapter 10 you will learn about different massage manipulations. The long gliding methods are best for application of lubricant. Keep the application even and very thin. It is easy to apply more, but it is difficult to remove excess. Keep a clean towel available in case this is necessary.

Do not pour lubricant directly onto the client. It is first warmed in the palms of the practitioner's hands by rubbing them together. Apply to one area at a time as opposed to the entire body. Avoid using lubricant on the face and hair as it disturbs make-up and hairstyles. The therapist's hands are to be cleaned before working in the area of the face. Some practitioners begin the massage with the face and head before any lubricant has been used.

Some clients may appreciate the lubricant being removed after the massage. An alcohol-based product will do this, but alcohol is drying to the skin. Rubbing the skin with an absorbent towel will remove most of the lubricant.

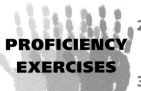

PROFICIENCY EXERCISES

1. Obtain the three basic types of lubricants—oil, cream, and powder. Give a massage with each type. Which do you prefer to use?
2. Find a practice client with a hairy body, and again practice using the different types of lubricant. Which one was the easiest to use? Which one did the client prefer?
3. Have a fellow student give you a massage using all three types of lubricant on different parts of the body. When receiving the massage, compare and see which type you prefer.

4. Practice giving a massage with as little lubricant as possible. See if you can give a massage with only one tablespoon of oil or cream.

THE MASSAGE ENVIRONMENT

SECTION OBJECTIVES

Using the information presented in this section, the student will be able to:

1. Design an efficient massage therapy environment.
2. Organize an office and massage room.

When most people think of massage, they picture a quiet, private room with low lighting and soft music. Therapeutic massage can be done almost anywhere and under most any conditions, so the ability to be flexible is another needed professional skill. Successful massage practices have been developed in noisy public locations such as airports, in a client's home, in the work place, and outdoors at sporting events or retreats. No matter where the massage is done, the most important aspect is to present and deliver the highest standard of professional care to the public.

Conditions for massage areas that need to be considered are the room temperature and fresh air supply. It is suggested that the massage room be kept at 75°F. Massage produces a vasodilation effect, which brings the blood closer to the surface and allows internal heat to escape, cooling the client. It is impossible for the client to relax if he or she is cold. The massage therapist is active, fully dressed, and can become warm while doing the massage. Some therapists will put an electric blanket on the table to keep the clients warm. A piece of lambswool may be used because it traps and retains body heat. Placing a hot water bottle at the feet and another at the neck or wherever comfortable for the client may increase body temperature. The massage practitioner's uniform needs to be cotton or a cotton blend to wick moisture and perspiration. It should have short sleeves and be loose fitting to help keep the therapist from becoming too warm.

The room should have access to fresh air, but a window that opens to the outside is not always available. A small fan in the room pointed at the ceiling or the wall keeps the air moving without causing a draft on the client.

Clients will require privacy for removal of clothing in preparation for the massage treatment. If the massage room is separate from other public areas, the client can be left alone to get ready for the massage. Sometimes a screen or curtained area can be used to divide one large room into two distinct areas.

A Typical Massage Room, Home Office, or Clinical Setting

It is necessary to designate a massage site separate from the business location. People do associate behavior with locations and expected activities at those locations. It is important that these two activities remain separate in the client's mind. The interaction that takes place when appointments are made and money is taken is very different from the one that takes place during a massage.

The business or reception area should be near the entrance, but privacy must be provided when taking the client history. If other clients are nearby, this area needs to be separate from the massage room. An appointment book, calendar, forms, receipts, pencils, phone, as well as a chair and a small table should all be set up in this area. Reading material should be available for clients. Clients will return for a massage because they appreciate the quality of the service and a professional personality. Thoroughly plan the image your massage environment is to convey to the public.

If the reception and business area is a separate room from the massage area, it can be small, about eight feet by eight feet (64 square feet). A room for massage should be ten feet by ten feet (100 square feet). The massage area should be located farther from the door or in an adjacent room (Fig. 9.8). Make sure that there is a place to hang clothes, an enclosed cabinet for storing linens and lubricants, and a place for the body supports. A hamper for used linens must be covered and located away from the massage table. Hand washing and bathroom facilities need to be easily accessible. If there is no sink in the massage room, then a hand cleanser must be available. If there is not direct access to the bathroom, make sure the client uses the facilities before the massage session begins. It is also important to have a plan for the client to get to the restroom if needed during the massage. This can get tricky if the only way to the facilities is to go down a public hall past offices that share restroom facilities.

If the two areas are in the same room, then a space at least twelve feet by twelve feet (144 square feet) is needed to provide the necessary working area (Fig. 9.9).

The Public Environment: Sports Massage, Demonstration Massage, On-Site or Corporate Massage

The massage therapist travels to this location as opposed to the client coming to the practitioner's setting. These massage sessions normally last

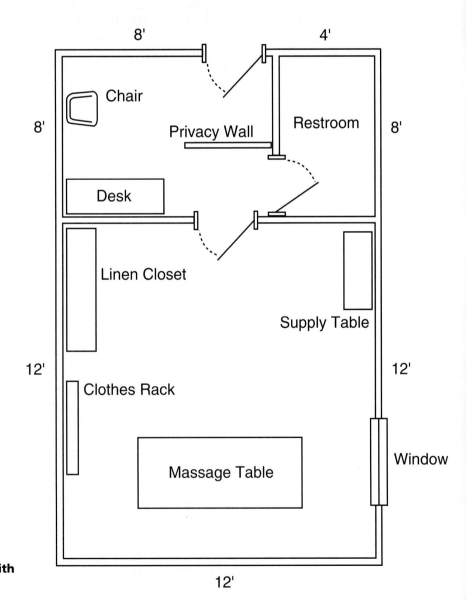

Figure 9.8
Sample layout of massage office with separate office and massage area.

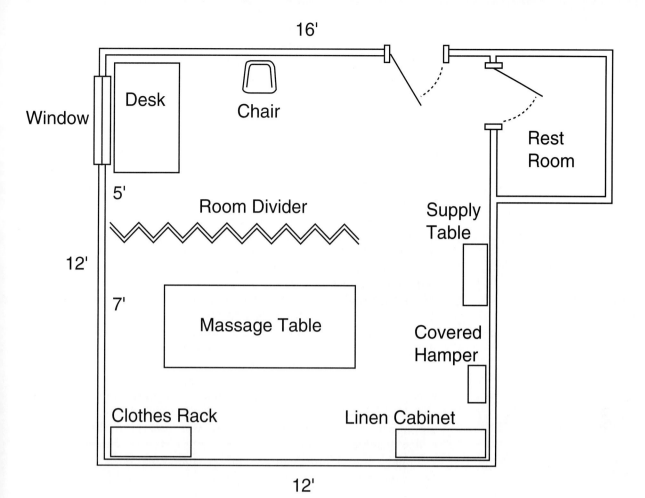

Figure 9.9
Sample layout of massage office all in one room.

less than thirty minutes with the client remaining fully clothed. There is often little control of noise, lighting, and other conditions. Clear enough space to set up the table or massage chair. Attempt to locate this area in a corner, which will give two walls to provide some privacy. It is still important to create both a business and a massage area. Find a flat surface, and use it to set up a portable office from a briefcase or similar carrying case, containing receipts, an appointment book, and handouts. A few steps away, set up the massage area. Although the use of linen and lubricants will usually be limited, it is still important to have access to them; they should be carried in a closed bag. Make provisions for hand washing or hand cleaning products to maintain hygiene and sanitation.

Residence On-Site

Because the massage takes place in the client's residence, it is the most difficult environment in which to maintain professionalism and professional boundaries. There are many reasons for providing on-site massage in the home including service and convenience for the client, especially if the person is housebound. A sixty or ninety minute massage is usually given. A portable table is most often used, but a massage chair or mat is acceptable as well. Find a private location for the massage, but avoid the bedroom and opt for a family room or den. If the only room available is a bedroom, try to have it be the guest room or a child's room instead of the client's bedroom. Make sure it is near an area where hands can be washed. Set up a business area using a briefcase as the office, and maintain the atmosphere. Avoid sitting at the kitchen table or in the living room as the professional role of the massage therapist may become confused in these traditional conversation locations.

Linens, body supports, and lubricants are needed. It may be wise to carry a small fan to keep the air moving and drown out noise from other areas. Never lock the door because a locked door invites secrecy and creates a difficult environment in which to maintain professionalism. Under rare circumstances it could constitute entrapment or be perceived by the client as a violation of the boundaries of the therapeutic relationship. Carry a sign to hang on the door that says, "Massage in session." If music is used, bring a portable cassette or compact disc player.

Outdoors

Outdoor massage is usually provided at a sports massage event or promotional activity. Some massage therapists also work on boats, at family picnics, on the beach, and at poolside. This is a very casual setting, and the massage practitioner must maintain behavior that reflects professional and ethical standards.

Special conditions are created by wind, sun, rain, and insects. Wind will blow the draping, but picnic table clips can be used to prevent problems. Instructing clients to wear a swimsuit or other loose clothing and shifting to an over-the-clothing massage style will also help. A firm and level location is needed for the table because tables that sink into the sand are dangerous. It is important to do massage in the shade to avoid sunburn. A roof or canopy would also be helpful for protection from possible rain. If the area is screened in, technically it is not outdoors. True outdoor massage has insects. Blend brushing away of insects into the massage as well as possible. If an area for washing hands is not convenient, use a special disinfectant hand cleanser. The portable office is set up in an area away from the massage setting (Fig. 9.10).

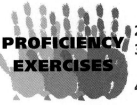

PROFICIENCY EXERCISES

1. **Arrange to give a massage in each of the four basic environments. What was different about each experience?**
2. **Put together a briefcase office.**
3. **On paper, design three different set-ups for a clinical massage environment. Locate the areas for the business and massage areas.**
4. **Design a plan for use of the restroom if it is located outside of the immediate massage area.**

ADDITIONAL EQUIPMENT

In addition to a massage table, draping material, and supports, it is desirable to have disposable tissues, a clock, and music available.

Music is used to distract the client from surrounding noise. A less recognized use of music is for interaction and modulation of the autonomic nervous system. Simple, soft music with a base beat of less than sixty beats per minute tends to activate a parasympathetic response, which results in a soothing and relaxing effect. Music with more than 60 beats per minute encourages sympathetic responses, which results in a stimulating and invigorating effect.

With music, a practitioner must consider the effect that needs to be created, and whether both the client and the massage therapist like the music being played. The best recommendation is for the massage therapist to choose a variety of music and then offer this collection for the client to choose from for the session. Make sure there is an assortment of styles, rhythms, and instruments, as well as a cassette player or other equipment. The volume needs to be kept soft but loud enough so the ears

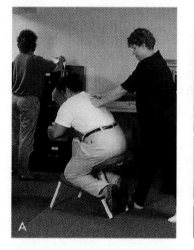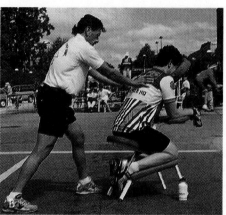

Figure 9.10
A, On-site massage in office setting. B, Outdoor sport massage setting using massage chair.

do not have to strain to follow the music. The music itself can be very helpful in pacing the massage. If the tunes are familiar, they can provide an idea of timing without having to constantly look at the clock.

Lighting

The massage area must be lit well enough to meet standards required for proper cleaning and for safety (see Chapter 5, sanitation requirements). Bright light is often harsh and glaring for the client. Indirect or natural light from a window is much better. If there are overhead lights in the massage area, use a lamp in the corner of the room. A dimmer switch is excellent because the lighting can be adjusted. Never work in a dark room or by candle light because an open flame is a safety hazard.

Candles, Scents, Incense, and Flowers

The massage practitioner will be working with a variety of people during a day, each one with different ideas of what is considered pleasant or offensive. Many clients are also environmentally sensitive and react to these amenities. The best recommendation is to avoid their use. Even if you remove a scented candle from the room, the smell lingers and can cause problems for a client.

Warm Hands, Hygiene, Chemicals, Perfume, and Pets

It is important for the massage therapist to attend to personal hygiene and avoid body odors because people are sensitive to these smells. Avoid heavy use of aftershave, perfume, scented cosmetic products, or hair spray. Clients will not comment on offensive breath or body odors; they just may not return. Because it may be difficult to recognize odors in ourselves, ask a family member or friend who will answer truthfully.

Many massage therapists will have a home office. If there are pets in the home, potential clients need to be informed in case of allergy or fear of animals. Pets should not be allowed in the business or massage areas.

Cold hands are a real problem for many massage therapists. Hands should be heated with warm water, on a hot water bottle, or by rubbing them together before touching the client.

If the massage therapist is a smoker, the smell of smoke can linger in the fabric, carpet, furniture, and on the massage therapist, which can be very distasteful to a nonsmoking client. Because it is difficult to remove the odor, the massage environment should be a nonsmoking area. Not smoking during professional hours prevents the smell on hands, clothes, hair, and breath.

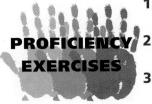

1. **Ask three people who will provide you with candid information on improvements in your hygiene and professional presentation.**
2. **Develop a music library of four different types of tapes. Mark each fifteen minute segment to assist with timing of the massage.**
3. **Do an evaluation of the massage area to see what potential items may cause allergic reactions in clients.**

DETERMINING THE CLIENT'S EXPECTATIONS AND OUTCOME

SECTION OBJECTIVES

Using the information presented in this section, the student will be able to:

❶ Interview a client to better understand the client's expectations of massage in general and the outcome for a massage session in particular.

❷ Obtain a history from the client to identify contraindications, determine the need for referral, and evaluate the outcome of the massage session.

❸ Obtain informed consent from the client before the massage session begins.

❹ Develop methods to help focus attention to the massage session.

Chapter 2 defined the scope of practice for therapeutic massage. It is important to carefully explain the limitations of massage to the client, to put into perspective the expectations, and to help define the outcome for the massage. It is important to do this before the massage begins.

Massage that is performed without the supervision of a licensed medical professional is considered a personal service. Personal service activities are more focused to the general well being of the client as opposed to the treatment of a specific disorder. At this time, the standards of training in the United States of five hundred to one thousand hours of education are more focused to the health-enhancing wellness and personal service approach to therapeutic massage. Many clients confuse these health services with a medical treatment. Massage can be an effective medical intervention but only with medical supervision and extensive additional education. Massage therapists in Ontario, British Columbia, and other Canadian provinces are educated more extensively than wellness personal service levels of training in the United States. With this additional education, they are able to use massage therapy intervention in the medical setting. Clients seeking basic wellness personal service massage for health enhancement need to understand the limitations of this level of education. The massage practitioner needs to educate the client so that the expectations of the effects of massage are for increased general well being and efficient body function. The practitioner needs to help the client understand the difference between the medical intervention of massage and the general effects of increased well being and health enhancement offered through receiving therapeutic massage. Refer the client whose expectations are focused around specific treatment of a medical condition.

The massage therapist must be concerned with how the client thinks a massage is to be given. If the client has never had a massage, then expectations will be determined by what has been heard, read, or observed. Because methods and applications of massage vary so much, the client may not expect the style of massage that is offered. The difference in what is expected and what is received may be confusing. The client's answer to a simple question such as, "What do you think a massage is like?" or, "Describe for me how a massage would be done" will give the massage practitioner an idea of what expectations the client has for the session. The massage practitioner should explain the different approaches that are used so the client is not lying on the table wondering why this massage is so different from what was expected.

If a client has had a massage before from someone else, it is natural to compare the different styles. It is important for the massage practitioner to explain the procedures and methods that are used so the client understands there are many ways to do massage. NEVER discount another massage therapist's methods or approach and say that your way is better. This is unethical behavior. The only exception to this rule is if the massage previously received was in violation of professional standards and ethics. It is important to explain to the client that massage therapists do not conduct themselves in a manner that violates professional codes of ethics. Using the example of the code of ethics in this textbook or one from one of the professional organizations can be a framework for the discussion (see Chapter 2).

The outcome for massage is what the client can anticipate in response from the benefits of the proposed massage plan. Each massage manipulation has an anticipated response. A client can be made aware of these benefits and any risks to the proposed massage session. Do not confuse expectations with outcome.

For example, the client has never had a massage before, but a friend in another city regularly receives therapeutic massage. The client explains that the massage the friend receives is for a chronic headache problem that seems to be related to daily stress and the massage helps a lot (expectation). When asked why this client came for a massage (the outcome), the explanation is that there are no real problems, although sometimes there are headaches, just like the friend. The client thinks a massage would feel good. The outcome is a basic massage that feels good, not a more specific approach to get rid of headaches.

The expectations are based on information from the friend. It is natural for the first-time client to consider this information, but the outcome is very different. If the massage therapist is not careful to differentiate the two, than the massage provided for the client may not meet the client's needs.

Some questions to ask in order to help determine the client's outcome are:
- Why do you wish to receive a massage?
- How do you want to feel after the massage?
- What do you think massage will do for you?
- What results do you want from the massage?

Then carefully go over all the client policies and procedures as discussed in Chapter 7. Never assume that a client understands the complexities of massage practice. Explain everything in detail.

HISTORY TAKING

Once the client understands the scope of practice of massage, the type of massage that will be provided to fit with his or her expectations, and the general outcome for the massage has been determined, then it is time to take a **history.** In actuality, the history-taking process and determination of client expectations and outcome are often the same.

For wellness massage covered in this book, the history serves three functions.
1. Determines contraindications (see Chapter 4).
2. Decides if the client needs to be referred.
3. Provides information for designing the massage.

Extensive assessment procedures, including the client history, are discussed in Chapter 11. This section will only discuss the process of obtaining a history.

Take a client history using a client information form (See Fig. 7.7, pg. 169). This form requests information such as name, address, phone numbers, age, occupation, medical and health information, names of *all* doctors or chiropractors, and any special situations. It usually contains a disclaimer stating that the massage therapist may not diagnose or treat any specific medical condition and that the massage is provided for the purposes of health enhancement and stress reduction.

A history can be taken simply by giving the client the form to fill out and then reading it before the massage to decide if there are contraindications or if the client needs to be referred. Chapter 11 teaches the use of the client information form as an interviewing tool. Sit with the client and ask the questions. Use the time to discuss the client's situation and get to know the client as a person. Do not hesitate to ask the client questions about any current condition or medication. Look up the medications in a *Physicians Desk Reference* or similar resource book. Use a medical dictionary to look up any conditions you do not understand. Also use the time to explain to the client why you need to know this information. Explain to the client what a contraindication is, and explain the benefits of massage.

Plan on approximately thirty minutes during the first client visit to take a history and obtain informed consent. This detailed process only needs to be done once. Because it is the responsibility of the massage therapist to maintain up-to-date records, it is suggested that the entire process of establishing appropriate client expectations, determining the client's outcome, and updating the history is done periodically. A general guide is once every three months for a regular client. If the client is not seen regularly (at least once a month), then there is a need to be more specific with reestablishing this very important link and obtaining this information from the client each visit. A new client information form may not be necessary, but a notation regarding updated information needs to be made.

It is possible that in some states or jurisdictions a specific, written treatment plan is required for each visit. It is the responsibility of the massage therapist to be in compliance with all regulations pertinent to the professional practice of therapeutic massage.

CLIENT FILES

The client information form, signed client policies and procedures (as described in Chapter 7), and all updates along with S.O.A.P. notes (a charting procedure) on each session with the client (described in detail in Chapter 11) become an important part of the client's file. Maintain these records in an organized and professional manner. Keep them in a secured and fire-resistant filing cabinet.

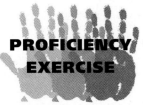

PROFICIENCY EXERCISE

- **Use your client information form to interview three of your fellow students. Make additions or corrections in the form based on these interviews.**

PRE-MASSAGE PROCEDURES

SECTION OBJECTIVES

Using the information presented in this section, the student will be able to:

1 Explain the general massage plan to a client.

2 Obtain informed consent from the client.

After the history-taking process, the client is ready to enter the massage room. It is recommended that the client be given an orientation of the area. Before leaving the client to prepare for the massage, it is important that the massage sequence be explained in step-by-step detail. The massage practitioner will need to obtain informed consent from the client for all massage procedures before the massage begins. This means that all procedures, benefits, possible risks, and projected outcome of the massage plan have been explained to the client, and the client understands and agrees with the massage plan.

Following is the step-by-step orientation process:

1. Take client to the massage area.
2. Show where clothes may be hung. Explain to the client to remove only the amount of clothing necessary and to leave on underclothing. If you have any other special requirements about clothing, now is the time it should be disclosed.

3. Show the massage table, how it is draped, and how the draping will work. Explain the requested starting position (prone, supine, side-lying) on the table.

4. If using a massage chair or mat, show how to use the chair or mat for proper positioning.

5. Ask about the use of music, and offer a few selections.

6. Reveal the restroom location and the procedure for getting there if it is not next to the massage area.

7. Briefly explain any charts you may have on the walls.

8. Ask about a lubricant. Show what you have and offer a choice. It is important for clients to choose the type of lubricant or have the option for no lubricant to avoid any misrepresentation by the massage therapist of diagnosing or prescribing.

9. Explain that you will leave the room to allow for privacy while the client undresses. The exception to this would be if a client is a very elderly person or a woman in an advanced stage of pregnancy who requests assistance (or any other special situation when the client would require the massage therapist's assistance). If staying in the room, explain how assistance will be provided and modesty maintained. This is usually done by holding up a sheet in front of the client or by using a screen.

10. Explain all sanitary precautions, and show these to the client.

11. Show the sign on the door stating that a massage is in session, and explain why the door is not locked.

12. Give a general idea of the massage flow. For example, explain that the massage will start on the back and take about ten minutes, and then the legs and feet will be done for fifteen minutes. Explain that any alteration in a basic pattern, such as if more time is spent on the neck, then less time will be available for doing the back.

13. Instruct the client to get on the table by sitting between the end of the table and the hinged area (if portable table) or in the middle of the table (if free standing table). Next, the client should lean on one side and roll to the supine or prone position. For the client to get off the table, it is just the opposite. The person rolls to one side, pushes up to a seated position, and sits for a minute to avoid any dizziness. Then, the client gets off the table. If there is any chance that the client may fall or need assistance getting on or off the table, stay in the room to help. Demonstrate the procedures if necessary, but do not use any draping materials placed on the table. It is unsanitary for anything or anyone to touch the drapes before the client uses them.

14. Ask if there are any questions.

15. Explain that while you are occupied with washing your hands and preparing for the massage, the client should get ready.

16. Tell the client how long you will be gone and that you will knock and announce yourself before entering the room.

Any modifications that need to be made because of the location and environment of the massage should to be taken into consideration. People can become anxious if they do not know how to do what they are supposed to do. Do not assume that a client remembers the instructions or has knowledge of what to do or expect. Explain all steps in detail.

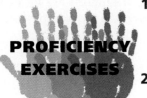

PROFICIENCY EXERCISES

1. **Get a massage from three different practicing massage therapists and evaluate their performance on history taking, setting realistic expectations, developing an outcome for the massage, obtaining informed consent, and informing you of the pre-massage information.**

2. **Develop a checklist of everything that the client needs to know before preparing for the massage.**

3. **Role play with three other students with one being the first-time client, one being the massage practitioner, and the other evaluating the performance. Practice using the checklist, explaining procedures to the client, and obtaining informed consent. Switch roles so that each student plays all three parts.**

FOCUS/CENTERING

While waiting for the client to prepare for the massage, it is important for the therapist to do the same. There are many ways to do this. Slow, deep breathing combined with stretching slows the mind and focuses the attention into the body. Looking at a nature scene or a painting is another way. Listening to music or performing some sort of repetitive behavior like washing your hands under warm water while visualizing the water carrying away all concerns for the next hour can become a trigger for focus. The goal is to be present in the moment for the client and not focused on lists of things that need to be done. If a routine sequence is developed, the practitioner will become calm and centered much faster.

PROFICIENCY EXERCISES

1. **Develop three different ways to focus attention before beginning the massage. Make note of your ideas for future reference.**
2. **Work with three students and teach each other ways to focus.**
3. **Discuss what works and what does not work in focusing.**

POSITIONING AND DRAPING THE CLIENT

SECTION OBJECTIVES

Using the information presented in this section, the student will be able to:

❶ Position, drape, and perform a massage session in four basic positions.
❷ Drape effectively with two basic styles.

The basic positions for massage are supine or face up, prone or face down, side-lying, and seated. The intent of this section is to learn to use body supports and proper draping for these basic positions.

It is possible that a client will be in all four of the positions during a massage session. Staying in one position for any longer than fifteen minutes may become uncomfortable. The exception would be a painful situation that limits the client's ability to move with ease.

Pillows or other supports, such as folded towels, blankets, or specially designed pieces of foam, are used for client comfort. They fill any gaps in the contours when the client is positioned and provide for soft areas to lean against. Supports are generally used under the knees, ankles, and neck. After the first trimester, a pregnant woman will most likely be comfortable in a side-lying position. If a client has a large abdomen, supports need to be used to lift the chest and support the abdomen. This can be done with foam with an area cut out for the abdomen. Women with large breasts may need a chest pillow. Side-lying positions require pillows or supports for the arms and a small support between the knees. Clients with lower back pain may be more comfortable with a support under their abdomens when lying prone.

Moving the client's position will require shifting the body supports. All supports need to be under the sanitary drape or protected with sanitary coverings that are changed after each client.

Practice efficient shifting of body supports. If supports are located under the sheets, simply fold the bottom sheet over the top to expose the supports and move them (Fig. 9.11).

Draping has two purposes:
1. Maintaining client privacy and sense of security. The drape becomes the boundary between the therapist and the client. It is a way to establish touch as professional. Respect for the client's personal privacy and

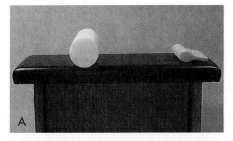
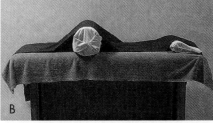
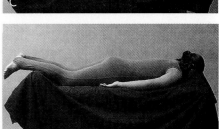

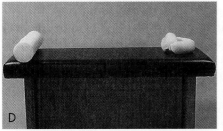
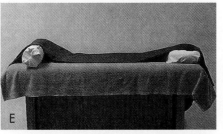
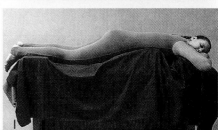

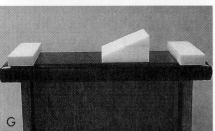
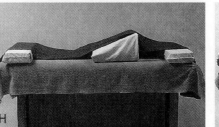
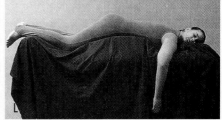

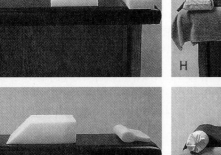
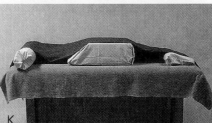
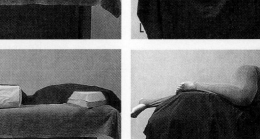

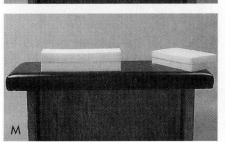
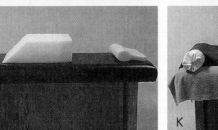

Figure 9.11
Use of support in five positions: A–C, supine. D–F, prone. G–I, large chest. J–L, low back support. M–O, sidelying. (For supporting a client with a large abdomen, see Fig. 12.5. The prenatal massage position incorporates use of supports for large abdomen.)

boundaries fosters an environment in which the client's welfare is being safeguarded.

2. Warmth.

There are many ways to drape. The main principles to follow during draping are:

- All draping material must be freshly laundered using a bleach or other approved solution. See Chapter 5 on sanitation. Disposable linen must be fresh for each client.
- Only the area being massaged is undraped.
- The genital area and the breast area of a woman are never undraped. (The exception is for specific medical massage under the supervision of a licensed medical professional. In Canada, breast massage for medical purposes has a specific process and consent process. These methods are

out of the scope of practice for the massage practitioner as defined in this text.)
- Draping methods should cover the client in all positions, including the seated position.

Using draping materials is a bit clumsy at first. To assure the modesty of the first few practice clients, have them leave all clothing on.

If the client uses a dressing area away from the massage table, then a robe, top sheet, or a wrap large enough to cover the body will be needed while walking to the massage area. If a wrap or top sheet is used, it can become the top drape once the client is on the table.

The two basic types of draping used are flat draping and contoured draping. In flat draping, the top sheet is placed over the client in the same manner that a bed is made, with a bottom sheet and a top sheet. Instruct the client to lie supine, prone, or side-lying between the drapes on the massage table. The entire body is covered. The top drape, and sometimes the bottom drape, is moved in various ways to cover and uncover the area to be massaged.

Important Note:

To ensure the privacy of male clients, the massage therapist needs to avoid smooth flat draping over the genitals while the male client is supine (face up). The penis may become partially erect resulting from parasympathetic activation or a reflexive response of the massage. This response is purely physiologic and does not necessarily suggest sexual arousal. Loose draping that does not lie flat against the body provides for a visual shield.

Contoured draping can be done with two towels or with a sheet and a towel. The drapes are wrapped and shaped around the client. This type of draping is very effective for securely covering and shielding the genital and buttock area. Placing the drape in the position may feel invasive, so having the client assist in placement of the drapes preserves a sense of modesty. A separate chest towel can be used to drape the breast area of a woman.

The following photographs will lead you step-by-step through several draping procedures. Practice them, and then combine the methods to fit the particular needs of the client.

An alternative to draping is to have the client wear a swimsuit or shorts and a loose shirt. The table or mat must be sanitarily covered with a bottom drape and a top drape needs to be available because the client may become chilled even if partially clothed. When working with a client who is wearing clothing or a swimsuit, it is still necessary to observe all the precautions for privacy and respect (Fig. 9.12).

These draping procedures will provide a starting point for modest and secure use of towels and sheets for proper and appropriate draping. Many other methods are available and can be developed.

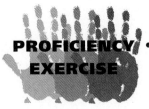

PROFICIENCY EXERCISE • **Obtain three different professional massages, and observe how the massage therapist drapes and uses body supports.**

AFTER THE MASSAGE

Once the massage is completed, the client will need to be left alone and allowed between five and ten minutes to rest. Reenter the massage area to help the client off the table if special needs exist (Fig. 9.13 on page 220).

To help a person off the table:
1. Reach under the client's neck and knees
2. Support the sheet loosely around the client's neck, and hold it so that it does not slip when the person is lifted

(Text continued on page 218.)

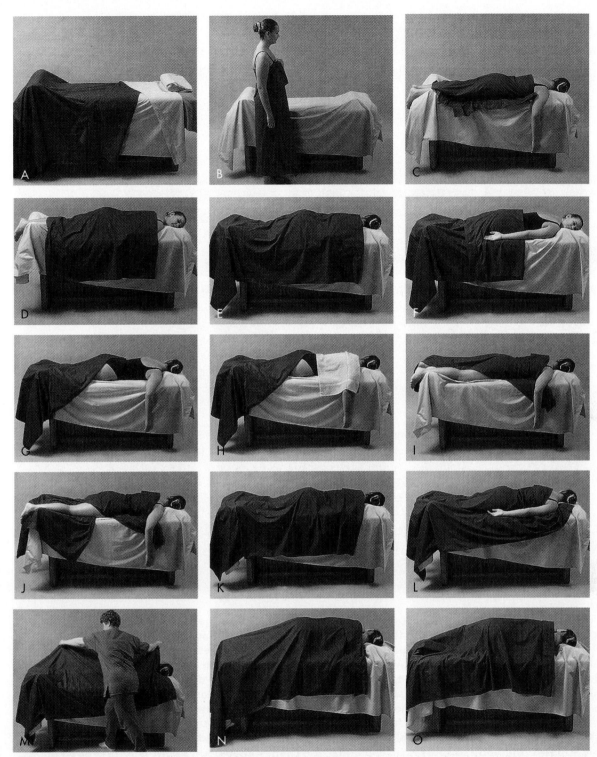

Figure 9.12
Samples of draping sequences using sheets and towels.
A, Basic table set up for draping. B, Client wrapped in top sheet. Top sheet is folded in half with fold at the top and end held in the front. C, Client lies in prone position and sides of drape are moved to the side of the table. D, Drape is spread to cover client. E, Client fully draped in prone position. F, Drape is folded back to provide access to back. G, Drape is folded again on the diagonal to provide access to gluteal region. H, A towel is used to drape the back while the gluteal region is massaged. I, Drape is repositioned to cover client and towel is removed. The end of drape is folded on the diagonal to provide access to the leg. J, Drape is positioned under the leg to be massaged to secure it. K, The client is re-draped. L, The arm is positioned over the drape and the drape is held secure by the arm. M, Position for holding the drape while client turns to side. Drape is held in the middle in a tent fashion. The massage therapist's knee secures the drape against the table. N, Client in side lying position with full draping. O, Client with top leg drawn up and supported with body support. *continued*

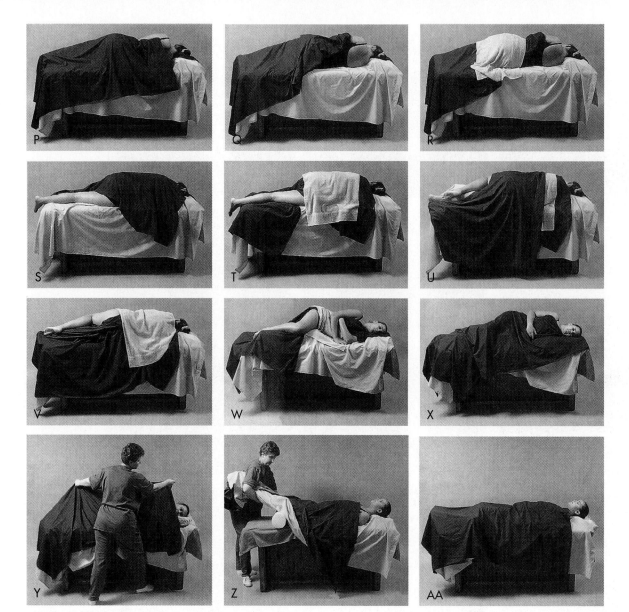

Figure 9.12 *continued*

P, Drape folded under top arm to provide access to arm. **Q,** Top corner of drape folded diagonally to provide access to back. **R,** Towel positioned to drape the gluteal area. **S,** Client with back redraped and end corner of drape folded diagonal to provide access to leg. **T,** Drape moved under exposed lower leg and towel used to drape gluteal area. Drape is secured under lower leg. **U,** Lower leg is redraped and opposite end corner of drape is folded diagonally to provide access to upper leg. **V,** Folded corner of drape is brought through the legs and secured under upper leg. Towel is used to drape the gluteal and abdominal area. **W,** Front view of this position. Notice that drape across the chest is secured under the client's head. **X,** Client is re-draped and towels are removed. **Y,** Drape is held in tent fashion and secured against the table with the therapist's knee as the client turns to supine position. **Z,** Both top and bottom drape are folded over client's legs to provide access to body support; the body support is placed under the client's knees. **AA,** Client is fully draped in supine position.

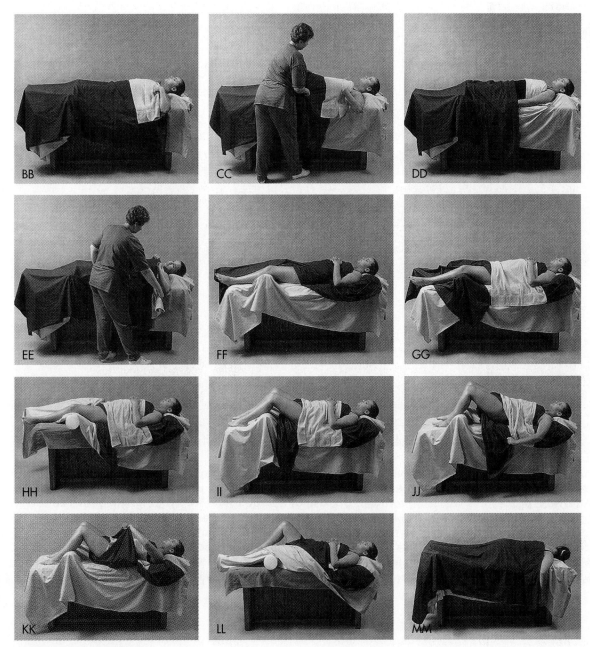

Figure 9.12 *continued*

BB, Towel is placed on the client's chest over the top drape. Client holds the towel in place. CC, The therapist pulls top of drape from under towel to provide access to abdomen. DD, Drape is repositioned over towel. EE, Towel is removed from underneath the drape. FF, The lower corner of top drape is folded diagonally to provide access to the client's leg. GG, Top drape is positioned under client's leg and secured by the leg. Towel is placed over the client's abdomen and groin area. HH, Lower corner of bottom drape is brought under leg diagonally and draped over opposite leg. This exposes the secondary sanitary bottom drape. Notice that client's leg does not touch the body support. This draping provides a secured groin covering while massaging, stretching, or providing range of motion to the leg. II, Alternate leg draping to provide access to both legs and to provide secure groin draping. Client bends knees and both end corners of drape are folded diagonally and positioned between the knees. The corners are spread at either side of the table. JJ, Client grasps each corner, lifts buttocks, and pulls drape under them. KK, Client or therapist can then tie ends together to secure the drape. LL, One leg is lower and the bottom drape is used to cover it, leaving only the area to be massaged exposed. MM, Client prone and fully draped. *continued*

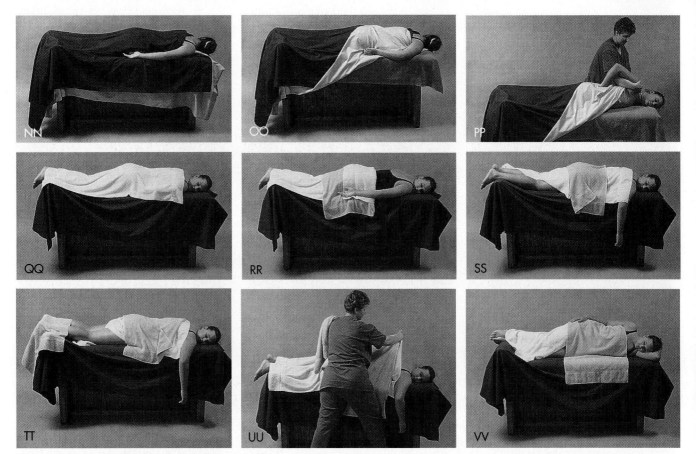

Figure 9.12 continued
NN, Client's arm is positioned outside of drape. **OO,** The corners of both the top and bottom drapes are folded diagonally under the arm and over the back. **PP,** Therapist secures the bottom drape while moving the shoulder and arm. Alternate procedures for using a towel. **QQ,** Use of a large towel for draping. **RR,** Bath size towel is placed over gluteal area for additional drape while top of towel is folded back to provide access to the client's back. **SS,** Back is redraped and end corners of towel are folded diagonally to provide access to legs. **TT,** Folded towel ends are placed between client's knees and additional towel is added to cover the feet. **UU,** Foot towel is removed, and large and small towel are secured against the table by the therapist's knee and lifted to allow client to turn to side position. **VV,** Large towel and bath size towel are repositioned over client.

3. Lift the client's torso off the table while swinging the knees around to the edge of the table
4. Stabilize the client for a moment in case of dizziness
5. Still holding the sheet, help the client to a standing position
6. Shift the position of the sheet so that the client can hold it securely

In rare instances, the client may need help with dressing. Let the client do as much as possible. Be very matter-of-fact and deliberate with any assistance.

If a client is left to get off the table alone, remind him or her of the following:

1. Roll to one side
2. Use the arms to push to a seated position
3. Sit for a minute before getting up
4. Leave the sheets on the table
5. Get dressed and return to the business area

After the client is dressed and ready to leave, make the next appointment or provide a reminder if it already has been made. If the fee is not

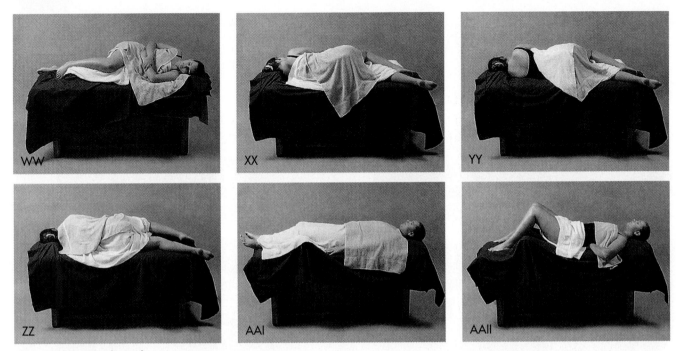

Figure 9.12 continued
WW, Large towel end corner is folded diagonally to provide access to top leg and brought under top leg to be secured between leg and support under bent knee. Additional bath towel is placed over gluteal region. XX, Back view. YY, Top end of drape folded diagonally to provide access to back. ZZ, Drape over gluteal area and bottom lower leg folded up to provide access to bottom leg. AAI, Client draped with towels in supine position. AAII, Client draped to provide access to abdomen and legs. Towel is used over large towel and held in place by client as therapist pulls the large towel under and folds it back to expose the abdomen. Bottom ends of large towel are diagonally folded in and placed between the client's knees with the ends at the side of table so that client is able to grasp the ends of the towel and pull it under them providing secure draping of the groin.

collected in advance, the client should pay at this time. Do not linger in conversation. The attitude in the business area is one of polite and courteous completion. It is often difficult to get a client to leave. After spending extended time in a comfortable and caring environment, the person may want to talk. It is difficult to break this pattern when business increases, so it is best to establish a consistent departure routine. People respond well to sameness. A client will get used to leaving and making the break from the massage therapist more easily if the sequence is always the same.

For example, the client approaches the desk and the massage therapist takes the money, writes a receipt, and confirms the next appointment. The massage therapist gets up from the desk and says, "I really enjoyed working with you today. I am glad that you continue to feel that the massage is beneficial. It will be nice to see you again in two weeks. Remember to do the stretches we talked about, keep track of any changes, and we will discuss them next time I see you." The massage therapist extends a hand for a warm handshake. In some situations, a quick friendly hug is appropriate **only** if initiated by the client. Professionally and respectfully accept hugs or physical contact initiated by the client. Then say good-bye while gesturing or looking toward the door. At this point, it is important for the massage therapist to make a move to leave the area or additional conversation may be initiated by the client.

After the client has left, the therapist needs to update all records, prepare the room for the next client, and attend to personal hygiene and stretching.

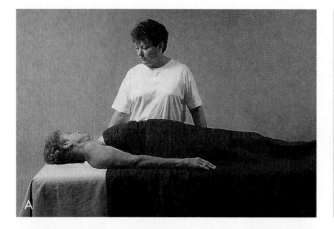
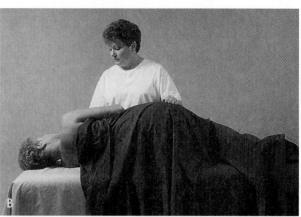
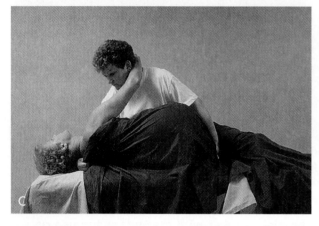
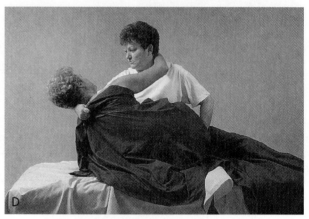
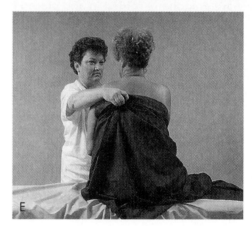

Figure 9.13
A, Assisting a client off of massage table. B, Client rolls to side and bends knees. C, Client wraps arm around therapist's shoulder. D, The therapist brings sheet under head and holds front and back portions together while other hand is behind client's knees, providing support. E, Therapist lifts client by standing up and leaning back while swinging the client's knees over the table to the seated position. Therapist then adjusts drape and assists client from table. The use of a foot stool for the client is helpful. (Please note, C and D are incorrect in that the client is grasping the therapist's neck rather than the shoulder.)

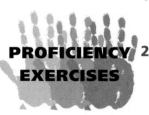

PROFICIENCY EXERCISES

1. Practice helping clients off of the massage table. Find ten different body shapes and sizes to work with, and notice the difference in leverage needed for each client.
2. Write down your departure routine, and practice with other students. What will you do to successfully end a massage session with a client who does not want to leave? Have one of the students in your practice group role play this situation, and see how successful your procedure works.

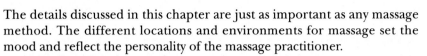

SUMMARY

The details discussed in this chapter are just as important as any massage method. The different locations and environments for massage set the mood and reflect the personality of the massage practitioner.

Careful consideration of equipment such as massage tables and body supports, supplies such as oils and linens, and music and other amenities provides not only the necessary equipment, but also a personalized approach.

Taking time to explain massage procedures to a client, taking a basic history, and learning and understanding the expectations and outcome for each massage will help to create an approach that is not only effective, but meets the needs of the client. Providing safe and respectful touch by using careful and modest draping procedures and positioning is very important.

This chapter has described professional skills that create the confidence, respect, and trust important to the successful application of therapeutic massage. Attention to these details is necessary in the professional massage practice.

REVIEW QUESTIONS

1. What matters need to be considered before the massage actually begins?
2. What is the most important piece of massage equipment?
3. How do you protect the massage therapist's hands?
4. What types of massage equipment provide a surface that supports the client while the massage is given?
5. What features should be considered when looking for a massage table?
6. What needs to be checked on the massage table to ensure client safety?
7. What are body supports?
8. What are drapes?
9. What types of draping materials are available?
10. What consideration needs to be made for clients with sensitive skin?
11. What sanitary measures must be taken with draping materials?
12. What is the purpose of lubricants?
13. What types of lubricants are used?
14. What are some important things to remember about lubricants?
15. What are some general considerations for creating a good massage environment?
16. What are the main types of massage environments?

17. What special consideration needs to be made for the use of music?

18. What consideration needs to be made concerning lighting in the massage room?

19. Why is a scentless environment so important?

20. What other considerations need to be made for client comfort?

21. Why must the massage therapist educate the client about appropriate expectations for the massage session?

22. What is the importance of a client history?

23. Why does the massage practitioner carefully explain all procedures to the client before the massage begins?

24. What are the basic massage positions for a client, and how are body supports used in these positions?

25. What are specific rules concerning draping?

26. How is the drape a type of boundary?

27. What are the two basic types of draping procedures?

28. How is a chest towel used?

29. How do you assist a client to a seated position?

30. What is the attitude of the massage practitioner at the conclusion of the massage?

31. After the client leaves, what activities does the massage therapist need to attend to?

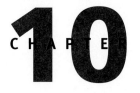
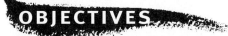 OBJECTIVES

After completing this chapter, the student will be able to do the following:

1 Explain the basic theory for physiologic effects of massage methods and techniques.

2 Organize the massage methods and techniques into basic flow patterns.

3 Perform a full-body massage using the methods and techniques presented.

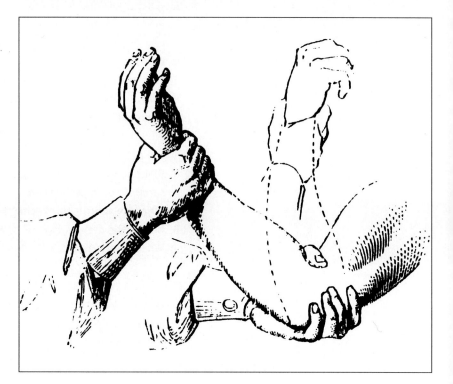

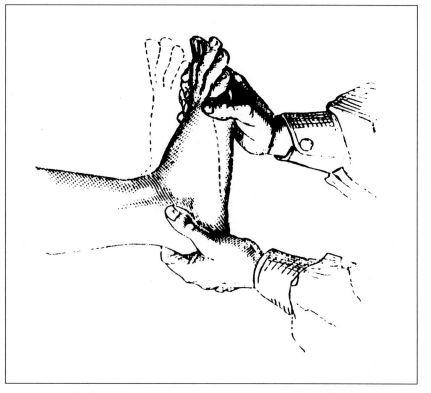

Passive mobilization of the soft tissues and joints for assessment and treatment.

INTRODUCTION

This core technical chapter includes definitions, descriptions, and directions for the applications and uses of all massage methods and techniques. Background concepts are given for each massage technique. As a massage therapy student, you must learn to think things through for variations of application. Massage routines offer limited benefits. Each session needs to be designed specifically for each individual client (see Chapter 11).

It is important to understand both why and where massage methods and techniques are used, and how to organize a process that uses the various therapeutic approaches efficiently. The next step is to examine each of the individual massage manipulations and techniques and to learn how to use them well. In the practice of therapeutic massage, the tools used by the practitioner are the fingers, thumbs, hands, forearms, and, for some methods like shiatsu, the knees and feet. Our focus will be on methods that use the fingers, thumbs, hands, and forearms. You should always stay mindful of how to best use your body when applying the tools of massage, as stated in Chapter 8.

The massage professional uses a structured, purposeful application of various forms of touch for specific reasons. Since the late 1800s these massage manipulations have used the French names of effleurage, petrissage, compression, vibration, tapotement, and friction. The current trend is to use English descriptions; both are acceptable.

Mosby's Medical, Nursing, and Allied Health Dictionary[9] defines *manipulation* as "the skillful use of the hands in therapeutic or diagnostic procedures . . . see also massage." The same reference defines *massage* as "the manipulation of the soft tissue of the body through stroking, rubbing, kneading, or tapping . . . " The word *manipulation* will be used in this chapter to indicate each of these methods.

It is important to differentiate between the soft tissue manipulations of the massage professional and the joint manipulations of the chiropractor, osteopath, or physical therapist. The massage professional does not perform specific, direct, joint manipulations. Massage techniques that incorporate passive and active joint movement within the physiologic barrier of the joint, as well as lengthening and stretching methods, may indirectly affect the range of motion of a joint through changes in the soft tissue. The focus of the massage professional is on the soft tissue and not the osseous structure of the joint. Often a combination of soft tissue work and specific joint manipulation is required. In these instances, the massage practitioner, with appropriate training, becomes part of the multidisciplinary team under the supervision of the health care professional. This type of approach provides the skills and expertise to best serve the client.

A NOTE TO THE READER:

Most models in this chapter are pictured in leotards or sportswear in order to enhance and clarify the various body positions. The properly groomed massage professional would wear a uniform as shown in Figure 5.1 on page 108.

PHYSIOLOGIC EFFECTS

Using the information presented in this section, the student will be able to do the following:

❶ Classify massage manipulations and techniques into three categories based on reflexive, mechanical, and chemical effects.

❷ Categorize the effects of massage methods and techniques into stimulating or inhibiting physiologic responses.

In general, massage manipulations and techniques either stimulate or inhibit a response. When thinking in terms of muscle, think of toning (causing it to contract) or relaxing (reduction of the neural stimulation causing contraction) the muscle. Connective tissue deals with tissue that is too hard, too soft, too thick, or too thin. Regarding circulation, there is rushing fluid flow and sluggish fluid flow. With nervous system activity, think of overactivity or underactivity. Simply stated, imbalances fall into two categories, "too much" or "not enough." Massage methods restore balance by inhibition of "too much" conditions and the stimulation of the "not enough" conditions.

All massage methods use forms of external sensory information that can stimulate or inhibit body processes, depending on their use. Some methods are better at stimulation and others are better at inhibition. Some work better with mechanical effects, others with reflexive effects, and still others are better at initiating chemical responses. In general, fast, specific applications of methods tend to stimulate, while slow general applications tend to inhibit.

It is not easy to generalize the mechanical, reflexive, or chemical effect of massage manipulations and techniques. It is often a combination of the effects coupled with the client's psychologic state and receptivity to the massage that causes the response. Begin the "thinking-things-through" process here:

- Methods that move through the skin to the underlying tissue tend to be more mechanical and will stimulate localized chemical responses.
- Massage manipulations and techniques that stay within the skin and superficial fascial layer tend to have a more direct effect on the nervous system. Many sensory nerves are located in the skin. These methods also tend to stimulate the release of hormonal and other body chemicals that provide for a general systemic (whole body) effect.
- Methods that move the body, causing muscles to contract and joint positions to change, deliver sensory input to the proprioceptors and are more reflexive in nature.
- Methods that stretch (pull on) soft tissues are reflexive, mechanical, and chemical in their effect.

QUALITY OF TOUCH

Using the information presented in this section, the student will be able to do the following:

❶ Evaluate massage manipulations based on seven criteria.

Gertrude Beard, one of the most respected educators for massage therapy, as an integral part of physical therapy described the components of massage as follows:

"The factors that must be considered as components in the application of massage techniques are: the direction of the movement, the amount of pressure, the rate and rhythm of the movements, the medium used, the frequency and duration of the treatment, the position of the patient and of the physical therapist."[2]

Beard's definition of "medium" had to do with the application of lubricants or other instruments used. The definition of "frequency" reflected how often per day or week the massage was given. From Beard's information and other sources, the following components for the quality of touch are considered in this textbook. Individual methods vary in relation to the depth of pressure, drag, direction, speed, rhythm, frequency, and duration.

Depth of pressure (compressive stress) can be light, moderate, deep, or variable. *Drag* is the amount of pull (stretch) on the tissue (tensile stress). *Direction* can move from the center of the body out (centrifugal) or from the extremities in toward the center of the body (centripetal). It can proceed from origin to insertion of the muscle following the muscle fibers, transverse to the tissue fibers, or in circular motions.

Speed of manipulations can be fast, slow, or variable. *Rhythm* refers to the regularity of application of the technique. If the method is applied at regular intervals, it is considered even or rhythmic. If the method is disjointed or irregular, it is considered uneven or non-rhythmic. *Frequency* is the rate at which the method repeats itself in a given time frame. In general, each method is repeated about three times before moving or switching to a different approach. *Duration* is the length of time that the method lasts or the manipulation stays in the same location.

BASIC FLOW

Using the information presented in this section, the student will be able to do the following:

1 Organize a massage sequence in four basic patterns.

2 Use a specific massage pattern on the abdomen.

Organization of the various massage manipulations and techniques must follow a cohesive pattern. During a full-body massage, all the soft tissues are addressed and the joints are moved within their physiologic ranges of motion. For purposes of learning, it is helpful to begin with four general patterns and then make modifications. The patterns presented cover the client beginning prone, supine, lying on his or her side, and seated. The sequence used on the abdomen always remains the same.

Pattern 1: Prone Position (Fig. 10.1)
Beginning point BACK. Ending point FACE.

Sequence:

Left side back
Left side gluteal region
Move to head and contact both sides of back
Neck
Move to right side
Right side back
Right side gluteal region
Right leg back
Move to feet
Contact both legs from back
Move to left side
Left leg back
(Turn client to supine position)
Right foot
Right leg front
Left foot
Left leg front
(Have client bend knees to prepare for abdominal massage)
(Abdominal pattern)
Left arm and hand
Left shoulder and upper thorax (chest)
Right arm and hand
Right shoulder and upper thorax
Neck
Head
Face

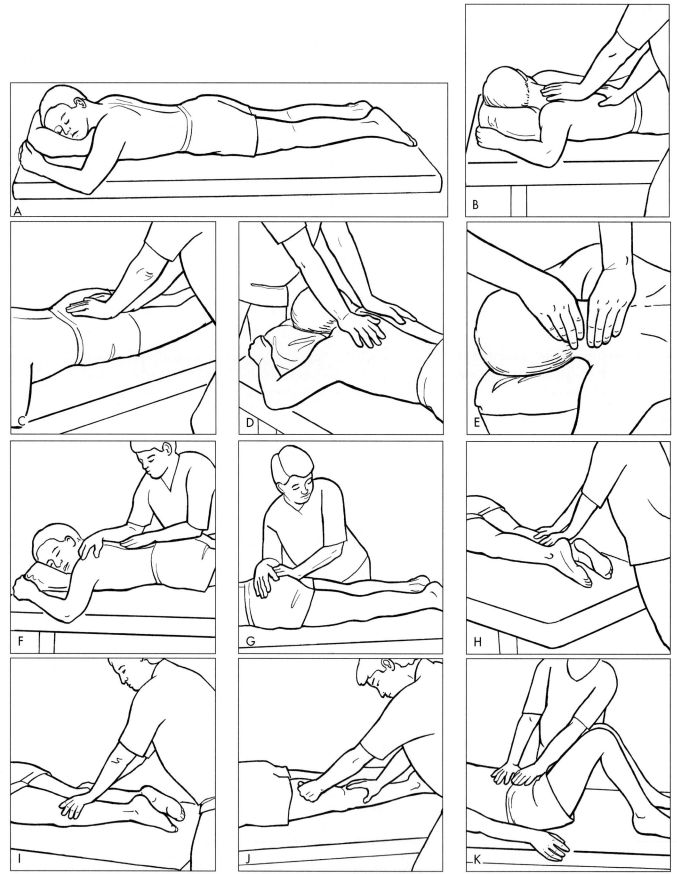

Figure 10.1   Pattern 1. A, Prone position Beginning point BACK. Ending point FACE. Sequence: **B,** Left side back. **C,** Left side gluteal region. **D,** Move to head and contact both sides of back. **E,** Neck. **F,** Move to right side. Right side back. **G,** Right side gluteal region. **H,** Right leg back. **I,** Move to feet. Contact both legs from back. **J,** Move to left side. Left leg back. **K,** Turn client to supine position.

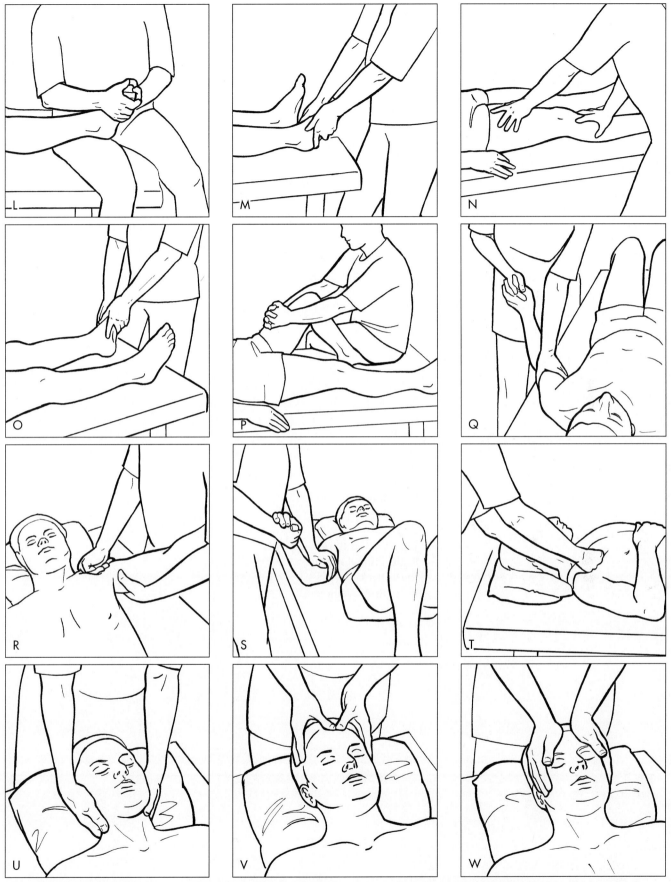

Figure 10.1 *continued*   L & M, Right foot. N, Right leg front. O, Left foot. P, Left leg front. Q, Left arm and hand. R, Left shoulder and upper thorax (chest). S, Right arm and hand. T, Right shoulder and upper thorax. U, Neck. V, Head. W, Face.

Pattern 2: Supine Position (Fig. 10.2)

Beginning point FACE. Ending point BACK.

Sequence:

Face
Head
Neck
Right shoulder and upper thorax
Right arm and hand
Left shoulder and upper thorax
Left arm and hand
(Have client bend knees to prepare for abdominal work)
(Left side for abdominal work [see special section for pattern for abdominal work])
Left leg in bent position
Front upper left leg
Medial upper left leg
Lateral upper left leg
Back upper left leg
Back lower left leg
Lateral lower left leg
Straighten left leg
Left foot
Right leg in bent position
Front upper right leg
Medial upper right leg
Lateral upper right leg
Back upper right leg
Back lower right leg
Lateral lower right leg
Straighten right leg
Right foot
(Turn client to prone position)
Right gluteal region
Right back
Left gluteal region
Left back
Neck
Head

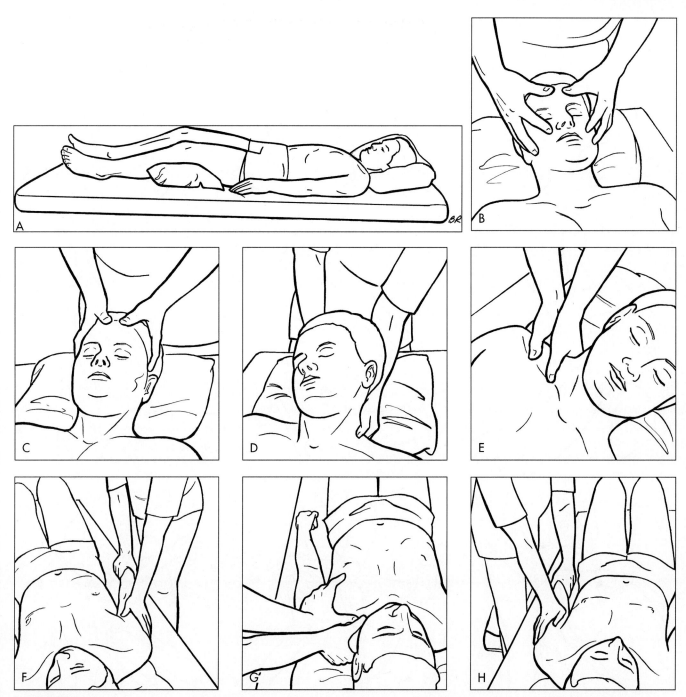

Figure 10.2
Pattern 2. A, Supine position. Beginning point FACE. Ending point BACK. Sequence: B, Face. C, Head. D, Neck. E, Right shoulder and upper thorax. F, Right arm and hand. G, Left shoulder and upper thorax. H, Left arm and hand. Have client bend knees to prepare for abdominal work. Left side for abdominal work (see special section for abdominal work pattern) see Figure 10–5. *continued*

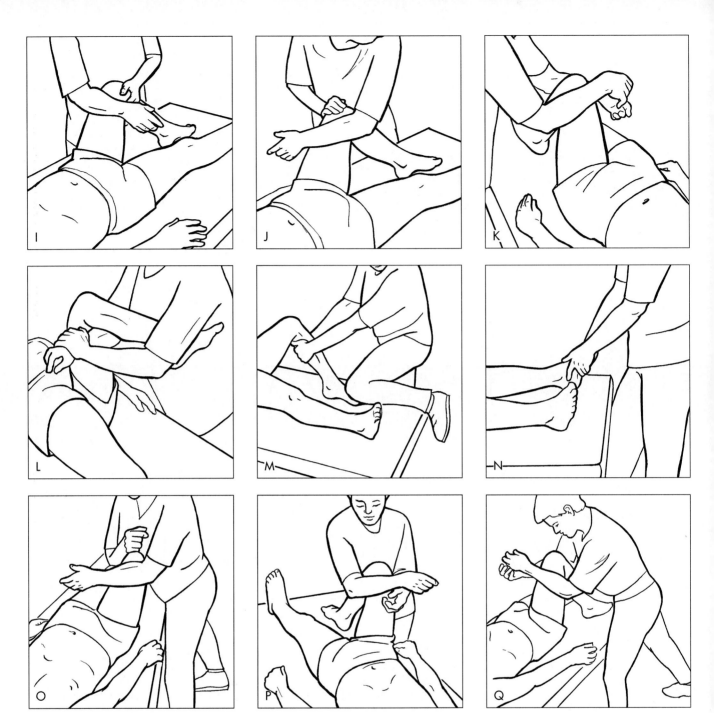

Figure 10.2 *continued*
I, Left leg in bent position. Front upper left leg. J, Medial upper left leg. K, Lateral upper left leg. L, Back upper left leg. M, Back lower left leg. Lateral lower left leg. N, Straighten left leg. Left foot. O, Right leg in bent position. Front upper right leg. P, Medial upper right leg. Q, Lateral upper right leg.

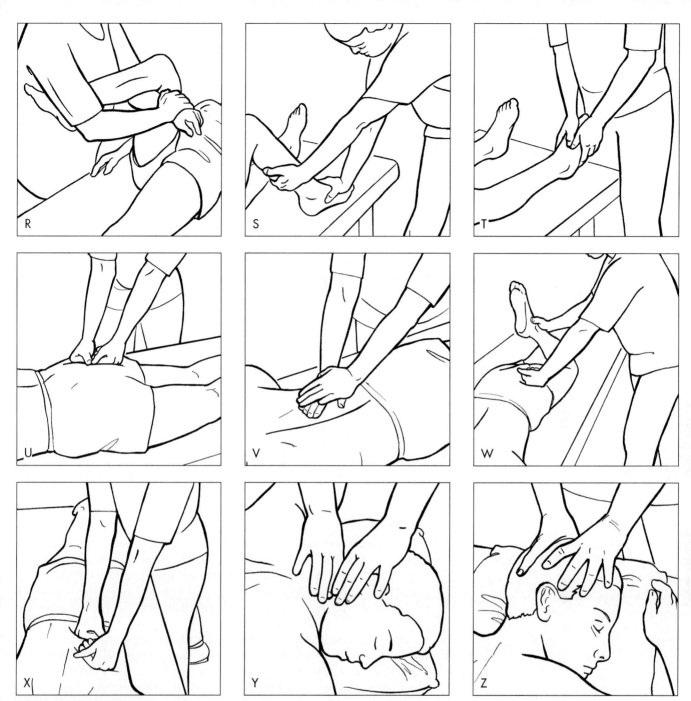

Figure 10.2 *continued*
R, Back upper right leg. S, Back lower right leg. Lateral lower right leg. T, Straighten right leg. Right foot. U, Turn client to prone position. Right gluteal region. V, Right back. W, Left gluteal region. X, Left back. Y, Neck. Z, Head.

Pattern 3: Side-Lying Position (Fig. 10.3)

Beginning point HEAD. Ending point HEAD.

Sequence:

(Client lies on left side with right knee bent and supported)
Right side head
Right side face
Right side neck
Right side shoulder and upper thorax
Right arm and hand
Right side back
(Abdominal pattern)
Right side gluteal
Right back leg
Right lateral leg
Left medial leg
Left foot
(Turn client to right side with left leg bent and supported)
Right foot
Right medial leg
Left lateral leg
Left back leg
Left side gluteal
Left side back
Left side arm and hand
Left side shoulder and upper thorax
Left side neck
Left side head
Left side face

Abdominal Pattern:

To encourage peristalsis and mechanical emptying of the colon, all massage manipulations must be directed in a clockwise fashion. To avoid any chance of impaction of fecal material, the manipulations begin in the lower right-hand quadrant at the sigmoid colon. The methods progressively contact the large intestine and eventually end up encompassing the entire colon area (Fig. 10.4).

Standing on the left side of the body when the client is in the supine position facilitates the body mechanics of the therapist. When the client is lying on his or her side, body mechanics for the massage practitioner and elimination patterns are most efficiently dealt with when the client is lying on the left side (Fig. 10.5). The direction of flow for emptying of the large intestine and colon is as follows:

1. Massage down the left side of the descending colon using short strokes directed to the sigmoid colon.
2. Massage across along the transverse colon to the left side using short strokes directed to the sigmoid colon.
3. Massage up the ascending colon on the right side of the body using short strokes directed to the sigmoid colon.
4. End at the right ileocecal valve located in the lower right-hand quadrant of the abdomen.
5. Massage the entire flow pattern using long, light to moderate strokes from the ileocecal valve to the sigmoid colon. Repeat the sequence.

It is appropriate to develop a combination of the prone, supine, and side-lying positions during the massage session. As you will remember from Chapter 9, client comfort is important when using positioning and supports. Clients may appreciate a positional shift during the massage to

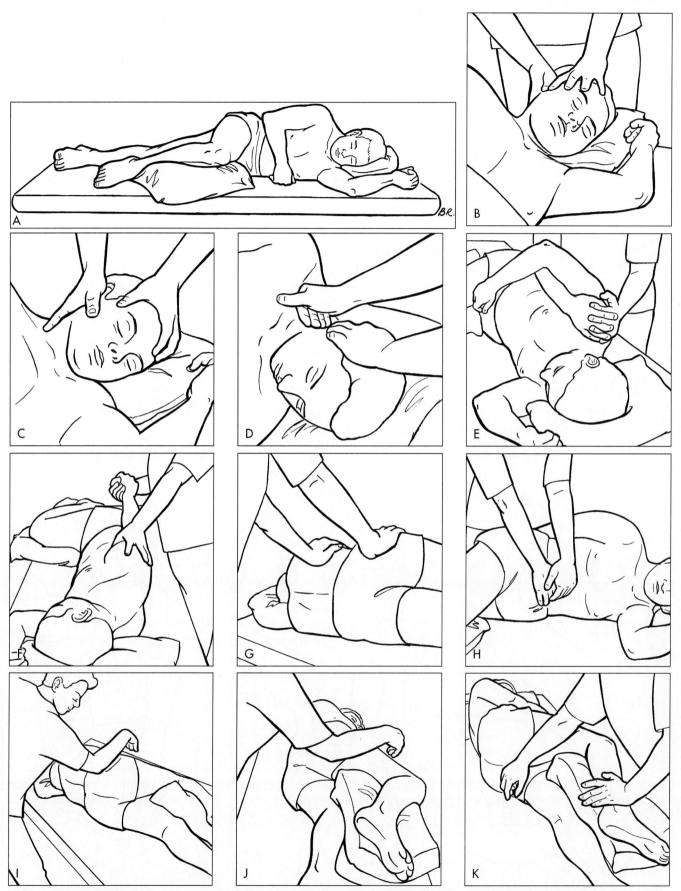

Figure 10.3 Pattern 3. A, Side Lying Position. Beginning point HEAD. Ending point HEAD. Sequence: B, Client lies on left side with right knee bent and supported. Right side head. C, Right side face. D, Right side neck. E, Right side shoulder and upper thorax. F, Right arm and hand. G, Right side back. H, Abdominal pattern. (see Figure 10.5) I, Right side gluteal. J, Right back leg. K, Right lateral leg. *continued*

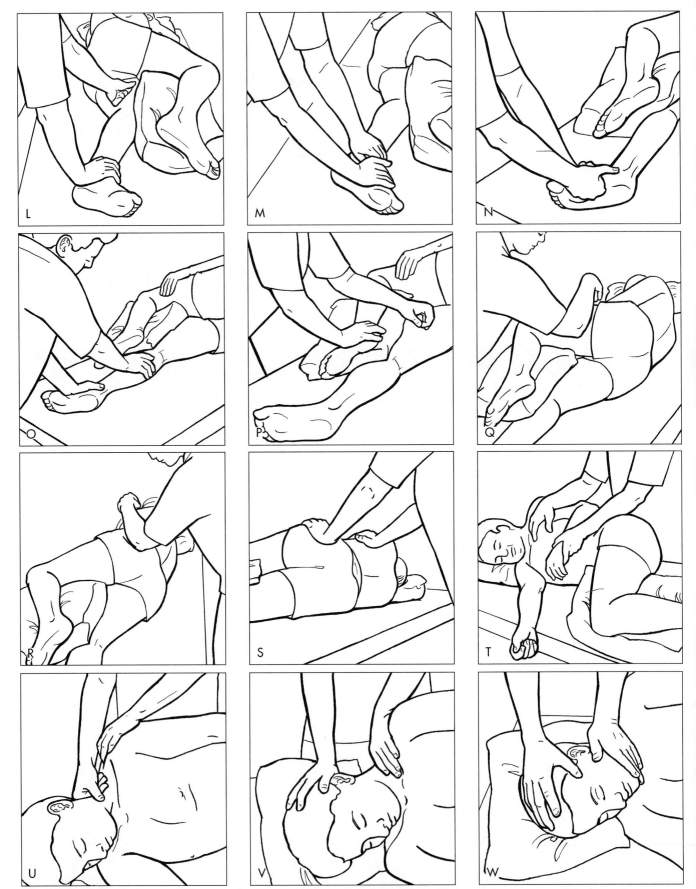

Figure 10.3 *continued* Pattern 3. L, Left medial leg. M, Left foot. N, Turn client to right side with left leg bent and supported. Right foot. O, Right medial leg. P, Left lateral leg. Q, Left back leg. R, Left side gluteal. S, Left side back. T, Left side arm and hand. U, Left side shoulder and upper thorax. V, Left side neck. W, Left side head. Left side face.

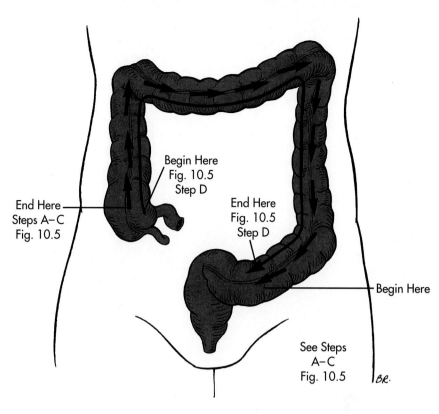

Figure 10.4
Colon with flow pattern arrows. All massage manipulations are to be directed in a clockwise fashion. The manipulations begin in the lower left-hand quadrant (on the right side as you view the illustration) at the sigmoid colon. The methods progressively contact all of the large intestine as they eventually end up encompassing the entire colon area.

Begin Here
Fig. 10.5
Step D

End Here
Steps A–C
Fig. 10.5

End Here
Fig. 10.5
Step D

Begin Here

See Steps
A–C
Fig. 10.5

BR.

Figure 10.5
Abdominal sequence. The direction of flow for emptying of the large intestine and colon is: A, Massage down the left side of the descending colon using short strokes directed to the sigmoid colon. B, Massage across along the transverse colon to the left side using short strokes directed to the sigmoid colon. C, Massage up the ascending colon on the right side of the body using short strokes directed to the sigmoid colon. End at the right side ileocecal valve located in the lower right hand quadrant of the abdomen. D, Massage entire flow pattern using long light strokes to moderate strokes from ileocecal valve to sigmoid colon. Repeat sequence.

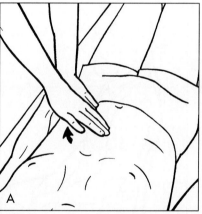

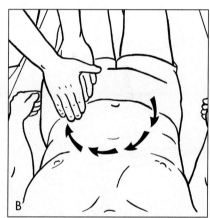

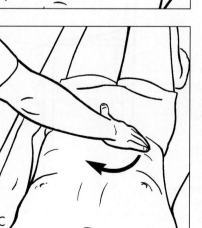

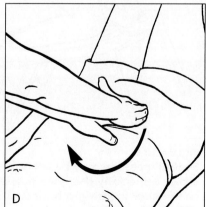

maintain general comfort levels. Inquire about client comfort approximately every fifteen minutes.

There is an additional flow pattern to consider for seated massage. It is important to be able to work efficiently when the client is seated. There are specially designed massage chairs that position the client comfortably and conveniently, but you should not be dependent on such specialized equipment. A regular straight-back chair can be used successfully (Fig. 10.6). Have the client sit facing the back of the chair. Use a pillow on the back of the chair so he or she can lean comfortably.

In this position, which is not used for full-body massage, the clothing is left on. The focus is usually on the upper body only, but with practice the legs and feet can be addressed as well.

Pattern 4: Seated Position (Fig. 10.7)
Begin at HEAD. End at FEET.

Sequence:

Head
Face
Neck
Shoulders
Back—both sides simultaneously
Left arm
Right arm
Left lower leg and foot
Right lower leg and foot

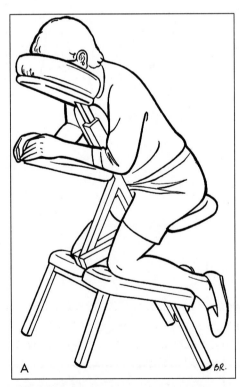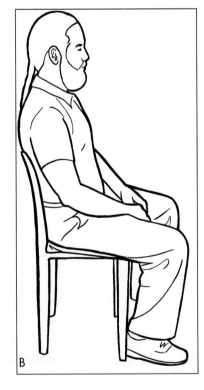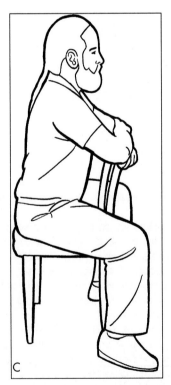

Figure 10.6
Seated massage may be performed in either a specially designed massage chair (A) or in straight back chairs without arms (B,C).

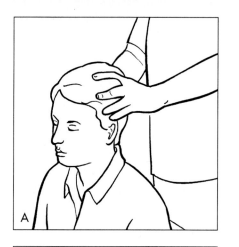

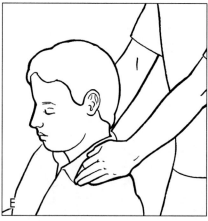

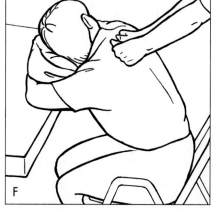

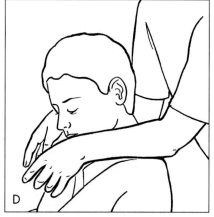

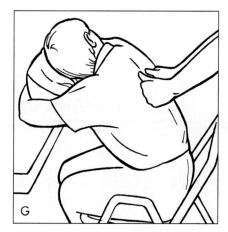

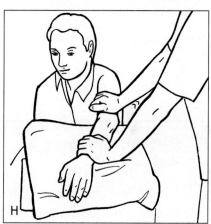

Figure 10.7
Pattern 4. Seated position.
Seated in regular chair. Begin at
HEAD. End at FEET. Sequence
A, Head. B, Face. C, Neck.
D & E, Shoulders. F & G, Back—
both sides simultaneously.
H, Left arm.

continued

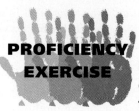

PROFICIENCY
EXERCISE

- **Practice efficiency of movement and ease of positional shift by walking through the patterns. Do not do any massage at this point. Only touch the areas and position the body. Use each massage method with an entire body focus for all four basic flow patterns.**

For example, first move around the entire body using pattern 1. The only technique used is the resting position. Then use the resting position for the entire sequence of patterns 2, 3, and 4. Repeat this exercise with effleurage, petrissage, compression, and other manipulations.

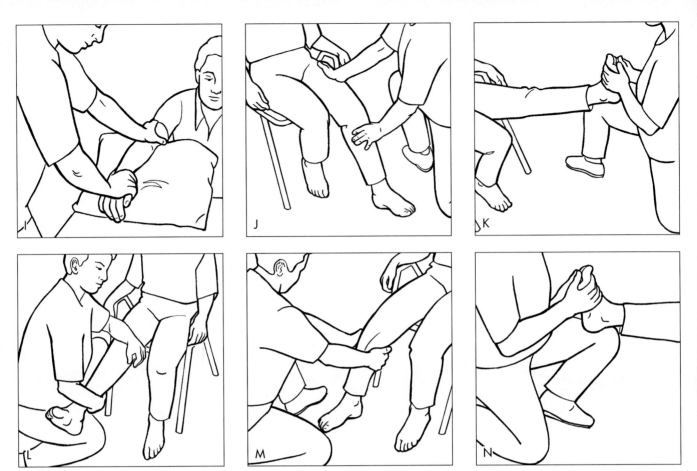

Figure 10.7 *continued*
I, Right arm. J & K, Left lower leg and foot. L, M, & N, Right lower leg and foot.

MASSAGE MANIPULATIONS

SECTION OBJECTIVES

Using the information presented in this section, the student will be able to do the following:

❶ Perform eight basic massage manipulations.

❷ Combine the eight massage manipulations into a basic full-body massage.

Albert Baumgartner, in his 1947 book *Massage in Athletics,*[1] quotes Plato as saying "Massage must be simple." Baumgartner also says that "Many endeavor to introduce improvements into the science of massage but fail to gain adherents to their preventive methods. It would be well to advise these witty inventors of the new sub-methods to keep their improvements to themselves."

The massage manipulations and techniques in this textbook are explained and organized in a manner that consolidates, condenses, and simplifies therapeutic massage methods based on what seems to be the consensus from the historical material and currently accepted terminology and theory. You are encouraged to return to the section on the basic physiologic effects of massage at the beginning of this chapter in order to gain a broader understanding of the methods and techniques described.

In 1879, the terms *effleurage, petrissage, friction,* and *tapotement* first appeared in the *VonMosegeil* (Proceedings of German Society for Surgery) to describe Mezger's methods. Since then, these terms have been found in almost every textbook of massage.[1] Kellogg described the resting position in terms of passive touch.[5] Most textbooks do not separate superficial stroking from effleurage, and many describe compression by classifying it as part of petrissage or pressure. Current trends separate the methods of compression into a distinct description. The majority of references agree on "tapotement" or "percussion," yet resources seemed evenly split between "vibration" or "shaking" being classified separately or together. "Friction" is classified many different ways but is usually defined in similar terms. This textbook refers to passive movements by the names developed through Mezger's work combined with current usage, and are listed in the massage manipulations section. Active movements or gymnastics, as defined by Taylor and others, are listed in the massage techniques section using current terminology.

Resting Position

The act of placing your hand on another person seems so simple, yet this initial contact must be made with respect and a client-centered focus. With this technique, we enter the client's personal boundary space, defined by sensitivity to changes in air pressure and movement picked up by the sensory receptors in the skin. The root hair plexus is one of the most sensitive receptors. Activation of the heat sensors indicates that something is close enough to cause physical harm. Because of these sensors, the fight or flight responses of the sympathetic autonomic nervous system are often activated with the initial contact. The *resting position* provides time for the client to become acclimated to the proximity of another human being. It gives the client time to evaluate, on a subconscious level, whether this touch is safe.

Due to the instinctual survival and protective mechanisms designed to protect humans from hand-to-hand combat, our physiologic safety zone is generally an arm's length. If another person is at this distance, the sensory mechanisms of sympathetic arousal are less sensitive than if the person is close enough to touch. This is why the first approach to touch by the massage professional is so important. This touch sets the stage for the first fifteen to thirty minutes of the massage, since it takes that long for the fight or flight response, which causes adrenalin to be released into the blood, to reverse itself.

The resting position also provides for stillness when intermixed with the other movements of massage. The body needs time to process all the sensory information during massage. Stopping the motions and simply resting the hands on the body provides for this moment of stillness.

The resting position is an excellent way to call attention to an area through stimulation of the cutaneous (skin) sensory receptors. Simple, sustained touch over an area of imbalance is often enough stimulation to cause a reflexive response. This position also adds body heat from the massage therapist to an area of the client's body. It is also an excellent way to re-establish contact with the client if the flow of the massage is interrupted and physical contact is broken.

In most circumstances, a slow, steady approach by the therapist with deliberate hesitation at the arm's-length boundary, coupled with a verbal announcement that you will begin touching, is the best way to avoid excessive sympathetic arousal. Most of the time the restorative parasympathetic state is what the massage practitioner seeks to activate for the client. Yet even in a situation in which the massage is designed to stimulate sympathetic activation, the first touch should be slow, gradual, and deliberate (Fig. 10.8).

An open, soft, relaxed, warm and dry hand is best. It is a signal to our survival mechanism that there is no weapon or intent to strike. A cool and clammy hand suggests sympathetic activation in the therapist. Subconscious survival mechanisms will recognize this and respond to perceived danger by tensing up for protection. Practice extending an open, relaxed hand. It is recommended that the massage professional rub his or her hands together to warm them, and then towel-dry them before touching.

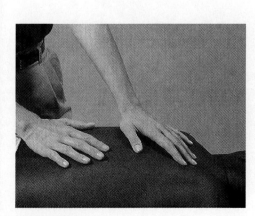

Figure 10.8
Opened relaxed hands.

The resting position should be applied slowly and gradually, in a confident and secure manner. As part of the survival mechanism, the body will innately respond to a hesitant touch by withdrawing. An unsure touch is difficult to interpret and is unsettling to the client. When the application of the resting position is mastered, it is easy to flow into the other methods (Fig. 10.9).

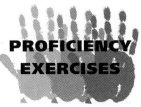

PROFICIENCY EXERCISES

1. **Purposeful touch may be simple, but it is not easy. Diligent practice is required. If you enjoy animals, practice your approach with them. They do not hide responses as people do. Practice using the resting position to touch a dog or cat while the animal is asleep, and see if you can do it without waking the animal.**
2. **Babies and young children are good for practice as well. Practice the resting position with a baby or child. Acceptance of the touch will be indicated by the child not startling or moving away.**

Effleurage/Gliding Strokes

The current term for *effleurage* is "gliding stroke." Effleurage originates from the French verb meaning "to skim" and "to touch lightly on." The most superficial applications of this stroke do this, but the full spectrum of effleurage is determined by pressure, drag, speed, direction, and rhythm, making this manipulation one of the most versatile.

The distinguishing characteristic of effleurage is that it is applied horizontally in relation to the tissues (Fig. 10.10). Increasing pressure adds a

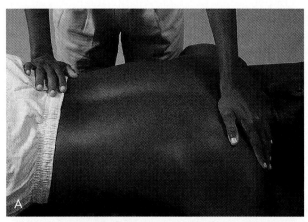
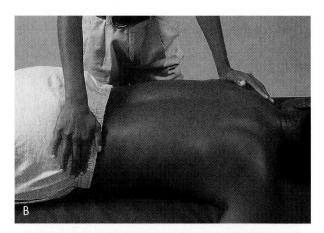
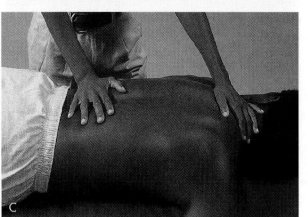
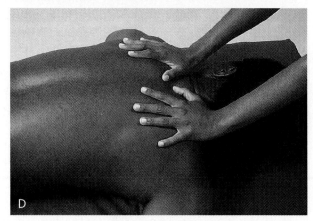

Figure 10.9
A-D, Four examples of the resting position on the back.

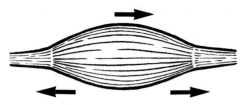

Figure 10.10
The focus of effleurage is horizontal.

compressive force and drag to the stroke. Light stroking is done with the fingertips or palm of the hand. Small body areas such as the fingers can be grasped and surrounded as effleurage is applied to the entire area. The surface contact increases with full hand and forearm application of the manipulations. Superficial applications, that stay within the skin and subcutaneous layer, tend to have a more reflexive effect, while deeper strokes have a more mechanical effect.

Effleurage that proceeds from the trunk of the body out using superficial pressure usually follows the dermatome distribution and is more reflexive in its effects. Strokes that use moderate pressure from the fingers and toes toward the heart following the muscle fiber direction, are excellent for mechanical and reflexive stimulation of blood flow, particularly venous return and lymphatics. Light to moderate pressure, with short, repetitive effleurage stroking following the patterns for the lymph vessels is the basis for manual lymph drainage (see Chapter 13).

During effleurage, moderate pressure extends through the subcutaneous layer to reach muscle tissue, but not so deep as to compress the tissue against the underlying bony structure. Moderate to heavy pressure that puts sufficient drag on the tissue will mechanically affect the connective tissue and the proprioceptors (spindle cells and Golgi tendon organs) found in the muscle. Heavy pressure produces a distinctive compressive force of the soft tissue against the bone.

The more superficial the stroke, the more reflexive the effect. Slow, superficial strokes are very soothing while fast, superficial strokes are stimulating. If a deeper stroke pressure with a slower rate of application is used, the effect will be more mechanical.

After the application of the initial touch or resting position, effleurage is often done next in sequence, especially if a lubricant is used. The long broad movement of this method is excellent for spreading the lubricant on the skin surface. The ease of the application makes this an effective manipulation to use repetitively while gradually increasing the depth of pressure. This is one of the preferred manipulations to warm or prepare the tissue for more specific bodywork. Because of the horizontal nature of the manipulation, the flow pattern of the massage can progress smoothly from one body area to another. It is a good method to use when evaluating for hard and soft tissue, hot and cold areas, or areas that seem stuck (see Chapter 11). Effleurage is the preferred method for abdominal massage (Fig. 10.11).

Do five massages and experiment with the suggestions below plus any other application of effleurage.

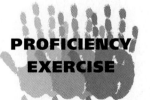

PROFICIENCY EXERCISE

- **Use finger stroking of the face following the direction of the muscle fiber. Have a chart of the facial muscles available.**
- **Using the forearm on the back, follow the muscle fiber directions from origin to insertion. Keep a muscle chart nearby.**
- **Use the palm of the hand or pads of the fingers to lightly stroke the dermatome pattern from the spine to the fingers and toes. This method is sometimes called *nerve stroking*. Have a chart of dermatome distribution available.**
- **Use the palm of the hand to glide from the toes and fingers along the main pathways of the superficial vein. Use an anatomy chart as needed.**
- **Grasp the fingers and toes and "milk" the tissue with effleurage.**
- **Use the forearm to effleurage the quadriceps, hamstrings, abductors, fascia lata, and iliotibial band of the thigh. Use a muscle chart to follow the fiber direction.**

- **Grasp the foot at the ankle with both hands and glide to the toes.**
- **Use the knuckles to glide on the bottom of the foot from the heel to the base of the toes.**
- **Use the thumbs to effleurage in a very specific pattern to gently separate the muscles in the hamstring and quadriceps groups.**
- **Use the four basic flow patterns and design an entire massage with only effleurage/gliding strokes.**

Petrissage/Kneading

Petrissage, from the French verb "petrir" meaning "to knead," requires that the soft tissue be lifted, rolled, and squeezed by the massage therapist (Fig. 10.12). Because skin and the underlying muscles cannot be lifted

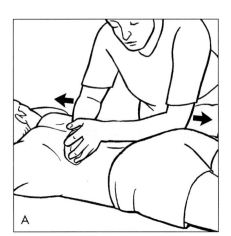
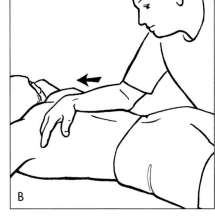
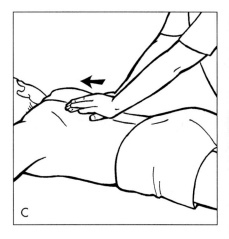
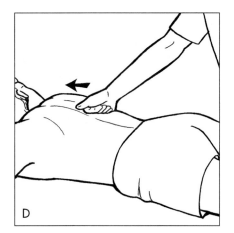
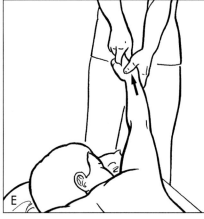
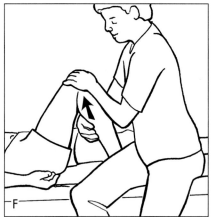
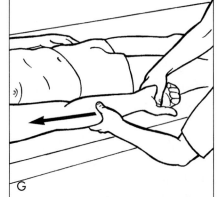
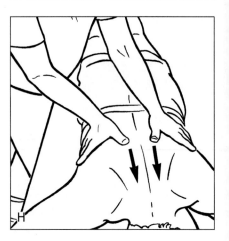

Figure 10.11
Examples of effleurage applications. A, Double forearm effleurage. B, Single forearm effleurage to back. C, Supported hand effleurage. D, Loose fist effleurage. E, Surrounding grasp effleurage. F, Single forearm effleurage to calf. G, Single hand effleurage. H, Double hand effleurage.

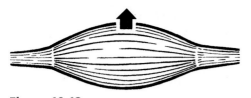

Figure 10.12
The focus of petrissage is vertical lifting up.

without first pressing into them, compression is sometimes classified as petrissage. This textbook has separated compression into a distinct manipulation, but it must be noted that the compression element is part of the process of lifting tissue. Just as effleurage is focused horizontally on the body, petrissage functions vertically. The main purpose of this manipulation is to lift tissue. Once lifted, the full hand is used to squeeze the tissue as it rolls out of the hand while the other hand prepares to lift additional tissue and repeat the process. (Fig. 10.13)

Petrissage is very good for decreasing muscle tone. The lifting, rolling, and squeezing action affects the spindle cell proprioceptors in the muscle belly. By squeezing the belly of the muscle (thus squeezing the spindle cells) the muscle feels less stretched. When lifting, the tendons are stretched, thus increasing tension in both the tendons and the Golgi tendon receptors, which have a protective function. The result of this sensory input is to reflexively relax the muscle to keep it from harm. Petrissage is a method of "tricking" the muscle into relaxation.

Petrissage is very good for mechanically softening the superficial fascia. This type of connective tissue, located under the skin, is similar to gelatin. It is a glycol (sugar) protein that binds with water. If gelatin is mixed with water and allowed to sit, it becomes thick and solidifies. If the gelatin is pressed into smaller pieces and stirred, it will soften, which is the effect of petrissage on connective tissue. The difference to the massage client is the same as comparing the stiffness of a brand new pair of shoes or jeans with the comfort of an old pair of jeans or a broken-in pair of shoes.

The fascia forms a major part of each muscle. Petrissage has the mechanical effect of softening and creating space around the actual muscle fibers, and making the tendons more pliable as well. The tension on

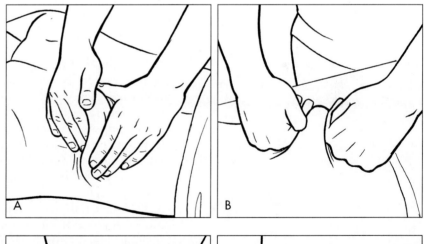

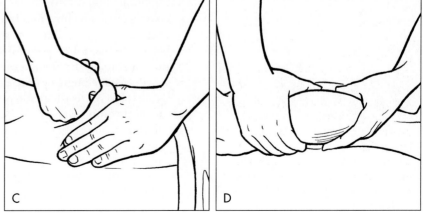

Figure 10.13
Examples of petrissage applications. A, Two hands with one hand pushing tissue into grasping hand. B, Two loose fists grasping and lifting tissue. C, Loose fist pushing tissue into grasping hand. D, Two grasping hands.

the tendon as it is pulled deforms the connective tissue and mechanically warms it. If you bend a piece of metal back and forth it will get warm. The effects of petrissage are similar. Instead of metal fibers, collagen fibers are bent and warmed in a similar way. When something is warm, the molecules that comprise it are moving faster and are further apart. The space, which is created at a molecular level, translates into a softer and more pliable structure.

A variation of this lifting manipulation is skin-rolling. In this technique, only the skin is lifted from the underlying muscle layer. Whereas deep petrissage attempts to lift the muscular component away from the bone, skin-rolling lifts only the skin. It has a warming and softening effect on the superficial fascia, causes reflexive stimulation to the spinal nerves, and is an excellent assessment method. Areas of "stuck" skin often suggest underlying problems. Skin-rolling is one of the very few massage methods that is safe to use directly over the spine. Because only the skin is accessed and the direction of pull to the skin is up and off of the underlying bones, there is no chance of injury to the spine, as there is when any type of downward pressure is used.

Additional variations of petrissage or kneading incorporate a wringing or twisting component once the tissue is lifted. Changes in depth of pressure and drag will determine whether the manipulation is perceived by the client as superficial or deep. By the nature of the manipulation, the pressure and pull peak when the tissue is lifted as far as it can be, and become less at the beginning and the end of the manipulation.

Although petrissage is very effective in softening and relaxing tissue, it is more difficult and energy-consuming for the massage practitioner to use. The fingers should be used as a unit along with the thenar eminence of the thumb. Excessive use of this manipulation should be avoided. It is better to use petrissage intermittently with effleurage and compression, which do not require such labor-intensive use of the hands. Constant attention must be paid to body mechanics. It is best to grasp the area and lift or pull by leaning back, using the whole body instead of only the arms.

Sometimes a client's tissue will not lift. This may be due to excessive edema (swollen tissue), a heavy fat layer, scarring that extends into the deeper body layers, and thickened areas of connective tissue especially over aponeuroses (flat sheets of superficial connective tissue). If applications of petrissage are attempted, they will be uncomfortable to the client. Shifting to effleurage and compression may soften the tissue enough so that petrissage can be used more effectively. Excessive body hair may interfere with the use of petrissage. The therapist must be careful not to pull the client's hair.

Petrissage must be rhythmic to feel correct. The speed of the manipulation is limited. If the tissue is lifted quickly or squeezed too fast, it is uncomfortable to the client. The speed and frequency of the application is determined by how much tissue can be lifted, and how long it takes for that tissue to be rolled and squeezed through the hand. This concept is hard to explain, but like milking a cow or goat, or kneading bread dough, the consistency of the material decides how it is kneaded.

Petrissage begins with palmar compression on a 45° angle to push the tissue forward. As the tissue bunches in front of the hand, the fingers, used as a unit combined with the palm of the hand, close over the mound of tissue. The tissue is then lifted, rolled, and squeezed through the hand. With skin-rolling, the wrist action is different. After the skin is lifted as high as it will go comfortably, the wrist rolls over instead of under the tissue. Except in very delicate areas such as the face, use of the fingers and thumbs to lift the tissue should be avoided since there is a tendency to pinch and cause discomfort to the client (Fig. 10.14).

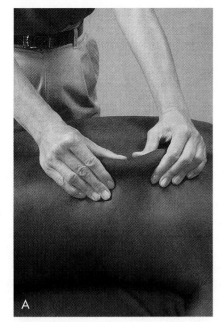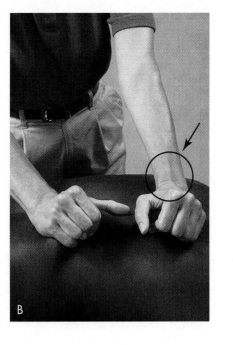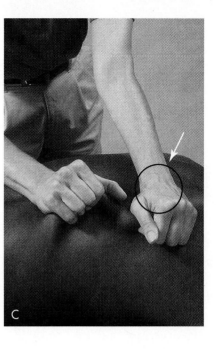

Figure 10.14
Comparison of petrissage and skin roll. A, Both petrissage and skin roll begin in the same position. B, Wrist goes under tissue with petrissage. C, Wrist goes over tissue in skin rolling.

To get a feel for the method, practice with some clay. Keeping the fingers pressed together, use them as one unit against the thenar eminence. Do not use the thumb itself. It is important to use as large a part of the palmar surface of the hand as possible. This upward pull should be extended until the end of the give to the tissue is felt. Kneading of this type works both on the skin and on the underlying muscular component including the tendons. In most cases only one hand at a time is used to lift, squeeze, and twist the tissue. Petrissage becomes continuous when a hand-over-hand rhythm is established. Two hands can also be used against each other on larger areas such as the hamstring muscle.

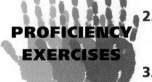

PROFICIENCY EXERCISES

1. **Knead a variety of sizes of bread dough. Small pieces can be used to practice the delicate applications used on the face and anterior neck while larger pieces can mimic big muscles such as the gluteals. Bread dough is good for practice because it is resilient (like body tissue) and will not allow you to petrissage too fast.**
2. **Petrissage an inflated balloon. If it slips out of your grasp, it is a sign that you just pinched your client. Using a balloon will help develop the use of the palm instead of the fingers.**
3. **For learning purposes only, practice using petrissage or kneading for an entire body massage using all four basic flow patterns. Notice that some parts of the body are more easily kneaded than others. Because of the repetitive use of the hand for petrissage, avoid extensive long-term use.**

Compression

Compression has developed as a distinct manipulation in recent years with the advent of sports massage and on-site corporate massage. It has always been the main method used in shiatsu and other oriental approaches. This manipulation is a way of working over the clothing or without lubricant. Very specific pinpoint compression is called direct pressure, or ischemic compression, and is used on acupressure points (motor points) and trigger points (Fig. 10.15).

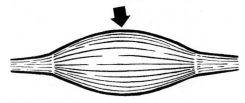

Figure 10.15
The focus of compression is a vertical pressing down.

Because compression uses a lift-press method, it is particularly suited for use when a lubricant is undesirable. It is also very good to use on bodies that are hairy since the manipulations do not glide on the skin, pull the tissue, or require lubricant.

Compression moves down into the tissues with varying depths of pressure. The superficial application resembles the resting position but uses more pressure. The manipulations of compression usually penetrate the subcutaneous layer, while in the resting position they stay on the skin surface. Much of the effect of compression results from pressing tissue against the underlying bone, causing it to spread and be squeezed from two sides, similar to flattening out a tortilla or a ball of clay, or pressing pizza dough into a pan. As with effleurage, the deeper the pressure, the more mechanical the effect will be. Likewise, the more superficial the pressure, the more reflexive the effect will be. Compression disconnects from the body with each lift, and then reconnects with each press in a piston-like fashion. It is different from effleurage and petrissage in that these manipulations maintain constant body contact in some form. Pressing rhythmically into connective tissue will soften it mechanically. Pressing tissue against the underlying hard bone will spread the tissue mechanically, enhancing the softening effect of the connective tissue component of the muscle.

Compression that takes all the slack out of the tissue then pushes or pulls in a 45° angle without slipping will produce a drag on the tissue. Compression used in the belly of the muscle will spread the spindle cells, causing the muscle to think it is stretching. To protect the muscle from overstretching, the spindle cell will signal for the muscle to contract. The lift-press application will stimulate the muscle and nerve tissue. These two effects combine to make compression a good method to tone muscles and stimulate the nervous system. Because of this stimulation, compression is a little less desirable for a relaxation or soothing massage. It is important to remember that not all people want to feel like a relaxed rag doll after a massage. If the client needs to be alert, then a stimulating massage is in order.

A muscle needs to contract or at least have the nerve "fire" (as occurs in a contraction) before it can relax. This is due to the threshold stimulation pattern of the nerve and its effects on the muscle tone. Nerves build up the energy needed to spark the nerve impulse. Sometimes the signals are enough to get everything ready to fire, but the signal is not strong enough to actually cause the contraction or discharge of the nerve. The result is that the muscle tenses up, but cannot quite contract. The automatic response of muscle fibers to contraction is a period of relaxation called the *refractory period.* If stimulation to the nerves can be increased just enough for the nerve to discharge, then the muscle contracts, and can reset to a normal resting length. Methods such as post-isometric relaxation are an example of this mechanism. Compression to the belly of the muscle and its effect on the spindle cell elicits this response on a smaller scale. Progressive relaxation (systematic, voluntary contraction or relaxation of muscles) uses this physiologic mechanism. Any sustained and repetitive use of a stimulation method that causes muscle fibers to maintain a contraction or contract repeatedly will eventually fatigue the muscle fibers. Compression used in this manner will initiate a relaxation response in mucles.

Compression proceeds downward, and the depth is determined by what is to be accomplished, where it is to be applied, and how broad or specific is the contact with the client's body. Compression can be used to replace effleurage if for any reason gliding strokes cannot or should not be used. Examples include working on areas where there is excessive body hair or where people are ticklish. Compression bypasses the tickle response by activating deep touch receptors. Compression does not slip or roll on the tissue.

Compression can be done with the point of the thumb or stabilized finger, palm and heel of the hand, fist, knuckles, forearm, elbow, and in some systems, the knee and heel of the foot (Fig. 10.16). When using the palm of the hand to do compression, hyperextension or hyperflexion of the wrist should be avoided by keeping the application hand in front instead of directly under the therapist's shoulder. Even though the compressive pressure is perpendicular to the tissue, the position of the forearm in relation to the wrist is about 120° to 130°. If using the knuckles or fist, the forearm is in a direct line with the wrist. Use of the thumb should be avoided, especially on large muscle masses or for extended periods of time. The tip or the radioulnar side of the elbow should not be used for compression. Since the ulnar nerve passes just under the skin and damage can result from extensive compression, the humerus side of the elbow should be used for compression. The massage therapist's arm and hand must be relaxed or neck and shoulder tension will occur. It is the bones of the forearm that do the work, not the muscles.

Deep compression presses tissue against the underlying bone. Because of the diagonal pattern of the muscles, the therapist should stay perpendicular or at a 90° angle to the bone, with actual compression somewhere between 45° and 90° to the body. Beyond those angles, the stroke may slip and turn into an effleurage.

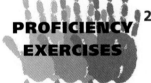

PROFICIENCY EXERCISES

1. **Blow up a series of balloons with different internal pressures. Fill some with water and others with gelatin and use these to represent the thickness or thinness of different tissue types. The use of balloons is great for practicing the angle and pressure of the manipulation. The best angle allows good firm compression into the balloon without it slipping out from under you.**

2. **Using pieces of foam with various densities, place them over different sized and shaped objects and determine how much pressure it takes to feel each object. Pay attention to the difference with the low-density foam compared with the high-density foam.**

3. **Design a complete massage for each of the basic flow patterns using only compression. Pay very close attention to how you can use compression manipulations in all of the variations to access the client's body successfully. Work to develop this skill and compression will serve you well.**

Vibration

Edgar Cyriax, one of the foremost authorities on massage and manual techniques, describes *vibration* as follows:

". . . Almost every author who attempts to describe the modus operandi for generating these vibrations prefaces his remarks by stating that they are extremely tiring to produce. After this he gives the information that they are generated by means of the operator tensing all the muscles of his arm (some even include the muscles of the shoulder) into a state of powerful complete tetanus. No wonder that this method is very fatiguing: no one can sustain such a contraction evenly for more than a minute or so owing to the great fatigue that must inevitably ensue. The correct technique for production of manual vibrations is to set up a small amount of alternating contraction and relaxation in some of the muscles of the forearm, those of the upper arm and the shoulder being kept quite passive (unless required for fixation purposes)."[3]

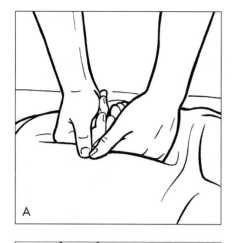

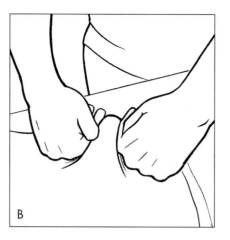

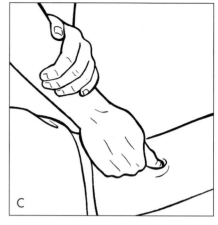

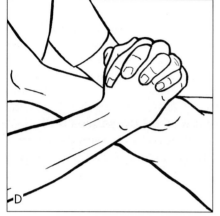

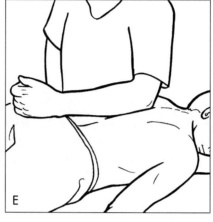

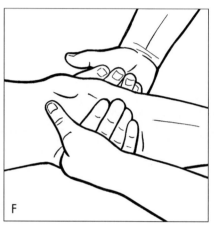

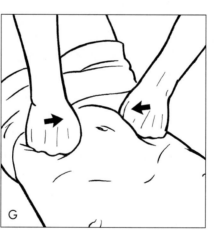

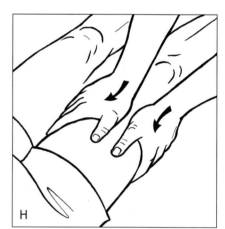

Figure 10.16
Examples of compression applica-
tions. A, Fist compression.
B, Stabilized hand compression.
C, Stabilized thumb compression.
D, Loose fist compression. E,
Forearm compression. F, Double
hand compression. G, Fists used in
lateral compression. H, Double
palm compression. I, Single palm
compression. J, Fist application of
compression to foot.

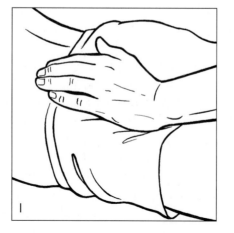

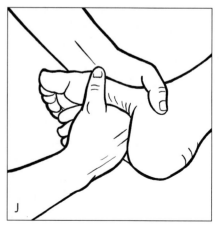

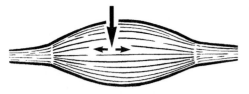

Figure 10.17
The focus of vibration is down and back and forth in an oscillating manner.

Vibration is a very powerful stroke, if it can be done long enough and at an intensity sufficient to produce reflexive physiologic effects. Manual vibration can be used successfully by the massage therapist to tone muscles by applying the technique at the muscle tendons for up to thirty seconds. The antagonist muscle pattern will relax through neurologic reciprocal inhibition.

Another use for vibration is to break up the monotony of the massage. If the same methods are used repeatedly, the body adapts and does not respond as well to the sensation or stimulation. Because vibration is used to "wake up" nerves, it is a good method to stimulate nerve activity. The nerves of the muscles around a joint also innervate the joint itself. Muscle pain is often interpreted by the client as joint pain and vice versa. Used specifically and purposefully, vibration is a great massage manipulation to confuse and shift the muscle/joint pain perception (Fig. 10.17).

All vibration begins with compression. Once the depth of pressure is achieved, the hand needs to tremble and transmit the action to the surrounding tissues. As described by Cyriax,[3] the muscles above the elbow should be relaxed. The action comes only from the alternating contraction/relaxation of the forearm muscles. Of all the massage methods, vibration may be the hardest to master.

To start with coarse vibration, place one hand on the client and compress lightly. Begin moving the hand back and forth using only the forearm muscles and limiting the motion to about two inches of space. Gradually speed up the back-and-forth movement, checking to make sure your upper arm stays relaxed. Then make the back-and-forth movement smaller until the hand does not move at all on the tissue but is trembling at a high intensity. This is vibration.

Because of the energy needed to do this manipulation, it should be used sparingly and for short periods of time. It is suggested that a forearm effleurage follow vibration since the action of the effleurage essentially massages and relaxes the therapist's arm, protecting it from repetitive use problems (Fig. 10.18).

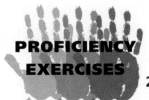

PROFICIENCY EXERCISES

- *The first two exercises to teach vibration were developed by a professional magician who is also a massage therapist and instructor. Many slight-of-hand movements required for his illusions use the same movements as vibration. Being able to perfect these two balloon exercises will enhance your vibration skills.*

1. **Using a clear 5″ balloon, put a penny inside, then blow up and tie the balloon. Grasp the tied end of the balloon (Fig. 10.19,A). Using wrist action only, circle the balloon until the penny begins to roll inside. Once you can do this, make the wrist circles smaller and smaller while continuing to roll the penny in the balloon. Eventually the action will be the movement required for vibration.**

2. **Use the same balloon and put the fattest part in the palm of your hand. Place your other hand on top of the balloon (pictured). Using just the bottom hand, use a coarse vibration to get the penny to jump and dance in the balloon. Once you can do this, make the movements smaller and smaller until you can make the penny dance with fine vibration movements (Fig. 10.19,B).**

3. **Combine all of the methods presented so far into a massage. Incorporate vibration at each tendon, paying attention to the results as the muscles contract or tone slightly in response to the stimulation.**

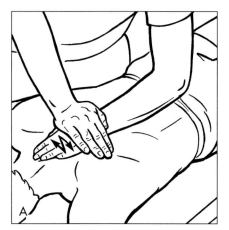
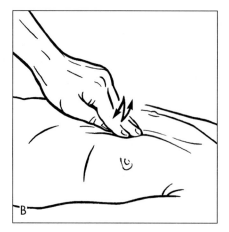
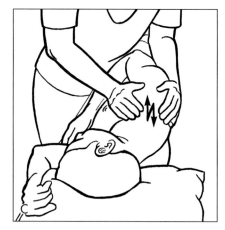

Figure 10.18
Examples of vibration applications.
A, Stabilized hand.
B, Stabilized fingers.
C, Double hand.

Shaking

Shaking is a massage method that is effective in relaxing muscle groups or an entire limb. Shaking manipulations confuse the positional proprioceptors so the muscles relax. The sensory input is too unorganized for the integrating systems of the brain to interpret, and going limp is the natural response in such situations. Shaking warms and prepares the body for deeper bodywork and works with joints in a nonspecific manner.

Rocking is a soothing and rhythmic form of shaking that has been used since the beginning of time to calm people. Rocking works though the vestibular system of the inner ear and feeds sensory input directly into the cerebellum. It is probable that other reflex mechanisms are affected as well. For rocking to be most effective, the body must move so that the fluid in the semi-circular canals of the inner ear are affected, initiating parasympathetic mechanisms.

Shaking is sometimes classified as a vibration even though the application is very different. Shaking begins with lift and pull components while vibration begins with compression. Either a muscle group or limb is grasped, lifted, and shaken. To begin to understand shaking, think of how a dog shakes when it is wet, shaking out a rug or blanket, what a dog or cat does when tugging on a toy, or the swish of a horse's tail.

The focus of the massage practitioner's shaking will be more specific and less intense than shaking a rug, but the idea is still the same. There is a lift and then a fairly abrupt downward or side-to-side movement that ends suddenly as if to throw something off. Even the most subtle shaking movements deliberately move the joint or muscle tissue to affect the receptors. Shaking is not a manipulation to be used on the skin or superficial fascia, nor is it effective to use on the entire body. Rather, it is best applied to any large muscle groups that can be grasped and to syn-

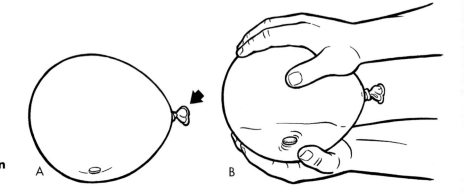

Figure 10.19
Balloon exercises for vibration.
A, Hold balloon where indicated by arrow. B, Hand placement for balloon exercise.

ovial joints. Good areas for shaking are the upper trapezius and shoulder area, biceps and triceps groups, hamstrings, quadriceps, gastrocnemius, and in some instances the abdominals and the pectoralis muscles close to the axilla. The joints of the shoulders, hips, and extremities also respond well to shaking. The larger the muscle or joint, the more intense is the method. If the movements are done with all the slack out of the tissue, the focus of the shake is very small and is extremely effective. The more focused and purposeful the approach, the smaller the focus of the shaking will be. You should always stay within the limits of both range of motion of a joint and "give" of the tissue. The goal is to see how small the shake can be and still have a physiologic effect.

Shaking should be used when the muscles seem extremely tight. This technique is reflexive in its effect, but there may be a small mechanical effect on the connective tissue as well owing to the lifting and pulling component of the methods (Fig. 10.20).

Rocking

Rocking is rhythmic and should be applied with a deliberate full-body movement. Rocking involves the up-and-down and side-to-side movement of shaking, but there is no flick or throw-off snap at the end of the movement. The action moves the body as far as it will go, then allows it to return to the original position. After two or three rocks, the client's rhythm can be sensed. At this point, the massage therapist works with the rhythm, either by attempting to extend gently the limits of movement, or by slowing down the rhythm. Nothing is abrupt: there is an even ebb and flow to the methods. All movement is flowing, like a wind chime in a gentle breeze or a porch swing on a hot summer night. Rocking is one of the most effective relaxation techniques of the massage therapist. Many

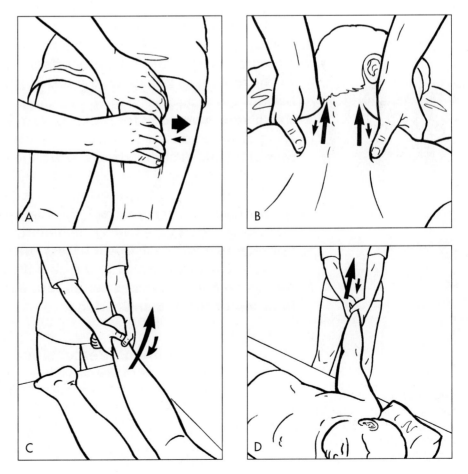

Figure 10.20
Examples of applications of shaking. A & B, Lift tissue and apply abrupt shaking movement as directed by large arrow and allow tissue to return in the direction of small arrow. C & D, Grasp area and pull out slack in tissues. Apply abrupt shaking movement in direction of large arrows and allow tissue to return in direction of small arrows.

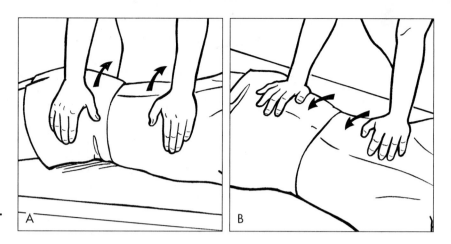

Figure 10.21
Rocking. A, Pull area toward therapist.
B, Rock area away from therapist.

parasympathetic responses are elicited by the rocking of the body during effleurage, petrissage, and compression.

With a tense and anxious client, begin with slightly more abrupt and bigger shaking manipulations. As the muscles begin to relax, switch to rocking methods. Rocking is reflexive and chemical in its effects, both at the whole-body and individual joint levels (Fig. 10.21).

Shaking focuses more on the soft tissue while rocking focuses on the joint receptors. Both methods, however, work on all the tissues through the stimulation of the nervous system, primarily the proprioceptors of the muscles and joints.

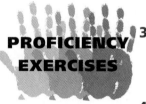

PROFICIENCY EXERCISES

1. **Lay a sheet on your massage table or other flat surface. Lift one end and practice shaking the sheet to achieve a wavelike motion in the sheet from one end to the other. Practice directing the ripple to various locations on the table.**
2. **Swing in a playground swing, using your legs to pump yourself. This exercise will give the full-body effect of the shake. Pay close attention to the feeling as you reach the top of the swing and begin to head back.**
3. **Using your own body for practice, systematically shake each joint, lying down to do the legs. See how small you can make the movement and still feel the effects. Grab the muscles of your arm and leg. Lift and shake the tissue, paying attention to the sensations.**
4. **Rock in an old-fashioned rocking chair, letting the chair rock you. See what happens when you rock the chair. Vary the speed to go faster and slower than the chair's movement.**
5. **Put on music with a 4/4 beat at less than sixty beats per minute. Pick up the sway of the music and rock with it.**
6. **Design an entire massage for all four basic flow patterns using a combination of shaking and rocking.**

Tapotement/Percussion

The term *tapotement* comes from the French verb "tapoter," which means "to rap, drum, or pat." Tapotement techniques require that the hands or parts of the hand administer springy blows to the body at a fast rate. The blows are directed downward to create a rhythmic compression of the tissue. Tapotement is divided into two classifications: light and heavy. The difference between light and heavy tapotement is determined by whether

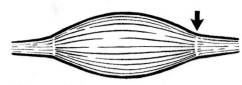

Figure 10.22
The focus of tapotement percussion is vertical, abruptly snapped down.

the force of the blows penetrates only to the superficial tissue of the skin and subcutaneous layers, or deeper into the muscles, tendons, and visceral (organ) structures such as the pleura in the chest cavity (Fig. 10.22).

Tapotement, or percussion, is a stimulating manipulation that operates through the response of the nerves. The effects of the manipulations are reflexive except for the mechanical results of tapotement in loosening and moving mucus in the chest. Children with cystic fibrosis are treated with tapotement, but therapy of this type is beyond the beginning skill levels of the massage therapist.

The strongest effect of tapotement is due to the response of the tendon reflexes. A quick blow to the tendon stretches it. In response, protective muscle contraction results. To obtain the best result, stretch the tendon first. The most common example of this reflexive mechanism is the knee-jerk or patellar reflex, but the response happens in all tendons to some degree. Knowing this is very helpful when preparing the muscles for stretching, e.g., if a client indicates that his or her hamstrings are tight and need to be stretched. With the client supine and the hip flexed to 90° and the knee flexed to 90°, tapotement on the stretched quadriceps tendon will cause the quadriceps to contract. As a result, the hamstrings will relax and be easier to stretch.

Tapotement is very effective when used at motor points. The repetitive stimulation causes the nerve to fire repeatedly, stimulating the nerve tract. Tapotement focused primarily on the skin affects the superficial blood vessels of the skin, initially causing them to contract. Heavy tapotement or prolonged lighter application will dilate the vessels due to the release of histamine, a vasodilator. While prolonged tapotement seems to increase blood flow, surface tapotement enhances the effect of cold application used in hydrotherapy.

When applied to the joints, tapotement affects the joint kinesthetic receptors responsible for determining the position and movement of the body. The quick blows confuse the system similar to the effect of joint-focused rocking and shaking, but the body muscles tense instead of relax. This method is useful for stimulating weak muscles. The force used must move the joint but should not be strong enough to damage the joint. For example, one finger may be used over the carpal joints while the fist may be used over the sacroiliac joint. Because of its intense stimulating quality to the nervous system, tapotement initiates or enhances sympathetic activity of the autonomic nervous system.

In tapotement, two hands are usually used alternately. When tapping a motor point, one or two fingers can be used alone. The forearm muscles contract and relax in rapid succession to move the elbow joint into flexion and then allow it to quickly release. This action travels down to the relaxed wrist, extending it; the wrist thus moves back and forth to provide the action of the tapotement. It is a controlled flailing of the arms as the wrists snap back and forth. The wrist must always stay relaxed. Beginning students usually want to use the wrists to provide the snap action. This is especially tempting when using small movements with the fingers, *but should not be done* because it will damage the wrist.

Heavy tapotement should not be done over the kidney area, or anywhere there is pain or discomfort. Proper methods are classified as follows (Fig. 10.23):

- *Hacking.* Applied with both wrists relaxed and the fingers spread, only the little fingers or the ulnar side of the hand strikes the surface in hacking. The other fingers hit each other with a springy touch. Point hacking can be done by using the fingertips in the same way. Hacking is used with the whole hand on the larger soft tissue areas such as the upper back and shoulders. Point hacking is used on smaller areas such as the individual tendons of the toes or over motor points.

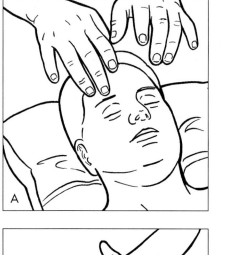
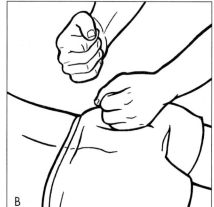
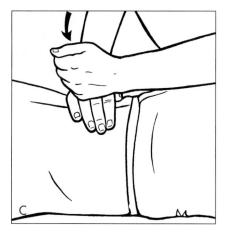
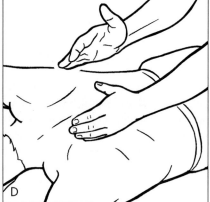
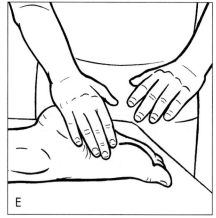
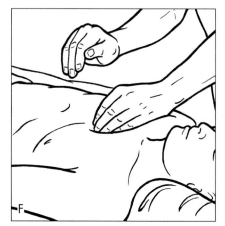

Figure 10.23
Examples of tapotement.
A, Finger tapping. B, Fist beating.
C, Beating over palm. D, Hacking.
E, Slapping. F, Cupping.

- *Cupping.* Fingers and thumbs are placed as if making a cup. The hands are turned over and the same action as hacking is done. Used on the anterior and posterior thorax, cupping is good for stimulation of the respiratory system and for loosening mucus. If the client exhales and makes a monotone noise while cupping is being done, enough pressure should used when the tone begins to break up from AAAAAAAAAAAAAHHHHHH to AH AH AH AH AH AH.

- *Beating and pounding.* These moves are done with a soft fist with knuckles down, or vertically with the ulnar side of the palm (pictured). Beating and pounding is done over large muscles such as the buttocks and heavy leg muscles.

- *Slapping (splatting).* The whole palm of a flattened hand makes contact with the body. This is a good method for release of histamine and its effects to the skin. It is also a good method to use on the bottom of the feet. The broad contact of the whole hand disperses the force laterally instead of down, and the effects remain in the superficial tissue. Kellogg[5] named this movement "splatting."

- *Tapping.* The palmar surface of the fingers alternately taps the body area with light to medium pressure. This method is good around the joints, on the tendons, on the face and head, and along the spine.

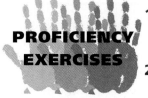

PROFICIENCY EXERCISES

1. **Play a drum or watch a drummer, paying attention to the action of the arms and wrist and the grasp of the drumsticks. Notice that the drummer holds the drumstick loosely.**
2. **Get a paddle ball or yo-yo and see what actions it takes to make these toys work. Play with a rattle or tamborine.**

3. Use the foam from the compression exercises and practice the different methods and pressures.
4. While shaking your hands very quickly, use hacking to strike the foam or a practice client. Without stopping, change hand positions so that all the methods are used.
5. Design a stimulating massage using all the basic flow patterns with various applications of tapotement.

Friction

One method of *friction* consists of small deep movements performed on a local area. This method was formalized by Cyriax and uses deep transverse friction massage while applying no lubricant. The skin moves with the fingers. Friction burns may result if the fingers are allowed to slide back and forth over the skin (Fig. 10.24). Friction manipulation prevents and breaks up local adhesions in connective tissue, especially over tendons, ligaments, and scars. This method is not used over acute injury or fresh scars. Modified use of friction, once the scar has stabilized or the acute phase has passed, may prevent adhesions from developing and may promote a more normal healing process. The Cyriax application also provides for pain reduction through the mechanisms of counter-irritation and hyperstimulation analgesia.

The movement in friction is usually transverse to the fiber direction; it is generally performed for thirty seconds to ten minutes, with some authorities suggesting a duration of twenty minutes. The result of this type of friction is the initiation of a small, controlled inflammatory response. The chemicals released during inflammation cause the reorganization of connective tissue. This type of work, coupled with proper rehabilitation, is very valuable. Due to its specific nature and direct focus on rehabilitation, the use of deep transverse friction is not suitable for the beginning-level massage practitioner. A modified application of friction, used to keep high-concentration areas of connective tissue soft and pliable, is appropriate for the beginner.

Connective tissue has a high water content. In order for the connective tissue to remain pliable, it must remain hydrated. Friction increases the water-binding capacity of the connective tissue ground substance. The method is the same, but the duration and specificity are reduced. The direction can be transverse or circular, pinpointed or more generalized, but the tissue under the skin is still affected. Friction is a mechanical approach best applied to areas of high connective tissue concentration such as the musculotendinous junction. Microtrauma from repetitive movement and overstretching are common in this area. Microtrauma predisposes the musculotendinous junction to inflammatory problems, connective tissue build-up, and adhesion. Friction is a good way to keep this tissue healthy. There is disagreement on whether an area that is to receive friction should be stretched or relaxed. Because both ways have merit, both positions should be included when frictioning.

Another use for friction is to combine it with compression. The combination adds a small stretch component. There is no slide to the movement. This application has a mechanical, chemical, and reflexive effect, and is the most common approach today. In many older textbooks, friction is a back-and-forth, brisk movement focused on the skin and subcutaneous tissue for dilation of the vessels of the skin. Excessive use will cause a friction burn on the skin similar to a rug burn. Historical literature on massage indicates that friction burns were done on purpose to produce long-term stimulation of the nerve. This is a method of counter-irritation, and is seldom used today.

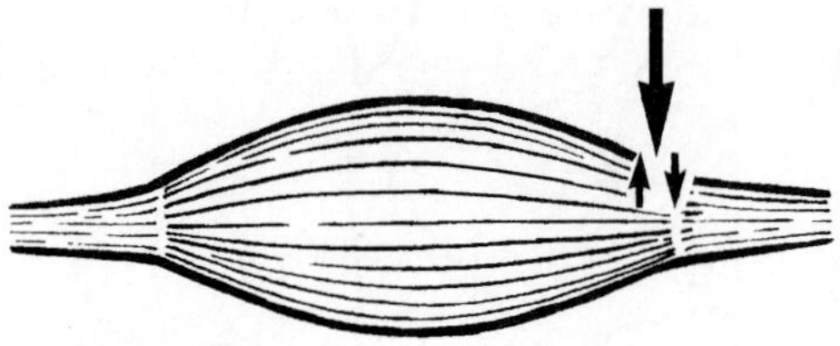

Figure 10.24
The focus of friction is a vertical pressing down, and then applying movement to underlying tissues.

The main focus when using friction is to move tissue under the skin. No lubricant is used since there must be no slide of the tissues. The area to be frictioned should be placed in a soft or slack position. The movement is produced by beginning with a specific and moderate to deep compression using the fingers, palm, or flat part of the elbow. Once the pressure required to contact the tissue is reached, the upper tissue is moved back and forth across the grain or fiber of the undertissue for transverse or cross-fiber friction, or around in a circle for circular friction.

As the tissue responds to the friction, gradually begin to stretch the area and increase the pressure. The feeling for the client may be intense, but if it is painful, the application should be modified to a tolerable level so the client reports the sensation as a "good hurt." The recommended way to work within the client's comfort zone is to use pressure sufficient for him or her to feel the specific area. Friction should be continued until the sensation reduces. Gradually increase the pressure until the client

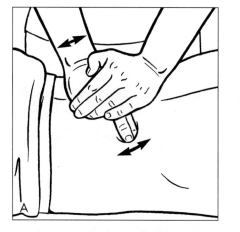

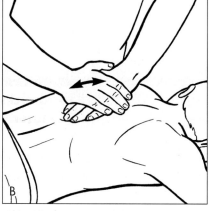

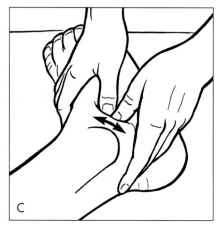

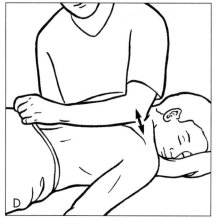

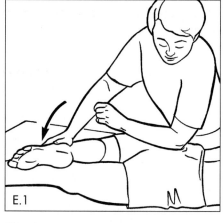

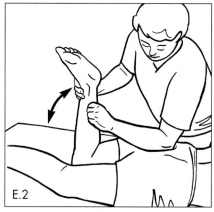

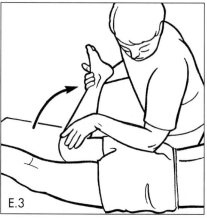

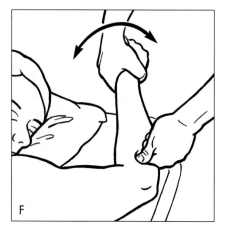

Figure 10.25
Examples of friction. A, Stabilized finger friction. B, Stabilized hand friction. C, Double thumb friction. D, Forearm friction. E (1–3), Forearm compression and movement of underlying tissue. F, Thumb compression and movement of underlying tissue.

again feels the specific area. Begin friction again and repeat the sequence for up to ten minutes. The area being frictioned may be tender to the touch for forty-eight hours after the technique is used. The sensation should be similar to a mild after-exercise soreness. The focus of friction is the controlled application of a small inflammatory response, causing heat and redness from the release of histamine and increased circulation. A small amount of puffiness occurs as more water binds with the connective tissue. The area should not bruise.

Another effective way to produce friction is a combination of compression and passive joint movement with the bone under the compression used to perform the friction. The process begins with a compression as just described, but instead of the massage therapist moving the tissue back and forth (or in a circle), the massage therapist moves the client's body under the compression. This automatically adds the slack and stretch positions for the friction methods. The result is the same. This method is much easier for the massage therapist to perform and may be more comfortable for the client as well. The movement of the joint provides a distraction from the specific application of the pressure and generalizes the sensation. Broad general methods can be used with a higher degree of intensity than a pinpointed specific focus (Fig. 10.25).

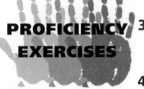

PROFICIENCY EXERCISES

1. **Put toothpicks laid in a haphazard fashion under a towel. Use fingertip friction to line up all the toothpicks.**
2. **Use a piece of rope a 1/2″ in diameter. Use friction to separate the fibers of the rope.**
3. **Access as many surface areas of the musculotendinous junction as possible. Gently friction across the grain of the fibers using fingers, palm, or ulnar side of elbow.**
4. **Using palmar or forearm compression on larger muscle groups, combine passive and active joint movement (see following section) to design a massage session.**

MASSAGE TECHNIQUES

SECTION OBJECTIVES

Using the information presented in this section, the student will be able to do the following:

❶ Use movement in a purposeful way to create a specific physiologic response.

❷ Explain the proprioceptive mechanisms and their importance in the physiologic effects of massage techniques.

❸ Move the synovial joints through the client's physiologic range of motion using both active and passive joint movement.

In *An Illustrated Sketch of the Movement Cure,*[10] George H. Taylor said:

The purpose of an active movement, is to convey to, and concentrate upon a selected point, the nutrition and energies of the system. Such a movement may accomplish a twofold purpose, that of supplying a part, and of relieving another part more or less distant.

The mode of effecting this purpose is as follows: The person to receive the application, is placed in an easy unconstrained position, sitting, lying, half lying, kneeling, or in a convenient position that will suitably adjust all parts of the body to the purpose. The body is fixed either by the hands of an assistant, or by means of an apparatus so as to prevent as much as possible any motion of all parts of the body, except the acting part. The patient is in some cases directed to move the free part in a particular direction, the effort to do so is resisted by the operator, with a force proportionate to the exertion made very nicely graduated to the particular condition of the part and of the system at large. The resistance is not uniform, but varies according to the varying action of muscles, as perceived by the operator. In other cases the operator acts while the patient resists. The action is the same, but in one case the patient's acting muscles are shortened; and in the other lengthened. The operator is a wrestle, in which a very limited

④ Incorporate muscle energy and proprioceptive neuromuscular facilitation techniques to enhance lengthening and stretching procedures.

portion of the organism is engaged. The motion must be much slower than the natural movement of the part engaged, which fact strongly fixes the attention and concentrates the will. The act is repeated two or three times with all the care and precision the operator can command, being cautious not to induce fatigue.

The use of movement as described in this next section follows the guidelines and recommendations described by Taylor. The principles of massage today are built on the same principles as those shown in the historical literature. The names may be different and the physiologic explanations more precise, but the methods are the same. The efficient use of massage techniques will reduce the need for repetitive massage manipulations. If used well, the neuromuscular mechanism can be activated and influenced quickly with less physical effort by the massage therapist (Box 10.1).

The techniques of passive and active joint movement, muscle energy, and proprioceptive neuromuscular facilitation work with the neuromuscular reflex system to relax and lengthen muscles. Stretching has both a reflexive and mechanical effect and is more focused on the connective tissue.

A working knowledge of the proprioceptive interaction between the prime mover and the antagonist is used to re-establish proper neurologic communication. All of the massage manipulations described previously affect proprioception reflexively. Sometimes the signals from a muscle can be continuously "on" or "off." Communication then becomes garbled and must be re-established. The focus of this section is to learn how to re-establish that all-important neurologic communication.

For example, if a client spends the day talking on the phone, holding the phone with the shoulder, the lateral neck flexors and shoulder elevators are in constant contraction while the other side of the neck is in constant extension. The neurologic signals sent to the muscles become confused and an energy imbalance results. An adaptation takes place so that when the neck muscle are used, there is painful resistance from the muscles whose proprioception is garbled. This type of interaction is responsible for most muscle tension. The following massage techniques specifically influence this essential proprioceptive mechanism.

Joint Movement

To understand joint movement, you must first understand the joint. A simplified review is included here. You are encouraged to consult anatomy and physiology resources for further clarification and understanding of individual joints (Fig. 10.26).

Box 10.1
SUMMARY OF "MOVEMENT CURE" ACCORDING TO TAYLOR'S INTERPRETATION

When using massage techniques:
1. Be specific.
2. Be mindful of patterns of "too much" and "not enough."
3. Position the client purposefully.
4. Stabilize the body so that only the focused target area is affected.
5. You may move the area or may cooperate in the effort with the client.
6. Be sure that the force and exertion are gradual and vary with the demand.
7. Remember that the purpose is to lengthen shortened tissue and tone weakened muscles.
8. You are a facilitator in the process.
9. Make sure the application is slow and purposeful.
10. Repeat the movement two or three times but not to fatigue.

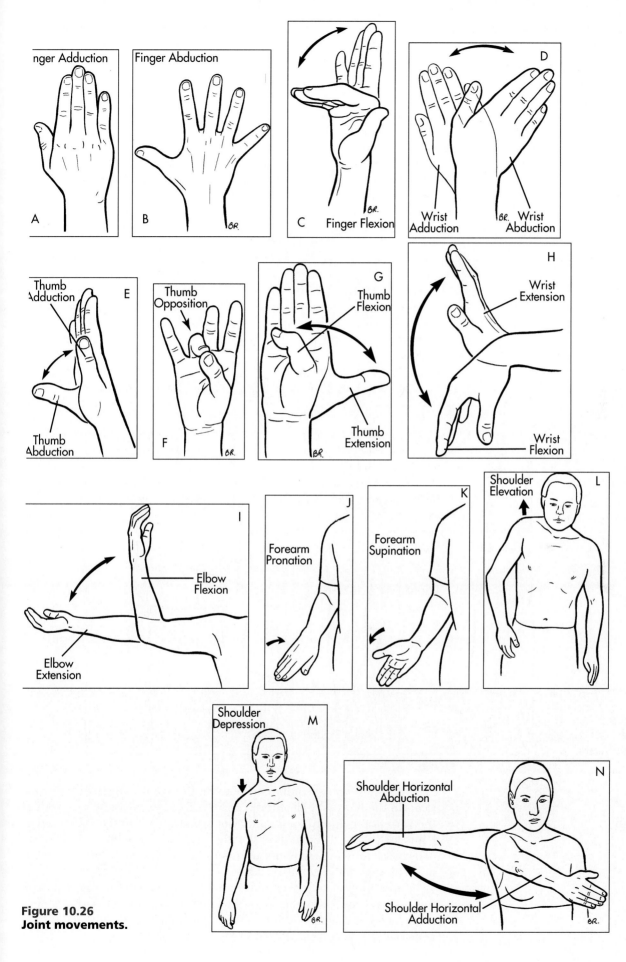

**Figure 10.26
Joint movements.**

continued

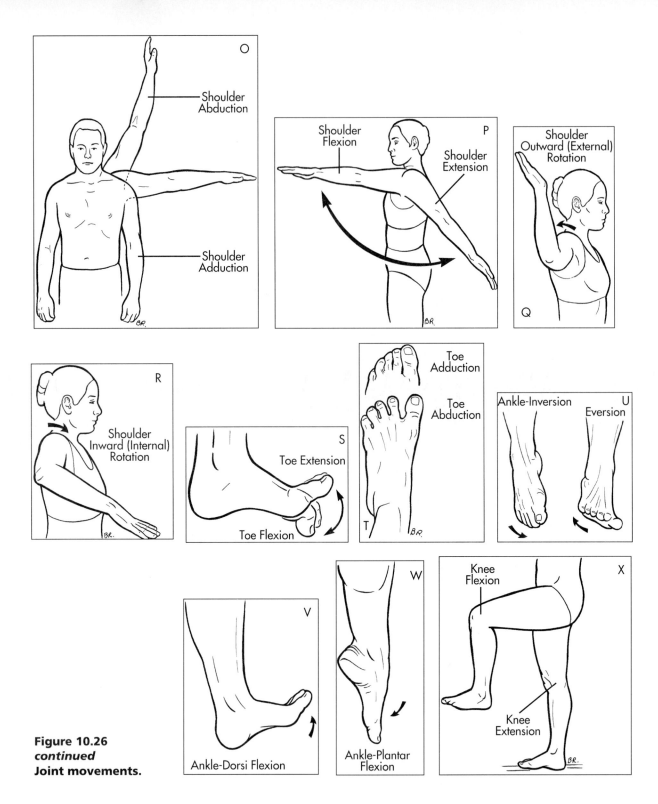

Figure 10.26
continued
Joint movements.

Joint movement techniques focus on the synovial or freely movable joints in the body (see Chapter 3, pg. 59). To a lesser extent, the joints of the vertebral column, hand, and foot are also considered, as are other joints such as the facet joints of the ribs, the sacroiliac joint, and the sternoclavicular joint. These joints are not directly influenced by muscles but move through indirect muscle action.

Joints allow us to move. Joint position and velocity receptors inform the central nervous system regarding where and how the body is positioned against gravity and how fast it is moving. This sensory data is the major determining factor for muscle tone patterns.

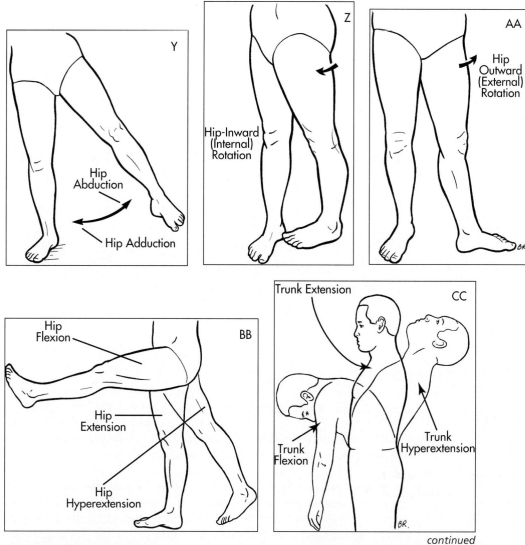

continued

Figure 10.26 *continued*
Joint movements.

We can control some joint movements voluntarily: we can move our limbs through various motions such as flexion, extension, abduction, adduction, and rotation. These are referred to as *physiologic* or *osteokinematic movements.* For normal physiologic movement, other types of movements *(accessory* or *arthrokinematic movements)* must occur owing to the inherent laxity or joint play that exists in each joint. This laxity allows the ends of the bones to slide, roll, or spin smoothly on each other. These essential movements occur passively with movement of the joint and are not under voluntary control.

A good example of joint motion is found on a door. The hinge holds the door both to the casing and away from the casing. In order for the door to open and close efficiently, the space must be maintained and the fit must be correct. In the body, ligaments act as the hinges. The door hinge must be oiled. In the joint, the synovial membrane secretes synovial fluid, produced on demand from joint movement. If a joint does not move, or is not moved, it will lock up like a rusty door hinge. If the fit of the door in the door casing is incorrect, or if the space is not maintained, the door will not open and close correctly. If the ligaments and connective tissue that make up the joint capsule are not firm enough to maintain joint space, the joint play is lost. If the ligaments and joint capsule are not pliable, then flexibility is lost. If the ligaments and joint capsule do not support the joint, then the fit is disrupted. Muscle contraction may pull the joint out of alignment. Muscle groups that flex and adduct the joints

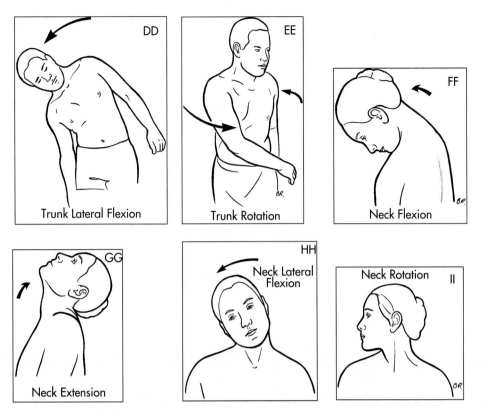

Figure 10.26 *continued*
Joint movements.

are about 30% stronger and have more mass than the extensors and abductors (see Chapter 11). If the body uses muscle contraction to stabilize a joint, the uneven pull between flexors and extensors, and adductors and abductors, will disturb the fit of the bones at the joint.

Joint-specific work, including any type of high-velocity manipulation, is beyond the scope of practice of the beginning massage professional. Because of the interplay between the joint proprioceptors, muscle tone, innervation of the joint, and surrounding muscles by the same nerve pattern, any damage to a joint can cause long-term problems. Working within the physiologic ranges of motion for each particular client is compatible with the scope of practice of the massage professional.

Joint movement involves moving the jointed areas within the physiologic limits of range of motion of the client. *Active* joint movement means that the client moves the joint by active contraction of muscle groups. *Active assisted* movement means that both the client and therapist move the area. *Passive* joint movement occurs when the client's muscles stay relaxed and the massage therapist moves the joint with no assistance from the client.

Whether active or passive, joint movements are always done within the comfortable limits of range of motion of the client. Anatomic barriers are determined by the shape and fit of the bones at the joint. Physiologic barriers are caused by the limits of range of motion imposed by protective nerve and sensory function. This type of barrier often displays itself as stiffness, pain, or a "catch." When using joint movement techniques, it is important to remain within the physiologic barriers and to gently and slowly encourage the joint to increase the limits of the range of motion.

When a joint is restricted or a muscle shortened, thus reducing the range of motion of its associated joint or region, there will always be a direction in which there is a limitation of movement. As the limit is reached, there will be a point beyond which comfortable movement is no longer possible. When a normal joint is taken to its limit, there is usually still a bit more movement possible, a sort of springiness in the joint. This is called a *soft end-feel*. When there is abnormal restriction, the limit does not have this spring, but like a jammed door or drawer, the joint is fixed at the barrier, and any attempt to take it further is uncomfortable and distinctly "binding" or jamming, rather than springy. This is called a *hard end-feel.* (see Chapter 11.) When doing passive joint movement, feel for the soft- or hard end-feel of the joint range of motion. This will become an important evaluation tool.

Joint movement becomes part of the application of muscle energy techniques and stretching methods. Because of this, the massage therapist should concentrate on the ability to efficiently and effectively use joint movement.

Joint movement is effective because it provides a means of controlled stimulation of the joint sensory receptors. Movement initiates muscle tone readjustment through the reflex center of the spinal cord and lower brain centers. As positions change, the supported movement gives the nervous system an entirely different set of signals to process. It is possible for the joint sensory receptors to learn not to be so hypersensitive. As a result, the protective spasm and movement restriction may lessen. Joint movement also encourages lubrication of the joint, an important addition to the lymphatic and venous circulation enhancement systems. Much of the pumping action that moves these fluids in the vessels results from compression against the lymph and blood vessels during joint movement and muscle contraction. The tendons, ligaments, and joint capsule are warmed from the movement. This mechanical effect helps keep these tissues pliable.

The illustrations provided show the "normal" range of motion for each joint. I have yet to encounter a "normal joint." Study the charts carefully, and use them to move each joint though its full range of motion, always being mindful to go slowly and stay within the limits of each client's physiologic barrier.

The client's body must always be stabilized, allowing only the joint being worked on to move. Occasionally, the entire limb is moved to allow for coordinated interaction among all the joints of the area, but the rest of the body is still stabilized. It is essential to move slowly because quick changes or abrupt moves may cause the muscles to form protective spasms.

Nerves stimulate muscles to contract, moving the joints. Nerves respond to sensory stimulation. If the signal is not quite strong enough the muscle may tense, but not contract. This is called *facilitation.* A facilitated area will respond to a lower-intensity sensory stimulation. If a threshold sensory signal does not occur, the nerve stays activated waiting to contact the muscle and discharge the tension. All massage therapists have had to deal with a leg or arm that is extremely stiff even though the client thinks it is relaxed. Most therapists will instruct the client to relax the muscles or use some other ineffective statement like, "Now just let me do it." The client cannot let go of the tension in the muscles because of the facilitation of the nerves. Systems that incorporate progressive relaxation recognize that a muscle will relax best if it contracts first. Active joint movement provides a mechanism to contract muscles, discharge the nervous system, and then allow for the normal relaxation phase to take over. A good approach is to have the client use active joint movement, pressing the area to be moved against the stabilizing pressure of the massage therapist. Then shake or rock the area to relax it.

Active Range of Motion

In active range of motion the client moves the area without any type of interaction by the massage therapist. This is a good assessment tool and should be used before and after any type of joint work because it provides information about the limits of range of motion and the improvement after the work is completed. This type of active range of motion is also great to teach as a self-help tool.

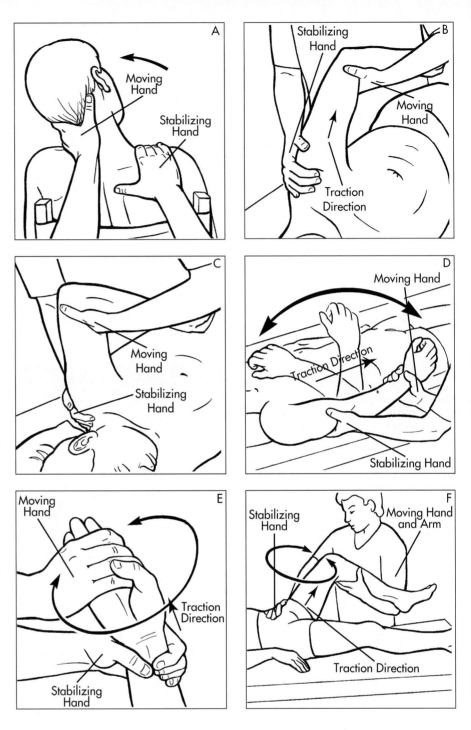

Figure 10.27
Examples of joint movement.
A, Neck. B & C, Shoulder joint.
Hand stabilizes at the shoulder joint while other hand produces a slight traction to the shoulder joint and moves shoulder through circumduction range of motion. (Circumduction—a circular movement of a jointed area.) D, Elbow joints. Stabilizing hand holds above elbow while moving hand produces a slight traction and moves joint through flexion and extension. Supination and pronation can also be achieved. E, Wrist joints. Stabilizing hand holds below wrist while moving hand produces a slight traction and moves joint through circumduction. F, Hip joint. Stabilizing hand holds above hip while moving hand and arm produces a slight traction and moves joint through circumduction.

A second type of active joint movement is sometimes called active assisted range of motion. In this movement, the massage practitioner firmly grasps and holds the end of the bone just distal to the joint being addressed. The massage therapist leans back slightly to place a small traction on the limb to take up the slack in the tissue, then instructs the client to push slowly against a stabilizing hand or arm while moving the joint through its entire range. A tap or light slap against the limb to begin the movement works well to focus the client's attention. Another method is to stabilize the entire circumference of the limb and instruct the client to pull gently or move the area. The job of the massage practitioner is to keep a gentle traction to prevent slack in the tissue, keep the movement slow, and give the client something to push or pull against, discharging the nervous system so the area can relax (Figure 10.27). The counterforce

**Figure 10.27 *continued*
Examples of joint movement. G, Hip joint alternate position. Stabilizing hand holds at opposite anterior superior iliac spine while moving hand moves hip through flexion and extension. No traction is produced in this position. H & I, Pelvis. Stabilizing hand and arm holds legs at calf while moving arm and hand moves pelvis to a side lying, "figure eight" pattern. J, Knee. Stabilizing hand holds above knee while moving hand produces a slight traction and moves joint through flexion and extension. K & L, Ankle. Stabilizing hand holds below above ankle while moving hand produces a slight traction and moves joint through circumduction.**

applied by the massage professional does not exceed the pushing or pulling action of the client but instead matches it. Once this is done, the client's body is more apt to accept passive range of motion.

Because the protective system of the joints does not like to be out of control, it takes time to prepare the body for passive range of motion. Shaking, rocking, and the active joint movement sequence previously described work well for this purpose.

If a client is paralyzed or very ill, only passive range of motion or joint movement may be possible. Some clients do not wish to participate in active joint movement and prefer to take a very passive role during the massage. Client participation is not necessary.

Hand placement with joint movement is very important. Make sure that the area is not squeezed or pinched. One hand should be placed close to the joint to be moved in order to act both as a stabilizer and for evaluation. The therapist's other hand is placed at the distal end of the bone and is the hand that actually provides the movement. Proper use of body mechanics is essential when using joint movement. The stabilizing hand must remain in contact with the client and must be placed near the joint being affected. Another method for placement of the stabilizing hand is to move the jointed area without stabilization and observe where the client's body moves most in response to the range of motion action. Place stabilizing hand at this point. Avoid working cross-body. Stand with thighs against the table while facing the client, positioned distal to the joint. Usually, the hand closest to the joint is the stabilizing hand. The actual movement comes from the massage practitioner's whole body, not from the shoulder, elbow, or wrist. The movements are rhythmic, smooth, slow, and controlled.

Before joint movement begins, the moving hand lifts and leans back to produce the slight traction necessary to put a small stretch on the joint capsule. If this is not done, the technique is much less effective. When tractioning is mastered and the joint is moved simultaneously, the size of the movement becomes smaller and the effect increases. It is not necessary or desirable to have the client's limbs flailing about in the air.

When incorporating joint movement into the massage, follow these basic suggestions:

- If possible do active joint movement first. Assess range of motion by having the client move the area. Then have the client move the area against your stabilizing force to increase the intensity of the signals from the contracting muscles, which discharges the nervous system.
- Incorporate any or all of the previously discussed massage methods.
- Once the tissue is warm and the nervous system relaxed, do the passive range of motion/joint movement.

During a massage session, strive to move every joint approximately three times. Each time, take up any slack in the tissues and gently encourage an increase in the range of motion.

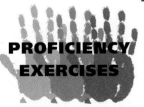

PROFICIENCY EXERCISES

1. **Using Fig. 10.26 for reference, move each of your joints through a normal range of motion, one at a time, using a variety of speeds. Notice the difference when you move slowly.**
2. **Pretend that a piece of plastic wrap is a joint. Hold one end tightly in your "stabilizing" hand. Now move the plastic wrap around, but do not stretch it or put any drag on the "tissue." Use your "moving hand" to traction the plastic wrap. Pull on it as far as it will go without stretching the tissue. Pretend to assess range of motion from this point and feel the difference. Lastly, pull the plastic wrap just a little more. Feel the pliability and do the joint movement from this position. Feel for the difference in effect.**
3. **Design and perform a massage incorporating joint movement using each of the basic flow patterns.**

Muscle Energy and Proprioceptive Neuromuscular Facilitation: Techniques to Lengthen Neurologically Shortened Muscles

Proprioceptive neuromuscular facilitation (PNF) techniques developed out of physical therapy during the 1950s. The first book on the subject, written by Margaret Knott and Dorothy Voss, was *Proprioceptive Neuromuscular Facilitation.*[6] The system was formalized as a rehabilitation method for spinal cord injury and stroke. It used maximal contraction and rotary diagonal movement patterns to re-educate the nervous system.

In recent years, the massage profession has begun to use pieces of the system to enhance stretching, primarily in athletes. The diagonal movement patterns incorporate cross-body movement used in repatterning for children born with various types of damage to the motor areas of the brain. Popularized as *cross-crawl,* the movements cause left and right brain hemispheres to function simultaneously by movement of one leg and the opposite arm into flexion and adduction to cross the midline of the body and then switching to the same movement with the other leg and arm. These types of movements reflexively stimulate the gait or walking pattern and are a valuable addition to any massage system (Fig. 10.28).

Muscle energy methods emerged from the osteopathic profession. Dr. T.J. Ruddy developed a technique he called *resistive induction.* Dr. Fred K. Mitchell is acknowledged as the father of the system that is now called *muscle energy technique.* He built on Dr. Ruddy's method and turned it into a whole-body approach.[4] Dr. Karel Lewit, author of *Manipulative Therapy in Rehabilitation of the Locomotor System,*[7] discusses the importance of methods that use post-isometric relaxation. Dr. Leon Chaitow, author of *Soft Tissue Manipulation* and many other books (see Chapter 1), synthesized these gentle methods, which fall within the scope of practice of therapeutic massage when used for general body normalization. Only those methods applicable to general massage are presented here. The system has much to offer and the diligent student of therapeutic massage will seek out additional training at more advanced levels. The majority of the information in this section is adapted from Dr. Chaitow's books and workshop notes.

The main difference between muscle energy and PNF is the origin of thought, the intensity of the muscle contraction, and how specific is the approach. For the purposes of this textbook they can be thought of as the same thing.

Muscle Energy Techniques

Muscle energy techniques involve a voluntary contraction of the client's muscle in a specific and controlled direction, at varying levels of intensity, against a specific counterforce applied by the massage practitioner. Muscle energy procedures have a variety of applications and are considered active techniques in which the client contributes the corrective force. The amount of effort may vary from a small muscle twitch to a maximal

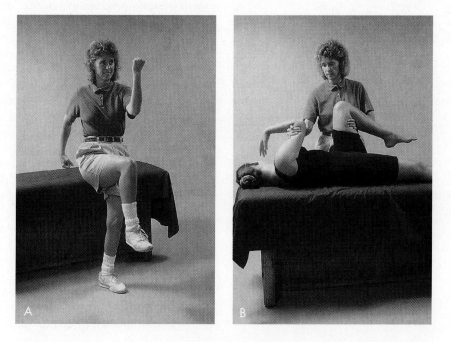

Figure 10.28
Cross crawl. A, Demonstration of cross crawl. B, Application of cross crawl with client on the table.

muscle contraction. The duration may last from a fraction of a second to several seconds. All contractions begin and end slowly, gradually building to the desired intensity. There is no jerking in the movement.

The focus of muscle energy techniques is to stimulate the nervous system to allow a more normal resting length. To describe what happens, the proper term *lengthening* is used because lengthening is more of a neurologic response that allows the muscles to stop contracting and to relax. Stretching is a mechanical force applied to the tissue.

Positioning

Muscle energy techniques are focused to specific muscles or muscle groups. It is important to be able to position muscles so that the origin and insertion are either close together or in a lengthening phase with the origin and insertion separated. There are resources that diagram specific positions for each muscle so that this can be accomplished. An alternate approach is to study muscle charts and understand the configuration of the muscle patterns. Practice isolating as many muscles as possible, keeping in mind that proper positioning is very important. When practicing, make sure that the muscles can be isolated regardless of whether the client is in a supine, prone, side-lying, or seated position (Fig. 10.29).

Counterpressure is the force applied to an area that is designed to match the effort or force exactly (isometric contraction) or partially (isotonic contraction). This holding force can be applied with the hand(s) of the person doing the exercise (the massage practitioner) against an immovable object, or against gravity where appropriate. The response of the method is specific to a certain muscle or muscle group referred to as the *target muscle*. The massage therapist uses three different types of muscle contractions to activate muscle energy techniques.

In an *isometric contraction,* the distance between the origin and the insertion of the target muscle is maintained at a constant length. A fixed tension develops in the target muscle as the client contracts the muscle against an equal counterforce applied by the massage therapist, preventing shortening of the muscle from the origin to the insertion. This is a contraction in which the effort of the muscle, or group of muscles, is exactly matched by a counterpressure, so that no movement occurs, only effort.

An *isotonic contraction* is one in which the effort of the target muscle or muscles is not quite matched by the counterpressure, allowing a degree of resisted movement to occur. With a concentric isotonic contraction, the massage therapist applies a counterforce but allows the client to move the origin and insertion of the target muscle together against the pressure. In an eccentric isotonic contraction, the therapist applies a counterforce but allows the client to move the jointed area so origin and insertion separate as the muscle lengthens against the pressure.

Isokinetic contractions require the client to move the joint through a full range of motion, using maximum muscle strength, against partial resistance supplied by the massage therapist. This is a multiple isotonic movement.

There are two neurophysiologic principles that explain the effect of the techniques as a result of physiologic laws being applied, not from mechanical force as in stretching. The first is postisometric relaxation (PIR; "tense and relax"), which occurs after an isometric contraction of the target muscle is over. The target muscle is lengthened passively to its comfort barrier (first point of resistance short of the client perceiving any discomfort). The isometric contraction involves minimal effort lasting seven to ten seconds. Following this contraction (which will have loaded the Golgi tendon organs and the musculotendinous junction and reflexively inhibited the extrafusal fibers of the muscle spindles) the muscle is in a refractory state and can be lengthened easily to a new resting

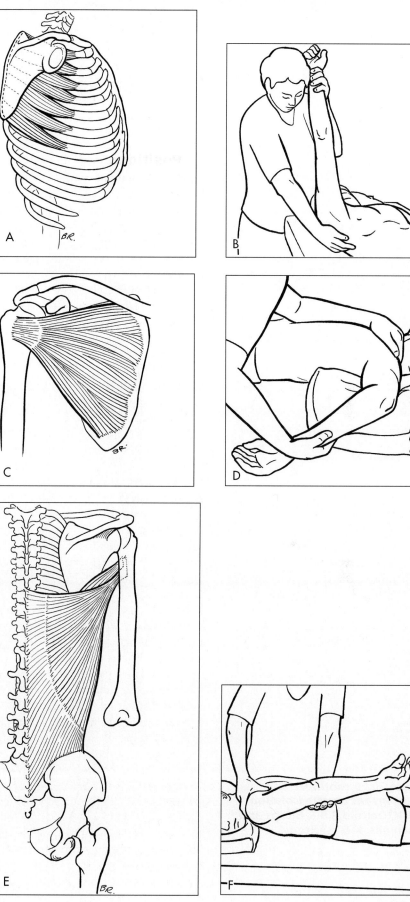

Figure 10.29
Positions for muscle isolation.
A & B, Serratus anterior.
C & D, Subscapularis.
E & F, Latissimus dorsi.

continued

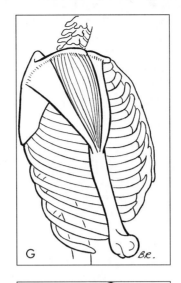

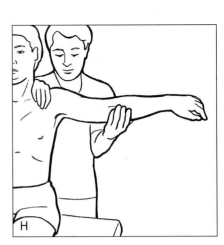

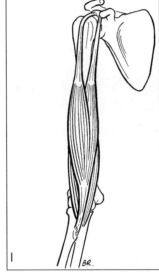

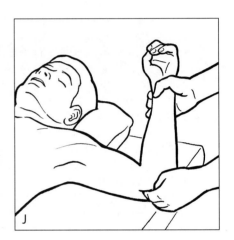

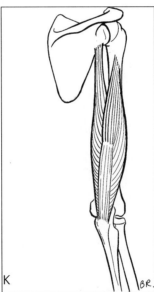

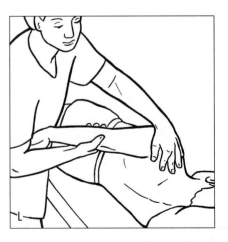

Figure 10.29 *continued*
**Positions for muscle isolation.
G & H, Deltoid. I & J, Biceps and
brachialis. K & L, Triceps.**

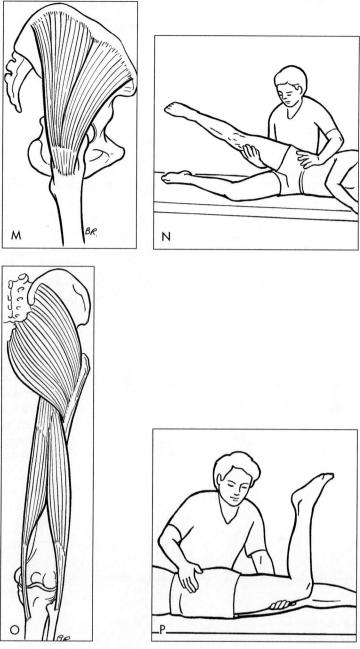

Figure 10.29 *continued*
Positions for muscle isolation.
M & N, Gluteus medius.
O & P, Gluteus maximus and
hamstrings.

continued

length. Repetitions continue until no further gain is noted. Post-isometric relaxation, which occurs after an isometric contraction of a muscle, results from the activity of the Golgi tendon bodies. It is in the brief latent period of ten seconds or so after such a contraction that the muscle can be lengthened painlessly, further than it could before the contraction.

Post-isometric Relaxation/
Tense and Relax Techniques

Procedure (Fig. 10.30)
1. Lengthen the target muscle to barrier. Back off slightly.
2. Tense the target muscle for 7–10 seconds.
3. Stop contraction and lengthen the target muscle. Repeat steps 1–3 until normal full resting length is obtained.

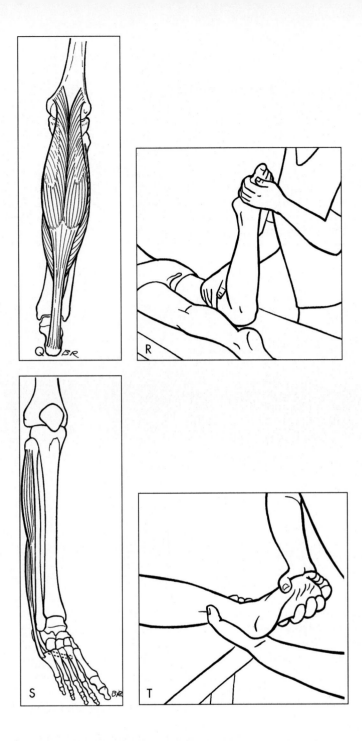

Figure 10.29 *continued*
Positions for muscle isolation.
Q & R, Gastrocnemius and soleus.
S & T, Peroneus.

Reciprocal Inhibition

The second principle is that of reciprocal inhibition (RI), which takes place when a muscle contracts, causing its antagonist to relax in order to allow for more normal movement. Generally, an isometric contraction of the antagonist of a shortened target muscle allows the muscle to relax and be taken to a new resting length. Such contractions usually begin in the mid-range rather than near the barrier of resistance and last seven to ten seconds. Reciprocal inhibition relaxes a target muscle as the tone increases in its antagonist. This works through the central nervous system, which cannot allow both the prime movers and the antagonists to be tightening at the same time in this reflex arc pattern.

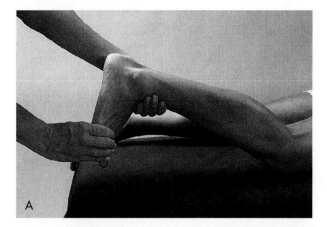

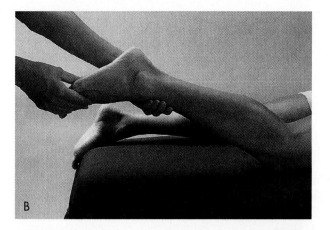

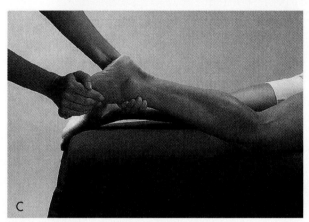

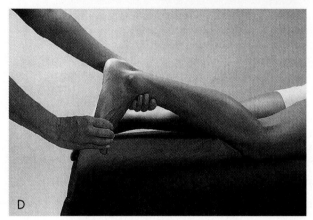

Figure 10.30
Post-isometric relaxation (PIR)/tense and relax techniques. Procedure: 1, Lengthen the target muscle (gastrocnemius/soleus) to barrier. (A) Back off slightly. (B) 2, Tense the target muscle for 7–10 seconds. (C) 3, Stop contraction and lengthen the target muscle. (D) Repeat steps 1–3 until normal full resting length is obtained.

Procedure (Fig. 10.31)

1. Isolate the target muscle by putting it in passive contraction (massage therapist moves the origin and insertion of the muscles together using joint positioning).
2. Contract the antagonist muscle group (the muscle in extension).
3. Stop contraction and slowly bring the target muscle into a lengthened state, stopping at resistance.
4. Place the target muscle slightly into contraction again.

Repeat steps 2 through 4 until normal full resting length is obtained.

"Make a Soft Muscle" Concept

Reciprocal inhibition is a great way to soften a muscle so that it can be massaged at its deeper levels. Any massage therapist knows what it is like to massage a hard muscle, especially when trying to get to tissue under that muscle. The following procedure reflexively makes a soft muscle, which in turn makes massage much easier.

Procedure (Fig. 10.32)

1. Isolate a target muscle or muscle group into passive contraction.
2. Place the hand that will massage the "soft muscle" on the target muscle. Place the other hand or other stabilizing object on the antagonist muscle group (the one that is stretched out at this point).
3. Have the client actively contract the antagonist muscles against the stabilization. The target muscle will be inhibited reciprocally and will become a "soft muscle." It will be easier to massage and the therapist will be able to reach the deeper areas.

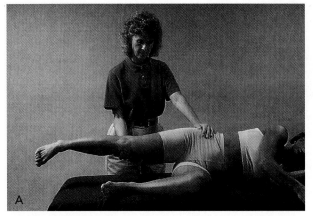
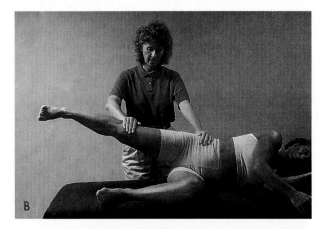

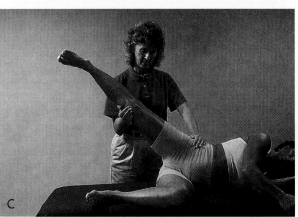

Figure 10.31
Reciprocal inhibition. Procedure: 1, Isolate the target muscles (adductors) by putting them in passive contraction (massage therapist moves the origin and insertion of the muscles together using joint positioning). (A) 2, Contract the antagonist muscle group (the muscle in extension). (B) 3, Stop contraction and slowly bring target muscle into a lengthened state, stopping at resistance. (C) 4, Place the target muscle slightly into contraction again. Repeat steps 2 through 4 until normal full resting length is obtained.

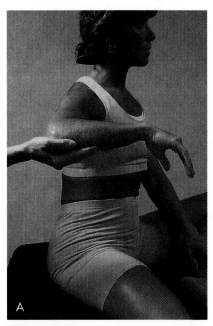
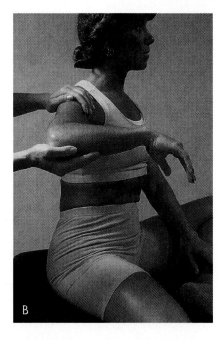
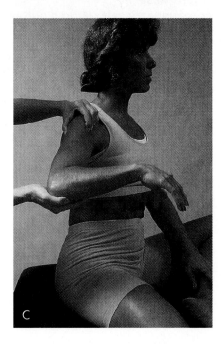

Figure 10.32
"Make a soft muscle concept." Procedure: 1, Isolate target muscle (deltoid) or muscle group into passive contraction. (A) 2, Place the hand that will massage the "soft muscle" on the target muscle. Place the other hand or other stabilizing object on the antagonist muscle group (the ones which are stretched out at this point). (B) 3, Have the client actively contract the antagonist muscles against the stabilization. (C) The target muscle will be reciprocally inhibited and become a "soft muscle". It will be easier to massage and the massage will be able to reach the deeper areas.

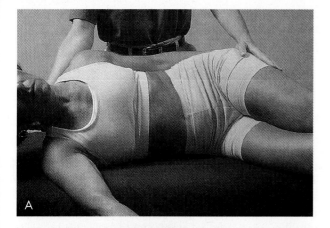
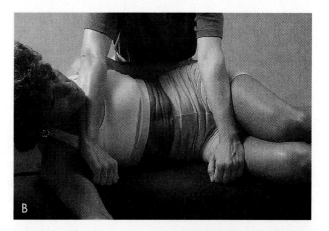
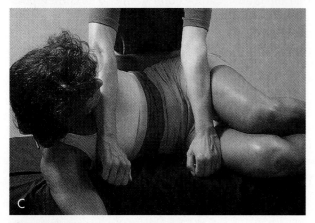
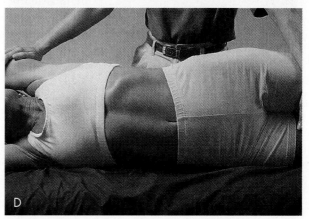

Figure 10.33
Procedure: 1, Isolate the target (abdominals) muscle by putting it into a passive contraction. (A) 2, Apply counter pressure for the contraction. (B) 3, Instruct the client to rapidly contract the target muscle in very small movements for about 20 repetitions. (C) 4, Slowly lengthen the target muscle. (D) 5, Repeat steps 2–4 until full normal resting length is obtained.

Pulsed Muscle Energy Procedures

Pulsed muscle energy procedures involve engaging the barrier and using small, resisted contractions (usually twenty in ten seconds), which introduces mechanical pumping as well as PIR or RI (depending on the muscles used.

Procedure (Fig. 10.33)

1. Isolate the target muscle by putting it into a passive contraction.
2. Apply counterpressure for the contraction.
3. Instruct the client to rapidly contract the target muscle in very small movements for about twenty repetitions.
4. Slowly lengthen the target muscle. Repeat steps 2 to 4 until full normal resting length is obtained.

Note: All contracting and resisting efforts should start and finish gently.

Muscle energy techniques usually do not use the full contraction strength of the client. With most isometric work, the contraction should start at about 25% of the strength of the muscle. Subsequent contractions can involve progressively greater degrees of effort but never more than 50% of the available strength.

Many experts use only about 10% of the available strength in muscles being treated in this way, and find that they can increase effectiveness by using longer periods of contraction. Pulsed contractions are also effective with minimal strength.

The use of coordinated breathing to enhance particular directions of muscular effort is helpful. As a general rule during massage, all muscular effort is enhanced by breathing in as the effort is made and exhaling on the lengthening phase.

Direct Applications

There are instances when the client does not wish to or cannot participate actively in the massage. The principles of muscle energy techniques can still be used by direct manipulation of the spindle cells or Golgi tendons. Pushing together in the direction of the fibers on the belly of a muscle weakens the muscle by working with the spindle cells. As the fibers of the muscle are pushed together, the spindle cells (which sense muscle length) think that the muscle is too short. The proprioceptive response is to relax the muscle fibers so that the muscle can be comfortable in its chosen position. Pushing together on the belly of the muscle is a way to relieve a muscle cramp. This is sometimes called *approximation*.

Separating the muscle fibers on the belly of the muscle and in the direction of the fibers strengthens the muscle. This time the spindle cells think the muscle is too long and signal the brain's proprioceptive intelligence to shorten the muscle so that the muscle can do the job appointed.

The same responses can be obtained by using the Golgi tendon organs except that the manipulation of the proprioception signal cells is reversed. Manipulation of the proprioception is at the ends of the muscle where it joins the tendons. To weaken the muscle, pull apart on the tendon attachments of the target muscle. This tells the body's proprioception center that tension on the tendon is excessive and the muscle should loosen in order to be in balance. To strengthen the muscle, push the tendon attachments together. This signals the body that there is too little tension on the tendon (in relation to the tension within the muscle belly). The muscle, in turn, contracts.

Direct Manipulation of Spindle Cells to Initiate Relaxation

Lengthening Response

Procedure (Fig. 10.34)
1. Place the target muscle in comfortable extension.
2. Press the spindle cells together on the target muscle.
3. Pull the spindle cells apart on the antagonist muscle.
4. Lengthen the target muscle.

Repeat steps 2 through 4 until normal full resting length is obtained.

Direct Manipulation of the Golgi Tendons to Initiate a Tense and Relax Response

Procedure (Fig. 10.35)
1. Place the target muscle in comfortable extension.
2. Pull apart on the tendon attachments of the target muscle.
3. Push the tendon attachments together on the antagonist muscle.
4. Lengthen the target muscle.

Repeat steps 2 through 4 until normal full resting length is obtained.

Positional Release/Strain-Counterstrain

Strain-counterstrain was formalized by Dr. Lawrence Jones and involves using tender points to guide the positioning of the body into a space where the muscle tension can release on its own. The tender points are often located in the antagonist of the tight muscle due to the diagonal balancing process the body uses to maintain an upright posture against

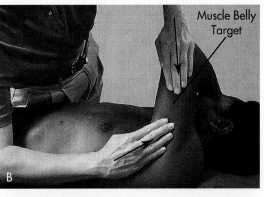

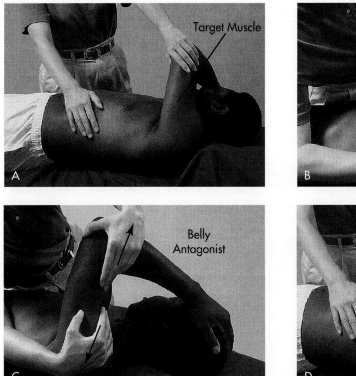

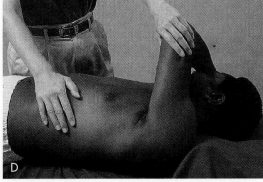

Figure 10.34
Direct manipulation of spindle cells to initiate relaxation lengthening response. Procedure: 1, Place the target muscle (triceps) in comfortable extension. (A) 2, Press the spindle cells together on target muscle. (B) 3, Pull the spindle cells apart on the antagonist muscle. (C) 4, Lengthen the target muscle. (D) 5, Repeat steps 2 through 4 until normal full resting length is obtained.

gravity (see Chapter 11). Strain-counterstrain methods are used on painful areas, especially recent strains, either before, after, or instead of muscle energy methods. Positional release is a more general method that allows the beginning therapist to do similar work.

Repositioning of the body into the original strain allows proprioceptors to reset and stop firing danger signals. By moving the body into the direction of ease (i.e., the way the body wants to go and out of the position that causes the pain), the proprioception is taken into a state of safety. By remaining in this state for a period of time the neuromuscular mechanism is allowed to reset itself. The massage therapist then gently and slowly repositions the area into neutral. The positioning used during positional release is a full-body process. An injury or loss of balance is a full-body experience. Areas distant to the tender point must be considered during the positioning process. It is very possible that the position of the feet will have an effect on a tender point in the neck.

Procedure (Fig. 10.36) The following is the sequence for generalized positional release.
1. Locate the tender point.
2. Gently initiate the pain response with direct pressure. Remember the sensation of pain is a guide.
3. Slowly position the body until the pain subsides.
4. Wait at least thirty seconds or longer until the client feels the release, lightly monitoring the tender point.
5. Slowly lengthen the muscle.
Repeat steps 1 through 5 until full normal resting length is obtained.

Positional release techniques are important because they gently allow the body to reposition. They are also one of the most effective ways of dealing with tender areas regardless of the pathology. Sometimes it is impossible to know why the point is tender to the touch, but if it is there will be a protective muscle spasm around it. Positional release is an excellent way to release these small areas of muscle spasm.

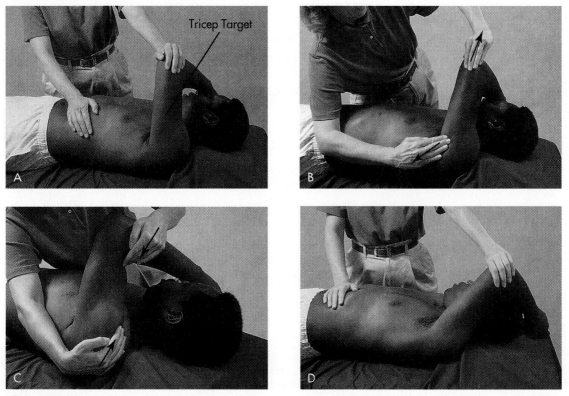

Figure 10.35
Direct manipulation of the golgi tendons to initiate a tense and relax response. Procedure: 1, Place the target muscle (triceps) in comfortable extension. (A) 2, Pull apart on the tendon attachments of the target muscle. (B) 3, Push the tendon attachments together on the antagonist muscle. (C) 4, Lengthen the target muscle. (D) 5, Repeat steps 2 through 4 until normal full resting length is obtained.

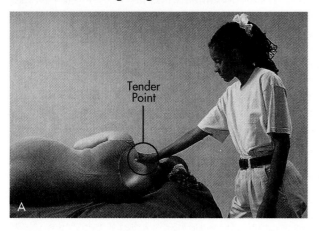

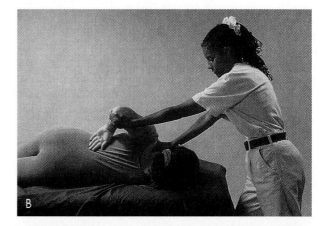

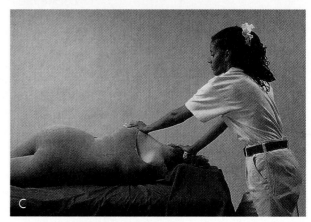

Figure 10.36
Positional release/strain-counterstrain. Procedure: The following is the sequence for generalized positional release. 1, Locate the tender point. 2, Gently initiate the pain response with direct pressure. Remember the sensation of pain is a guide. (A) 3, Slowly position the body until the pain subsides. Ease off on the pressure. 4, Wait at least 30 seconds or longer until the client feels the release. (B) 5, Slowly reposition into extended position. (C) 6, Repeat steps 1 through 5 until full normal resting length is obtained.

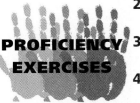

PROFICIENCY EXERCISES

1. **Design a progressive relaxation sequence for yourself using the concept of Post-isometric Relaxation (PIR).**
2. **Design a lengthening sequence for yourself using the pulsed muscle contraction.**
3. **Design a complete massage using petrissage and compression on "soft muscles."**
4. **Experiment with positional release concepts to relax sore spots on your body.**
5. **Design a complete massage incorporating all of the muscle energy/PNF methods presented.**

Stretching

Stretching is a mechanical method of pulling tissue to reduce tensile stress, which affects tendons, ligaments, areas of connective tissue concentration such as the lumbar dorsal fascial and the connective tissue component of muscles. Stretching and lengthening are different. The connective tissue component cannot be accessed until the muscle is lengthened. Without stretching, any neuromuscular lengthening will be restricted by shortened connective tissue. Before any stretching, lengthening must be done or the muscles of the area may form protective spasms. It is possible and often desirable to lengthen without stretching, but it is always necessary to lengthen before stretching. Chronic situations may develop changes in the surrounding connective tissue and may require stretching. Acute situations tend to be more neuromuscular in origin and lengthening is usually sufficient.

Longitudinal stretching pulls connective tissue in the direction of the fiber configuration. Cross-directional stretching pulls the connective tissue against the fiber direction. Both accomplish the same thing, but longitudinal stretching is done in conjunction with movement at the joint. If this is not advisable, if ineffective in situations of hypermobility, or if the area to be stretched is not effectively stretched longitudinally, then cross-directional stretching is a better choice. Cross-directional stretching is focused on the tissue itself, and is not dependent on joint movement. The tensile stress on connective tissue from stretching warms it and increases the water-binding properties of the ground matrix (the gelatin material of connective tissue). The result is softer and more pliable tissue.

Muscle energy and PNF techniques prepare muscles to stretch. Reciprocal inhibition neurologically interrupts the signal and "turns muscles off" by contracting the opposing muscle groups. Sustained or pulsed contractions may be used. "Tense and relax" or post-isometric relaxation takes advantage of the automatic relaxation of a muscle after contraction. Sustained or pulsed contraction may be used. Direct manipulation manually affects a muscle without client participation. Either effleurage, tapotement, or vibration to Golgi tendons or compression to the spindle cell mechanism may be used.

(For the purposes of this textbook, the term *static stretching* refers to stretching a muscle with no previous preparation. A static stretch can fatigue the muscle, causing it to relax. It is the least effective method of muscle stretching.)

The direction of ease is how the body allows for postural changes and muscle shortening or weakening depending on its balance against gravity. Although inefficient, the patterns developed serve a purpose and need to be respected. It seems logical to locate a shortened muscle group or a rotated movement pattern and use direct methods to reverse the pattern. However, this may not be the best approach. Protective sensory receptors

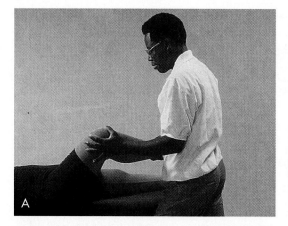
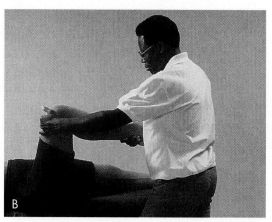
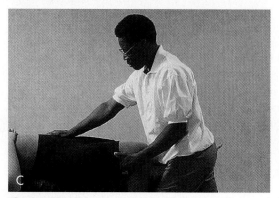
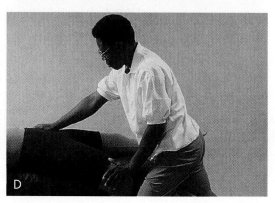

Figure 10.37
Longitudinal stretch. Procedure:
1, Position target muscle (quadriceps group) in "direction of ease."
Stabilize and isolate muscle group.
(A) 2, Choose a method to prepare target muscle to stretch. (In this example post isometric relaxation is used with client contracting the quadriceps against the stabilizing force of the massage therapist.) (B) 3, Once prepared, stretch the muscle to physiological barrier or wherever protective contraction is engaged. Stay in line with muscle fibers. Exert effort with one inhalation. Stretch on the exhalation. (C & D).

will prevent any forced stretch out of a pattern. Instead the pattern must be exaggerated and coaxed into a more efficient position.

For example, a client has shortened pectoralis muscles that pull the shoulders forward, giving a gorilla-like appearance. Instead of pulling the pectoralis muscles into a stretch by forcing the arms back, curl the shoulders and arms more into adduction, providing slack and space to the receptors in the pectoralis muscles.

Longitudinal Stretching
Stretch sequence (Fig. 10.37):
1. Position the target muscle in the "direction of ease." Stabilize and isolate muscle group.
2. Choose a method to prepare the target muscle to stretch (i.e., post-isometric relaxation, reciprocal inhibition, pulsed muscle energy, direct application).
3. Once prepared, stretch the muscle to its physiologic barrier or wherever protective contraction is engaged. Stay in line with muscle fibers. Exert effort with the inhalation. Stretch on the exhalation.
   The following two approaches are used for the actual stretch phase:
- Hold the stretch at the barrier for at least ten seconds to allow for the neurologic reset. This is the lengthening phase. Feel for secondary response (a small give in the muscle). Take up slack and hold for twenty to thirty seconds to reset the stretch reflex mechanism and to create longitudinal pull on the connective tissue. It is vital that you hold the muscle stretch as instructed to allow for changes in the connective tissue component of the muscle.

- Active isolated stretching uses different techniques to obtain the maximum length in a muscle. The muscle must be positioned properly to obtain lengthening. First, identify and isolate the muscle, making sure it is not working against gravity in this position. The client is reminded to exhale during the stretching phase of this technique. The muscle is then lengthened to its barrier, moved slightly beyond this point, and stretched gently for one to two seconds. The muscle is then returned to its starting position and this action is repeated. The client will benefit from doing a contraction with the antagonist while lengthening the target muscle. As in all proper lengthening and stretching movements, attention must be paid to the stretch reflex; bouncing is never done because it initiates this reflex.

Alternate Method for Longitudinal Stretching

If only a small section of muscle needs to be stretched, if the muscle does not lend itself to stretching with joint movement, or if the joints are so flexible that not enough pull is put on the muscles to achieve an effective stretch to the tissues, this method should be used.

Procedure (Fig. 10.38)

1. Locate the fibers or muscle to be stretched.
2. Place hands, fingers, or forearms in the belly of the muscle or directly over the area to be stretched.
3. Contact muscle with sufficient pressure to reset the neuromuscular mechanism.
4. Separate fingers, hands, or forearms or lift tissue with pressure sufficient to stretch muscle. Take up all slack from lengthening, then increase the intensity slightly and wait for the connective tissue component to respond (up to thirty seconds).

Note: All requirements for preparation of muscle and direction of stretch remain the same as described above.

Dr. Janet Travell popularized spray-and-stretch concepts. The reason the cold spray worked was that it stimulated cold receptors blocking other sensory signals so the proprioceptors were inhibited momentarily, allowing the muscle to relax. The cold spray used was a type of refrigerant that is no longer available because it damages the ozone layer. An ice pop (made by freezing water in a paper cup with a wooden stick inserted) can be used. Move the ice pop on the skin from origin to insertion along the path of the muscle that is to be stretched. Move at a speed of about one inch per second, and stretch the muscle.[11]

Using a form of tapotement, see what happens when the skin over the muscle along the same pathway as the ice pop massage is snapped quickly with a move like shooting marbles. If a tendon is tapped quickly, the muscle will contract. Use this method to assist in stretching. Apply the tap to the antagonist muscles so that they contract reflexively. As a result, the muscle you wish to stretch is inhibited reciprocally, allowing for a relaxation response and the ability to stretch with reduced protective muscle spasm.

Cross-Directional Stretching

Cross-directional tissue stretching uses a pull-and-twist component:

Procedure

1. Access the area to be stretched by moving against the fiber direction.
2. Lift or deform the area slightly and hold for thirty to sixty seconds until the area gets warm or seems to soften.

For skin and superficial connective tissue:

1. Locate area of restriction

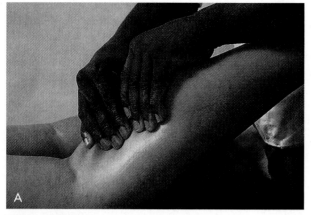
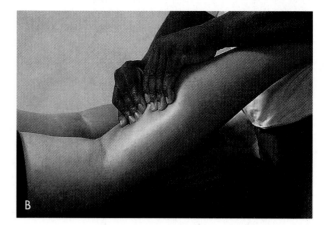

Figure 10.38
Alternate method for longitudinal stretching. Procedure: 1, Locate fibers or muscle to be stretched. 2, Place hands, fingers, or forearms in the belly of muscle or directly over area to be stretched. 3, Contact muscle with sufficient pressure to reset the neuromuscular mechanism. (A) 4, Separate fingers, hands, or forearms or lift tissue with pressure sufficient to stretch muscle. Take up all slack from lengthening first. Then increase intensity slightly and wait (up to 30 seconds) for connective tissue component to respond. (B)

2. Lift and pull (like taffy), first moving into the restriction and then pulling and twisting out of it, keeping a constant tension on the tissue (remember the plastic wrap exercise). Go slow. Take up slack until the area warms and softens.

To get to deep fascial planes it is necessary to have an understanding of the cranial sacral mechanisms and the deep structures involved. Entry level training does not explore this level of work. The approaches of cranial sacral therapy and advanced soft tissue systems such as myofascial release, deep tissue work, and soft tissue manipulation provide instruction in these very valuable methods. It is important to realize that we are one body with all its parts interconnected. Therefore, all stretching affects deep connective tissue. It is impossible to separate the body into layers. The only difference is the access point. A house may have three or four doors, each of which will let you into the house. Where you enter may be different, but once in you can have an influence on all the areas.

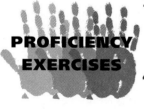

PROFICIENCY EXERCISES

1. **Petrissage (knead) extra flour into bread dough so that the consistency is quite firm. Practice stretching the dough. Feel for the give of the tissue as opposed to the tissue breaking.**
2. **Design a lengthening and stretching sequence for yourself that accesses the major muscle groups and connective tissue areas. Pay attention to the difference in the feel of neuromuscular lengthening with its quick release and connective tissue stretching with its softer, slower give.**
3. **Have a fellow student assume various stretch positions. Tell him or her to stretch as far as is comfortable and hold. Take the area and stretch it 1/8″ further and hold it. Pay attention to that feeling, and talk with the student to get feedback.**
4. **Practice tapping antagonist tendons and using ice massage on a client as you position the body for various stretches. Be willing to experiment. If you do, you will become your own best teacher.**
5. **See how many massage manipulations and techniques you can combine and do at once (e.g., joint movement combined with compression; effleurage combined with a stretch; tapotement combined with a stretch; petrissage combined with muscle energy methods, especially the "make a soft muscle" concept.**
6. **Design a massage for each of the basic flow patterns that combines at least two methods or techniques for every application.**

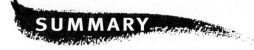

SUMMARY

In this chapter you have had the opportunity to design and give many different types of massage. Now that you have all the individual skills to give a great massage, your job is to practice using them in combination. The next chapter on designing the massage will help you to develop general assessment skills. The information gathered during the assessment will help you to decide what massage manipulations and techniques to use.

Massage manipulations and techniques can be combined to produce an infinite number of moves. Students must give themselves permission to practice and improvise. As you practice, ask the client how a particular application of a technique or massage manipulation feels. Always be open to thinking things through and do not be afraid to experiment with new techniques.

REVIEW QUESTIONS

1. What are the three effects of massage methods and techniques on the body? Explain each one.
2. Which massage methods seem to be more mechanical?
3. Which methods seem to be more reflexive?
4. What are the seven aspects of quality of touch?
5. What is the importance of variation of the quality of touch concepts as to variety in speed, rate, rhythm, and duration?
6. What is the importance of a basic flow pattern?
7. Why is the pattern for the abdominal massage always the same?
8. Why do you think that the similar trends, applications, and methods continue to make up the body of knowledge of therapeutic massage?
9. What are the major differences between massage manipulations and massage techniques?
10. What are the main uses for the resting position?
11. How does the massage therapist first approach the client?
12. What is the distinguishing characteristic of effleurage?
13. Why should deeper applications of effleurage/gliding always move slowly?
14. What are some specific uses of the effleurage/gliding massage manipulation?
15. What are the distinguishing qualities of petrissage/kneading?
16. Why should the massage therapist use petrissage sparingly?
17. What conditions interfere with the use of petrissage?
18. What are the physiologic effects of compression?
19. What are some things to remember to protect the therapist's hands and arm while doing compression?
20. Where is the best anatomic location to do vibration? Why?
21. How is rocking different than shaking?
22. What is the strongest physiologic effect of tapotement/percussion?
23. Where does the movement for tapotement come from?
24. What are the distinguishing characteristics of friction?
25. How long does friction need to be done to accomplish the desired results?
26. Describe two methods to apply friction.
27. Why does the use of joint movement and muscle energy techniques make massage manipulations more effective?
28. What are the three types of proprioceptors affected by movement techniques? What do they detect?
29. What are the two different types of joint movement described in this text?
30. What is the physiologic range of motion barrier?
31. Explain hand placement for joint movement?
32. What are the major uses of PNF/muscle energy techniques?
33. Describe the concept of lengthening.

34. **What is the importance of positioning?**
35. **What are the types of muscles contraction used for muscle energy techniques? Explain each one.**
36. **What is post-isometric relaxation (PIR)?**
37. **What is reciprocal inhibition (RI)?**
38. **How do pulsed muscle energy methods differ from the other methods described?**
39. **What is the target muscle?**
40. **How much strength is required during the contraction for the muscle energy method to work?**
41. **When is direct application of spindle cells and Golgi tendons used?**
42. **When is positional release/strain-counterstrain used?**
43. **Define stretching.**
44. **Why must lengthening methods be used before stretching?**
45. **Do all areas need to be stretched?**
46. **What are the two basic types of stretch?**
47. **What is direction of ease and why is it important?**

REFERENCES

1. Baumgartner AJ: *Massage in athletics,* Minneapolis, 1947, Brugess Publishing Company.
2. Beard G: A history of massage technic, *Physical ther Rev* 32: 613–624, 1952.
3. Cyriax E: Some misconceptions concerning mechano-therapy, *Br J Physical Med* October 1938, 92–94.
4. Greenman PE: *Principles of manual medicine,* Baltimore, 1989, Williams and Wilkins.
5. Kellogg JH: *The art of massage,* Battle Creek, MI, 1929, Modern Medicine Publishing Co.
6. Knott M and Voss D: *Proprioceptive neuromuscular facilitation,* New York, 1956, Harper and Row.
7. Lewit K: *Manipulative therapy in rehabilitation of the locomotor system,* ed 2, Oxford, 1991, Butterworth-Heinemann Ltd.
8. McNaught AB and Callander R: *Illustrated physiology,* ed 4, New York, 1983, Churchill Livingstone.
9. Anderson KE, Anderson LE, Glanze D, eds: *Mosby's Medical, Nursing, and Allied Health Dictionary,* 4/E, St. Louis, 1990, Mosby–Year Book.
10. Taylor GH: *An illustrated sketch of the movement cure: Its principle methods and effects,* New York: 1866, The Institute.
11. Travell JG and Simons DG: *Myofascial pain and dysfunction The trigger point manual,* Baltimore, 1984, Williams and Wilkins.

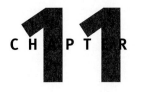

CHAPTER 11

DESIGNING THE MASSAGE

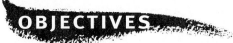

OBJECTIVES

After completing this chapter, the student will be able to:

1 Conduct an effective client interview.
2 Conduct a basic physical assessment.
3 Interpret assessment information, and develop a treatment plan.
4 Document information in a SOAP notes charting format.

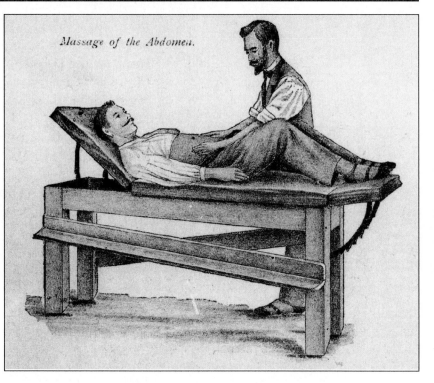

Massage of the Abdomen.

Massage approach employing manual vibrational therapy to stimulate peristalsis and relieve constipation. (Bettmann Archive)

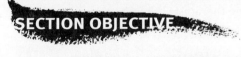

INTRODUCTION

The massage professional does not simply perform a step-by-step massage routine. However in the initial learning process, it is important for students to understand the value of sequence and general flow of the massage pattern. Massage routines are a learning method. Once the student grasps the concepts, the routine must evolve to meet the unique needs of the individual client. If the student can only perform a routine and does not understand how to modify and alter the application of therapeutic massage, there will be limits in his or her ability to best serve the client. People do not usually fit into a routine sequence of massage techniques. For the best results, the concepts learned from doing the routines need to be designed to fit individual needs of the client, instead of trying to make the client fit the routine.

Rather than providing the structure of a precise, systematic step-by-step routine, this text teaches the student to design a massage. There is no right way to do a massage and only a few wrong ways. If the general guidelines given in this chapter are followed, and the student is willing to think the massage through and modify the plan as he or she goes, the massages provided for the clients will meet the desired outcome. It is common to be clumsy with massage applications at first. Skills will evolve with experience and practice. Very few, if any, people do something the best way on their first attempt. Expertise is a never-ending process of learning, modification, and change. By working with a client-centered focus, allowing the client's needs to direct the massage, and not forcing any type of response, the client should experience beneficial results.

While learning the massage methods and techniques, many routines are practiced. In the Proficiency Exercise sections in Chapter 10, the student had to design several massage sessions to learn how to use a particular method. There were exercises that required that the student learn to combine methods. Basic flow patterns were given in order to teach an organized approach to the massage. Now it is time to use each method in a purposeful way and to blend all the methods into the massage.

SEQUENCE AND FLOW

Using the information presented in this section, the student will be able to:

❶ Design a basic full-body massage.

The basic full-body massage is a common approach in massage. The session lasts about one hour. The purpose of the massage is to affect the whole body, with some specific attention to problem areas. No matter what type of massage approach is used, the first, and maybe the most important massage manipulation to use is the resting position, or the first touch. As explained in the previous chapter, it must be done with skill and sensitivity.

The next massage manipulations chosen are used for general, broad applications and to connect all the other methods. This is the same concept as soup broth. The broth itself is the medium that all other massage manipulations and techniques float in, just like the vegetables contained in the broth of vegetable soup.

Methods used for general broad applications are *effleurage* or gliding strokes, compression, and rocking.

The most common massage manipulation chosen is the *effleurage* or gliding stroke. This manipulation is effective for:

- Applying lubricant
- Covering a large surface area efficiently
- Making changes between manipulations
- Moving from one area to another
- Creating a soothing approach for the massage

Compression is effective in situations when:

- Lubricant is not used
- People are hairy or ticklish
- The client prefers a more stimulating massage

Rocking is very effective when:

- Lubricant is not used
- Excessive rubbing or pressing on the skin or underlying tissue is not desirable
- Clients desire a soothing massage with generalized body responses

It is beneficial to blend these three methods to provide the general base of the massage.

The massage has a sense of wholeness with a beginning point and an ending point. The basic flow patterns from Chapter 10 provided the basis for this sense of structure. There needs to be a general sense of continuity to the massage. In simple words, the massage needs to flow, to feel connected like one continuous experience made up of all the applications of the massage methods in response to the individual client's needs. The general massage has to stimulate all of the sensory nerve receptors, contact all of the layers and types of tissues, and move all of the major joints of the body. There are a million ways to give a massage, and the choices made each time a massage is given develop from an understanding of the principles and practice of massage therapy. Each massage is different because the client is different each time, even if that client has been seen for many massage sessions.

The focus of the session depends on the needs of the client. To understand what those needs are, the massage practitioner must be able to take a general history and do a basic assessment of the client. Based on the information gathered in the history and assessment process, the therapist will then design the best massage for the individual client by picking and choosing what methods, rhythm, pacing, pressure, intensity, and amenities, such as music, to use.

The manipulations and techniques described in Chapter 10 were chosen for a specific type of reflexive (sensory stimulation), chemical, or mechanical response. The physiologic effects of each manipulation is explained in Chapter 10. Review this information. *Effleurage* or gliding strokes have many applications. The same is true for all the other methods. Assessment is how the massage therapist gathers the necessary information to begin to design the massage.

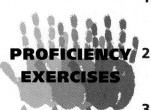

PROFICIENCY EXERCISES

1. **Design a general massage that combines *effleurage* or gliding strokes, compression, and rocking. Use only these methods to get the feel of "making a nice broth in which to build the massage soup."**

2. **Return to Chapter 10 and list each method that has a reflexive response. Then repeat this exercise for mechanical and chemical effects.**

3. **Design four different one-hour massage sequences on paper. Within the four massage patterns, be sure to use all the methods and tech-**

niques from Chapter 10. Find at least two other students and trade papers. Perform the other person's massages; attempting to follow another's sequence teaches many things. When you are finished, list what you learned from the experience, and share the list with your partners in the exercise.

4. Find at least three different massage professionals who were trained in different schools. Receive a massage from each. Report your objective and subjective observations in response to the basic sequence and flow of each massage. (Hint: review Chapter 4.)

ASSESSMENT

SECTION OBJECTIVES

Using the information presented in this section, the student will be able to:

❶ Use a SOAP note process during the assessment and charting procedure.

❷ Effectively interview a client by developing rapport skills, observation skills, and listening skills.

❸ Do a basic physical assessment, gait assessment, 13 level palpation assessment, and muscle testing assessment.

It is important to remember that the massage professional is not equipped to diagnose or treat any specific medical condition except under direct supervision of a licensed medical professional. The interpretation of the information gathered in the assessment section is for three purposes.

1. To determine if the client should be referred to a medical professional
2. To obtain informed consent from the client as well as active input from the client to be incorporated into the development of the massage plan
3. To design the best massage for the client

In reality, the assessment and application of massage technique is almost the same. During the actual massage, it is not uncommon to use massage manipulations and techniques to evaluate and assess the tissue and then use the same manipulation and technique, altered slightly in intensity, to normalize the situation (adaptation). For teaching purposes, the two approaches have been separated. One of the most difficult things to teach is pure assessment. Students rush into adaptation techniques without taking the time to discover the pattern that the client is presenting. The student must learn to separate assessment information obtained during the massage and learn to evaluate this information before attempting to alter the condition presented by the client.

Assessment is a skill. The ability to incorporate this skill enhances the quality of treatment given by the massage professional. Assessment is the collecting and interpretation of information provided by the client, the client's consent advocates (parent or guardian), and the referring medical professionals, as well as from information gathered by the massage practitioner.

In more clinical settings, assessment done by the massage professional is considered in the total treatment plan developed in cooperation with the client's health care team. Therefore, the massage practitioner needs to understand and practice standard assessment and charting procedures. Charting is a process of recording the ongoing massage program for a client. The SOAP-notes procedure used by nurses, physical therapists, and other health care professionals is discussed in this textbook. The procedure has been adapted for use by massage professionals. This text has also attempted to incorporate as many variations as possible. Whatever SOAP-notes procedure ultimately is used, it must be consistent in the charting of assessment information, the massage treatment plans, and the client's responses and progress during the massage sessions. SOAP notes are completed after each massage session with a client. The accumulation of these records becomes a paper trail of the client's massage treatment progress. This information is useful to review the client's progress and to develop future massage sessions.

SOAP Notes

The acronym SOAP stands for *subjective* assessment/information, *objective* assessment/information, *application,* and *plan/progress.* The SOAP notes process is a method of gathering and processing information. Regardless of the actual form used, the process evolves into a virtually automatic way of thinking.

Subjective Assessment

Subjective assessment is information provided by the client during the interview and history-taking process. The client's goals and desired outcome for the session are also a part of subjective assessment.

Objective Assessment

Objective assessment is the information that the massage therapist gathers from the assessment and history-taking process. The massage therapist also needs to state the goals for the session and be sure that the client's goals match.

From the subjective and objective information, the massage therapist, in cooperation with the client and with the client's informed consent, designs the massage session.

Application

The application section is a record of what was done during the session. It is a general list of methods used, any specific work that was done, and what the responses are to the work.

Plan/Progress

The plan/progress section includes information concerning the focus of the next massage session, areas that may need attention, evaluation of the progress, what applications seem to be working or not working, any self-help information that is shared, and other details that will influence future sessions.

The sample form is modified for the student to use to enhance learning. The added sections for techniques used, information learned, areas to be done differently, and comments received from the client provide for a self-assessment process as a learning experience. It is suggested that this process be used for a minimum of one hundred hours of massage—the more, the better. The form can also be modified for professional practice (Fig. 11.1).

SOAP NOTES STUDENT PRACTICE FORM					
Date ____ Name of Student	Practice Client's Name	Subjective Evaluation	Objective Evaluation	Application	Plan/Progress
Techniques Used	Information Learned	Focus on Improvement for Next Session	What Worked Well	Client Comment	

Figure 11.1
SOAP notes student practice form.

This modified version of SOAP-note charting is an excellent way to learn as the client progresses. If the student should move into a clinical setting, the charting process would be more specific and formal. Most clinical settings will have their own forms and variations of the SOAP-note process.

ESTABLISHING RAPPORT

The client is the most important resource during the assessment process. The skills required of the massage therapist during this process are the ability to establish rapport, keen observation, successful interviewing methods, and active listening.

Rapport is the development of a relationship based on mutual trust and harmony. It is the responsibility of the massage professional to initiate a sense of rapport with clients.

It is best to begin establishing rapport by learning and using the person's name. The massage practitioner needs to show a genuine interest in the person that goes beyond the problem that the person presents. What happens to a person affects the whole being. Many people need time to sort their thoughts and feelings and develop their statements. The conversation should proceed slowly, and the client should never be rushed. By giving the person full attention and by observing what makes the client most comfortable, it will be easier to resist the urge to treat everyone in the same manner. If the massage professional uses words, voice tone, and body language that is similar to that of the client, rapport will be further enhanced.

HOW TO OBSERVE

During the initial conversation, it is important to pay very close visual attention to the client. If the practitioner has a visual impairment, information gathered from the interview and physical assessment replaces visual assessment. An effective therapist uses all of the senses—hearing, smelling, seeing, and intuition. Information is only gathered at this time, not interpreted.

The practitioner senses the general presence of the person at this time—how well the client moves and breathes. Does the client's presence suggest sympathetic or parasympathetic activation? Sympathetic activation is the display of restlessness, anxiety, fear, anger, agitation, elation, or exuberance. Parasympathetic activation is indicated by a general relaxed appearance, contentment, slowness, or depression. Normal approaches of therapeutic massage can either stimulate or relax; this needs to be considered when designing the massage. The client's general state should also be taken into account as the massage therapist talks and interacts with the client. It is important to understand the client's needs so that his or her desired health outcome is attained. If a client is active and exuberant (sympathetic activation), the initial massage approach and the energy level of the massage practitioner need to match the energy level of the client. If the focus of the session is to calm the client, the therapist will begin to slow down as the massage progresses and may introduce appropriate rhythmic approaches to provide a calming effect. If the client is tired or moderately depressed, the therapist needs to proceed slowly in the initial pace of the massage. During the session, the energy and activity level of the massage practitioner and the methods used can increase as the client's energy increases.

Paying attention to detail and the needs of the client provides essential information to a sensitive, well-trained therapist. The client will notice the difference between the massage therapist who takes the time to honor needed space and adjust to it and the practitioner who tries to make the client fit into a routine method of massage application.

The practitioner must pay attention to where and how a client indicates that there is a problem on his or her body. These gestures will often show if a client has a muscle problem, joint problem, or visceral problem. The section on interpreting assessment information will explain this in greater detail. Another important activity is to observe the client's body language and responses while discussing various topics. Everything the person does is important. There is a pattern to everyone's behavior, and all the pieces of information will combine to show that pattern.

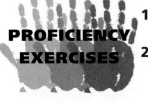

PROFICIENCY EXERCISES

1. **Watch people in a public place like a mall or airport. Is the general presence of a sympathetic or parasympathetic nature?**
2. **Ask ten people to explain a physical ache or pain to you. Watch their gestures carefully. What similarities do you notice in their explanations?**

INTERVIEWING

Open-ended questioning encourages conversation. It is important to avoid questions that can be answered with only one word. The point of the interview is to assist the client in communicating health history and revealing the reason for the massage. The question,"Have you ever had a professional massage before?" only requires the client to say "yes" or "no." A better question would be "What is your experience with therapeutic massage?" The second question requires the client to give more extensive detail when answering. When the client provides any information, it is important for the practitioner to restate what the client has said. The client will then have the opportunity to correct any information and be assured that the therapist was listening.

When speaking to the client, it is important to use words that the person can understand. Although professionalism is important, medical terminology does not have to be used. If a client uses a word that is unclear, the therapist should ask what he or she means. Asking for clarification enhances knowledge and understanding of the information obtained from the client.

There is specific information that needs to be obtained from the client. When encouraging conversation, it is easy to forget to ask the important questions. Using a client information form as a tool during the interview provides a framework for obtaining the necessary information. (see Chapter 7, Fig. 7.7).

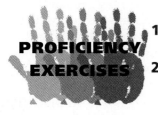

PROFICIENCY EXERCISES

1. **Using the sample client information form, practice asking three open-ended questions for each category.**
2. **During conversation with ten different people, practice restating information given to you in response to a question you asked.**

LISTENING

When listening, it is important to ONLY listen because listening cannot be done while thinking about what is going to be said, while writing, or when interpreting information. An active listener will nod or show other signs of interest to encourage the person to continue to speak. A client must also be allowed to finish a sentence and not be rushed or interrupted. Some people internally rehearse what they say before they say it. They will speak with pauses between their statements, and the practitioner must wait for the thoughts to be completed. If interrupted, the client will often forget what he or she was going to tell you. Other clients will talk nonstop. They may need to sort through their information by saying it aloud. When the client has completed a thought, it is important for the massage therapist to summarize and restate the information to ensure it was understood correctly. It is amazing how often information is misinterpreted. A competent professional will be very careful of any preconceived ideas and maintain an open mind until the assessment process is completed.

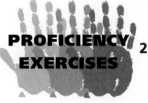

PROFICIENCY EXERCISES

1. Practice **LISTENING ONLY**. Keep a notebook with you, and mark down each time you begin to think of how you are going to respond to what the person is saying to you.
2. Carry around a tape recorder, and record general conversation. Before playing back the tape, write down what you think you heard. Then, play back the tape, and listen to what was actually said. This exercise is a real lesson in how little we hear when we listen.

PHYSICAL ASSESSMENT

When the subjective assessment is complete, the massage therapist may choose to do a physical assessment before beginning the massage. For a basic massage, the physical assessment is usually limited to the client showing to the massage practitioner any movements that feel restricted or may be causing pain. It is important to ask the client to point out any bruises, varicose veins, or areas of inflammation in order to avoid working over these areas. The massage therapist must ask the question, "Are there any areas that you feel I should avoid?" Be sure the information is indicated on the client information form and that these areas are avoided.

During physical assessment, the main considerations are body balance, efficient function, and basic symmetry. People are not perfectly symmetric, but the right and left halves of the body should be similar in shape, range of motion, and ability to function. The greater the discrepancy in symmetry, the more the potential for soft-tissue dysfunction. Assessment for a basic massage includes a general evaluation of the client's posture and gait (walking pattern). The ear, shoulder, hip, and ankle should be in a vertical line. If the gate reflexes are disrupted for any reason, there is a potential for many problems to develop. Common gait problems include functional short leg caused by muscle shortening, tight neck and shoulder muscles, aching feet, and fatigue. The massage therapist must have an understanding of basic biomechanics including posture, interaction of joint functions, and gait.

Posture Assessment—Standing Position

Three major factors influence posture: heredity, disease, and habit. These factors must be considered when evaluating posture. The easiest influence to adjust is habit. By normalizing the soft tissue and teaching balancing exercises, the massage practitioner can play a very beneficial role in helping clients overcome habitual postural distortion. Habits may be occupational, like a shoulder raised from talking on the phone, recreational (such as a forward-shoulder position in a bike rider), or sleep-related.

The influence of clothing, shoes, and furniture affects the way a person uses his or her body. Tight collars or ties restrict breathing and contribute to neck and shoulder problems. Restrictive belts, control top undergarments, or tight pants also limit breathing and will affect the neck, shoulders, and mid-back areas. Shoes with high heels or those that do not comfortably fit the feet will interfere with postural muscles. Shoes with worn soles will imprint the old postural pattern, and the client's body will again assume the dysfunctional pattern. It is important to change to shoes that do not have a worn sole if postural changes are to be maintained. Sleep positions can contribute to a wide range of problems. Furniture that does not support the back or is too high or too low perpetuates muscular tension.

When assessing posture, it is important for the massage therapist to notice the complete postural pattern. For every action there is a reaction. Most compensation patterns (reactions) are responding to gravitational forces. The body makes countless compensatory changes daily. This is normal and, in the absence of other pathology, seldom becomes problematic. However, if the client has had an injury, maintains a certain position for a prolonged period of time, or overuses a body area, the body's ability to return to a normal dynamic balance may not be efficient. The force of gravity and the balance of the body against it is the fundamental determining factor in one's posture or upright position. It is important to

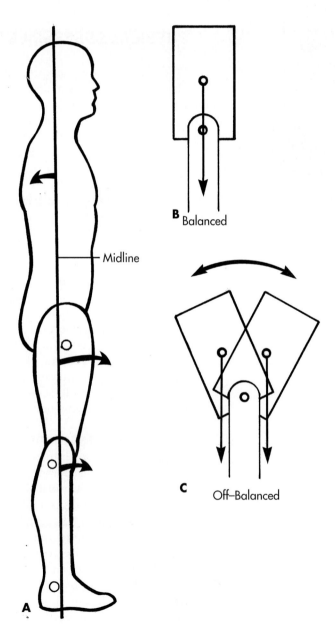

Figure 11.2
A, In normal relaxed standing, the leg and trunk tend to rotate slightly off the midline of the body, but maintain a counterbalance force. Balance is achieved in B and not in C. Any time the trunk moves off this midline balance point the body must compensate.

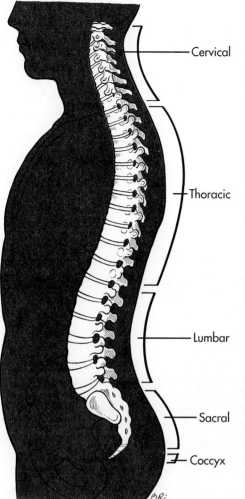

Figure 11.3
Normal spinal curves.

Cervical

Thoracic

Lumbar

Sacral

Coccyx

remember that even subtle shifts in posture demand a whole-body compensation pattern (Fig. 11.2).

The cervical, thoracic, lumbar, and sacral curves develop because of the need to maintain an upright position against gravity. In adults, the cervical vertebrae viewed laterally form a symmetric anterior convex curve. The thoracic vertebrae curve posteriorly, and the lumbar vertebrae reverse and curve in the anterior direction, with a posterior curve of the sacrum. There are a total of four curves. The sharp angulation above C1, the atlas that allows the head to be on a level horizontal plane, has also been considered a curve. Alteration in the normal spinal curves results in scoliosis, lordosis, or kyphosis (Fig. 11.3).

Mechanical Balance

A mechanically balanced, weight-bearing joint must be in the gravitational line of the mass it supports and fall exactly through the axis of rotation. Placement of the feet will influence the stability of the standing position by providing a base of support. The most common position is one leg in front of the other, with external rotation of the forward leg. It is common for people to have a functionally long and short leg. When standing, the long leg is often the front one. When seated with the legs crossed, the long leg is often on top.

The standing posture requires various segments of the body to cooperate mechanically as a whole. Passive tension of ligaments, fascia, and the connective tissue elements of the muscles support the skeleton. Muscle activity plays a small, but important role. Postural muscles maintain small amounts of contraction that stabilize the body against gravity by continually repositioning the body weight over the mechanical balance point. In relaxed symmetric standing, both the hip and the knee joints assume a position of full extension to provide for the most efficient weight-bearing position. The knee joint has an additional stabilizing element in its "screw home" mechanism. The femur rides backward on its medial condyle and rotates medially about its vertical axis to lock the joint for weight bearing. This only happens in the final phase of extension. The normal "screw home" extension pattern of the knee is not hyperextension, which causes a strain on the knee. The hamstrings are the major muscles that resist the force of gravity at the knee.[4,5]

At the ankle joint, bones and ligaments do little to limit motion. Passive tension of the two-joint (that is, the muscle crosses two joints) gastrocnemius muscle becomes an important factor. This stabilizing force is decreased if high-heel shoes are worn. The heel of the shoe puts the gastrocnemius on a slack. If these heels are worn constantly, the muscle and Achilles' tendon will shorten.

Body sway is limited by intermittent action of appropriate antigravity postural muscles. During prolonged standing, the average person shifts position frequently. The two basic positions used are the symmetric stance, with the weight distributed equally on both feet, and the asymmetric stance, in which nearly all the weight rests on one foot. The asymmetric stance is the most common, with the weight shifted back and forth between the feet. This allows for rest periods and shifting of the gravitational forces (Fig. 11.4).

When assessing the posture of a client who is in the standing position, it is important that the client be standing in the symmetric stance. The feet are about shoulder width apart. With closed eyes, most of the client's postural patterns are exaggerated because the client is not able to visually orient the body. Often the client will tip his or her head or rotate it slightly in order to feel balanced. This information indicates muscular imbalance and internal postural imbalances from positional receptors. Box 11.1 is a list of indicators for lack of symmetry.

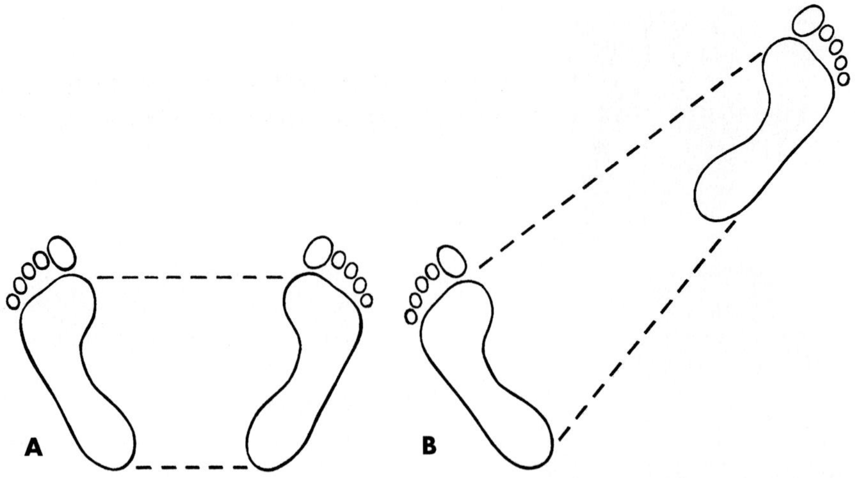

Figure 11.4
A, Symmetrical stance. B, Asymmetrical stance. The asymmetrical stance with the weight shifted from foot to foot is the most efficient standing position.

Box 11.1
LANDMARKS THAT HELP IDENTIFY LACK OF SYMMETRY

The following landmarks are helpful for comparison. Be sure to observe the client from the back, front, and left and right sides.

- The middle of the chin should sit directly under the tip of the nose. Check the chin alignment with the sternal notch. These two landmarks should be in a direct line.
- The shoulders and clavicles should be level with each other. The shoulders should not roll forward or backward.
- The arms should hang freely and at the same rotation out of the glenohumeral (shoulder) joint.
- The elbows, wrists, and fingertips need to be in the same plane.
- The skin in the thorax (chest and back) should be even and not look like it pulls or is puffy.
- The navel, located on the same line as the nose, chin and sternal notch, should not look pulled.
- The ribs should be even and springy.
- The abdomen should be firm but relaxed and slightly rounded.
- The curves at the waist should be even on both sides.
- The spine should be in a direct line from the base of the skull and on the same plane as the line connecting the nose and navel. The curves of the spine should not be exaggerated.
- The scapulae should seem even and move freely. A straight line should be able to be drawn from one scapula tip to the other.
- The gluteal muscle mass should be even.
- The tops of the iliac crests should be even.
- The greater trochanter, knees, and ankles should be level.
- The circumferences of the thigh and calf should be similar.
- The legs should rotate out of the acetabulum (hip joint) evenly in a slight external rotation.
- The knees should be locked in the standing position, but not hyperextended. The patellae (kneecaps) should be level and pointed slightly laterally.
- If a line is dropped from the nose it should fall through the sternum and navel and be spaced evenly between the knees, ankles and feet.
- The ankles should sit squarely over the feet without falling in or out.
- The feet should have even arches that are not overly exaggerated or flattened. The toes should contact the floor but not grip the floor.

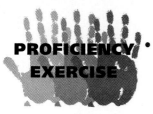

• **Using the information just presented and the form provided (Fig. 11.5), do a physical assessment of ten people.**

PHYSICAL ASSESSMENT FORM			
Chin in line with nose, sternal notch, navel:	Yes	No	Explain
Shoulders:	Level	Left High/Right Low	Right Forward/Backward
	Right High/Left Low	Both Rolled Forward	Left Forward/Backward
Clavicles:	Level	Other	
Arms:	Hang Evenly	Left Rotated	How
	Right Rotated	How	Other
Elbows:	Even	Other	
Wrists:	Even	Other	
Fingertips:	Even	Other	
Ribs:	Even	Other	Springy
	Other		
Scapula: Move Freely	Yes	No	Explain
	Even	Other	
Abdomen:	Firm	Other	
Hard Areas:	Yes	No	Explain
Waist:	Level	Other	
Spine: Curves Normal	Yes	No	Explain
Gluteal Muscle Mass:	Even	Other	
Iliac Crest:	Even	Right High	Left High
Legs: Muscle Mass Even	Yes	No	Explain
Rotation:	Even	Other	
Trochanter:	Even	Other	
Knees:	Even	Other	
Patella: Movable	Yes	No	Even
	Other		
Ankles:	Even	Other	
Feet: Relaxed	Yes	No	Explain
Arches:	Even	Other	
Toes:	Explain		
Skin: Moves Freely	Yes	No	Explain
Pulls:	Yes	No	Explain
Puffy:	Yes	No	Explain

Figure 11.5
Physical assessment form.

Gait Assessment

Understanding the basic body movements of walking will help the massage practitioner recognize dysfunctional and inefficient gait patterns. To begin, the therapist should do a self observation when walking, noticing the heel-to-toe foot placement. The toes should point directly forward with each step (Fig. 11.6).

Observe the upper body. It should be relaxed and fairly symmetric. There is a natural arm swing that is opposite to the leg swing. On each step, the left arm will move forward as the right leg moves forward and then vice versa. This pattern provides balance. The arm swing begins at the shoulder joint. The rhythm and pace of the arm and leg swing should be similar. Walking speed increases the speed of the arm swing. The length of the stride determines the size of the arm swing (Fig. 11.7).

Observe the client walk. Notice the general appearance. The optimal walking pattern is as follows:

1. The head and trunk are vertical with the shoulders level and perpendicular to the vertical line.
2. The arms swing freely opposite the leg swing.
3. Step length and timing is even.
4. The body oscillates vertically with each step.
5. The entire body moves rhythmically with each step.
6. At the heel-strike, the foot is approximately at a right angle to the leg.
7. The knee is extended, not locked, in slight flexion.
8. The body weight is shifted forward into the stance phase.
9. At push-off, the foot is strongly plantar flexed, with defined hyperextension of the metatarsophalangeal joints of the toes.
10. During the leg swing, the foot easily clears the floor with good alignment, and the rhythm of movement remains unchanged.
11. The heel contacts the floor first.
12. Then, the weight is rolled to the outside of the arch.
13. The arch responds by flattening slightly in response to the weight load.
14. The weight is then shifted to the ball of the foot in preparation for the spring off from the toes and the shifting of the weight to the other foot.

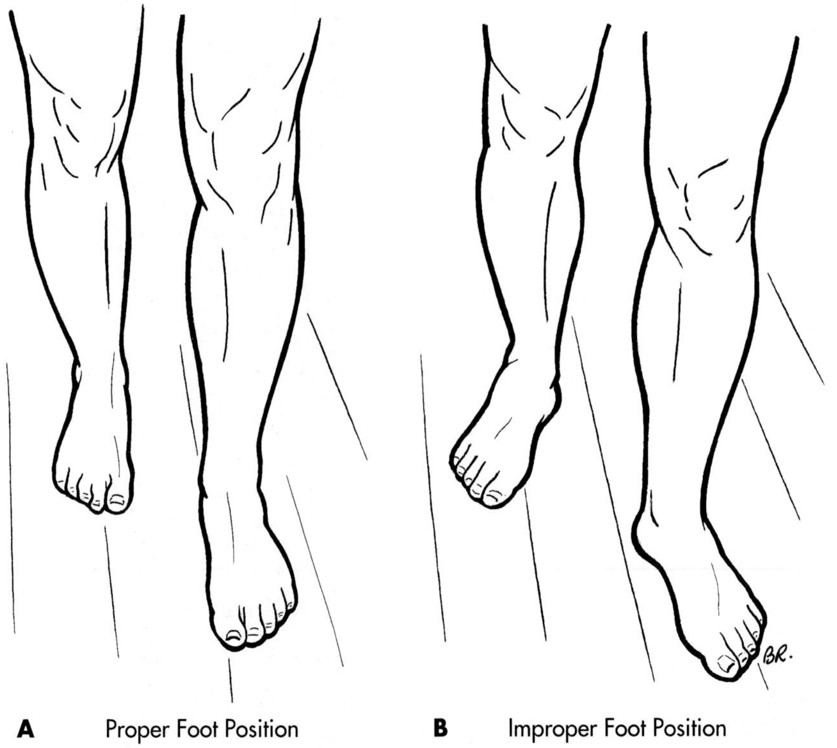

**Figure 11.6
Proper (A) and improper (B) foot position in walking.**

A   Proper Foot Position   **B**   Improper Foot Position

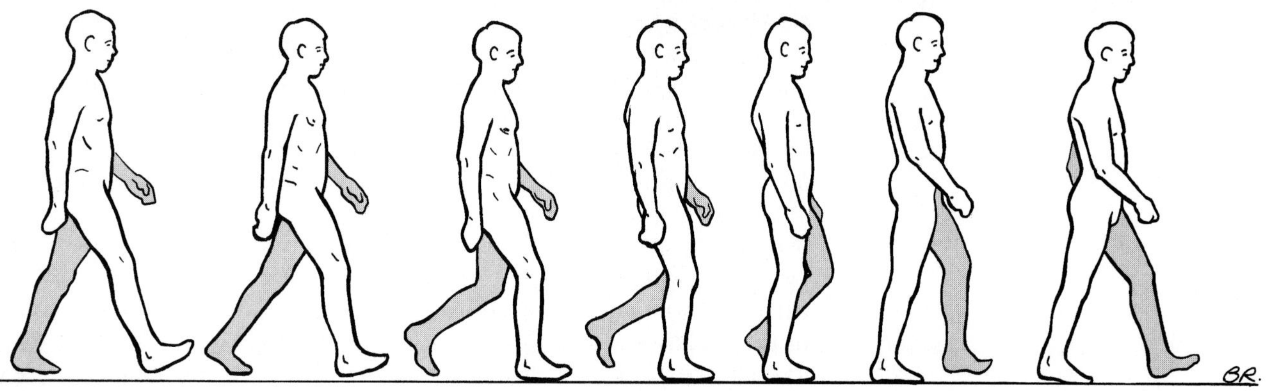

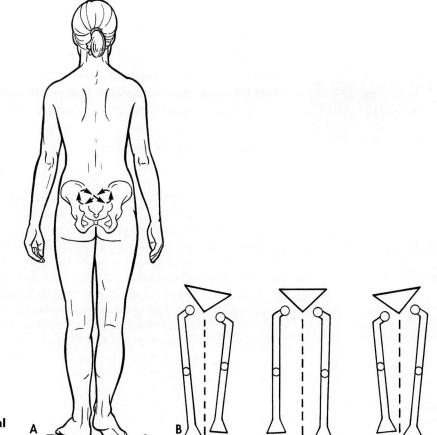

Figure 11.7
Efficient gait position.

During walking, the pelvis moves slightly in a laying-on-its-side figure eight pattern. The movements that make up this sequence are transverse, medial, and lateral rotation. The stability and the mobility of the sacral iliac joints play very important roles in this alternating side figure eight movement. If these joints are not functioning properly, the entire gait will be disrupted. The sacral iliac joint is one of the few joints in the body that is not directly affected by muscles that cross the joint. It is a large joint, and the bony contact between the sacrum and the ilium is broad. It is common for the rocking of this joint to be disrupted (Fig. 11.8).

The hips rotate in a slightly oval pattern beginning with a medial rotation during the leg swing and heel-strike, followed by a lateral rotation through the push-off. The knees move in a flexion and extension pattern opposite each other. The extension phase never reaches enough extension to initiate the normal knee lock pattern that is used in standing. The

Figure 11.8
A & B illustrate the mechanism of slight rocking movement of the sacral iliac joint.

ankles rotate in an arc around the heel at heel-strike and around a center in the forefoot at push-off. Maximum dorsiflexion at the end of the stance phase and maximum plantarflexion at the end of push-off is necessary.

Observing which areas of the body do not move efficiently during walking provides a good indicator of dysfunctional areas. Pain will cause the body to tighten and will alter the normal relaxed flow of walking. Muscle weakness or muscle shortening will interfere with the neurologic control between the prime mover and antagonist muscle action. Limitation of joint movement will result in protective muscle spasm. If the situation becomes chronic, both muscle shortening and muscle weakness will result. Changes in the soft tissue, including all of the connective tissue elements of the tendons, ligaments, and fascial sheathes, will restrict the normal action of muscle. Connective tissue usually shortens and becomes less pliable. Amputation will disrupt the normal diagonal balance mechanism of the body. It is obvious that any amputation of the leg will disturb the walking pattern. What is not so obvious is that amputation of any part of the arm will affect the counterbalance movement of the arm swing during walking. The rest of the body will need to compensate for the loss. The loss of any of the toes has a large effect on the postural information being sent to the brain from the feet. So often the little things are overlooked, when in fact they may be a major contributing factor to posture and gait problems.

It is possible to have soft tissue dysfunction without joint involvement. Any change in the tissue around a joint has a direct impact on the joint function. Changes in joint function will eventually cause problems with the joint. Any dysfunction with the joint will immediately involve the surrounding muscles and other soft tissue.

Any disruption of the gait will demand that the body compensate by shifting movement patterns and posture. Because of this, all dysfunctional patterns are whole-body phenomenons. Working only on the area of symptoms is ineffective and offers limited relief. Therapeutic massage with a whole-body focus is extremely valuable in dealing with gait dysfunction.

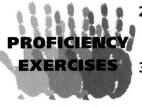

PROFICIENCY EXERCISES

1. **Watch people walk.**
2. **Pay attention to yourself when walking. Put on two different shoes, and notice what happens when you walk. Tie one arm to your leg, and pay attention to what happens when you walk.**
3. **Place your thumbs on a person's sacral iliac joints, and walk behind as that person walks. Feel for the movement. Notice if the figure eight pattern is even or lopsided.**

Assessment With Palpation

When dealing with palpation assessment, the main considerations for basic massage are the ability to differentiate between different types of tissue and the ability to distinguish differences of tissue texture within the same tissue types. Palpation includes assessment for hot and cold and observation of skin color and general skin condition. Palpation also assesses various body rhythms including breathing patterns and pulses.

The tissues that the massage therapist should be concerned with and should be able to distinguish are skin, superficial fascia, fascial sheaths, tendons, ligaments, blood vessels, and bone.

Before discussing actual palpation skills, it is important to understand what mechanism is being used to make palpation an effective assessment tool. The proprioceptors and mechanoreceptors of the hand receive stimulation from the tissue being palpated. This is the reception phase. These impulses are then transmitted through the peripheral and central nervous system to the brain where they are interpreted. The somatosensory area of the brain that interprets this sensory information devotes a massive area to the hand. The refined discriminatory sense of the hand can perceive very subtle shifts and changes. The interpretation ability is usually a sense of comparison. This tissue is softer than that tissue, or this feels rougher than that feels. Because comparison is a necessity, the practitioner must be careful to compare apples with apples. It is not logical to compare skin on the back with skin on the feet.

It is this same mechanism that makes self-massage less effective. It is difficult for the brain to decide which signals to pay attention to when the hand is doing the massage and trying to send sensory information, and the body area being massaged is also trying to decide what is happening. Because the hand sensory and motor areas in the brain are so large, it is possible that the information from the hand supersedes the information coming from the part of the body being self-massaged. The body seems to respond to the strongest set of signals. The result is that the brain pays attention to the hand and does not focus enough motor response to the area being massaged. The area being massaged by another person can respond without conflicting sensory input.

It is important to not limit a palpation sense only to the hand. Detection of movement, heat, and other sensations can be felt with the entire body. It is essential that the massage therapist's entire self becomes sensitive to subtle differences in the client's body. This is especially true with palpation skills. With palpation, what is going on must be felt and not thought about.

Varying depths of pressure must be used to reach all the tissue types and layers. Do not stay in one area too long or concentrate on a particular spot. The receptors in the therapist's hand or body will adapt, and what is subsequently felt or perceived is then lost. The practitioner's first impression should be trusted—if the area felt hot, then it probably was.

Palpation can begin many different ways. Once the skills are learned, this protocol will not need to be followed. It is best to begin with the lightest palpation and go on to the deepest levels because once the hands are used for deep compression, the light-touch sensors momentarily decrease in sensitivity.

The first level of palpation does not include touching the body. It detects hot and cold areas. This is done best just off the skin using the back of the hand because the back of the hand is very sensitive to heat. The general temperature of the area and any variations should be noted. It is important to move fairly quickly in a sweeping motion over the areas being assessed because heat receptors adapt quickly.

Very sensitive cutaneous (skin) sensory receptors also detect changes in air pressure and movement of the air. This is one of the reasons we can feel someone coming behind us when we cannot see them. The movement and change in the surrounding air pressure alerts us; this is a protective survival mechanism. Being able to consciously detect subtle sensations is an invaluable assessment tool. It is important to realize from where the information comes and why it can be sensed in order to avoid any idea that this ability is of an "extrasensory" origin. We are subconsciously aware of all the sensory stimulation that we have receptor mechanisms to detect. It is possible, with practice, to become consciously aware of these more subtle sensory experiences. Sensitivity or intuition is the ability to work with this information on a conscious level. The information received from near-touch assessment just above the skin will feel somewhat like putting two poles of a magnet together: there is a very subtle resistance. Areas that seem thick, dense, or bumpy, or those that tend to push the therapist away are hyperactive. Deeper palpation will often reveal muscular hyperactivity or hot spots. Areas that seem thin or feel as if there are holes are usually underactive.

The second level of palpation is very light surface stroking of the skin. First, determine if the skin is dry or damp. The damp areas will feel a little sticky, or the fingers will drag. This light stroking will also cause the root hair plexus that senses light touch to respond. It is important to notice if an area gets more goose bumps than other areas (pilomotor reflex). Although not palpation, this is a good time to observe for color, especially blue or yellow coloration. The practitioner should also note and keep track of all moles and surface skin growths, pay attention to the quality and texture of the hair, and observe the shape and condition of the nails.

The third level of palpation is the skin itself. This is done through gentle, small stretching of the skin in all directions and comparing the elasticity of these areas. Another palpation of the skin is for surface texture. By applying light pressure to skin surface, roughness or smoothness can be felt (Fig. 11.9).

The fourth level of assessment is a combination of skin and superficial connective tissue. A method such as *petrissage* or skin rolling is used to further assess the texture of the skin by lifting it from the underlying fascial sheath. The skin should move evenly and glide on the underlying tissues, and areas that are stuck, restricted, or too loose should be noted (Fig. 11.10).

The fifth level of palpation is the superficial connective tissue. This layer of tissue is found by using compression until the fibers of the underlying muscle are felt. The pressure should then be lightened so that the muscle cannot be felt, but if the hand is moved, the skin moves too. This area feels a little like a very thin water balloon. The tissue should feel resilient and springy like gelatin. Superficial fascia holds fluid. If there is surface edema, it will be in the superficial fascia. This water-binding quality is what gives this area the water balloon feel, but it should not be boggy, soggy, or pitting edema (where the dent from the pressure stays in the skin). Connective tissue separates as well as connects. The superficial connective tissue separates and connects the skin and the muscle tissue. It provides for gliding of the skin over the muscles during movement.

Just above the muscle, and still in the superficial connective tissue, lie the more superficial blood vessels. The vessels are distinct and feel like soft tubes. Pulses can be palpated, but if pressure is too intense, the feel of the pulse will be lost. Feeling for pulses helps find this layer of tissue.

In this same area are the more superficial lymph vessels and lymph nodes. Lymph nodes are usually located in joint areas and feel like small,

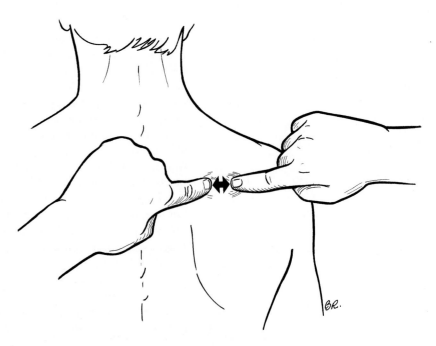

Figure 11.9
Skin stretching assessing for elasticity. Areas that seem tight compared to surrounding skin may indicate dysfunctional areas.

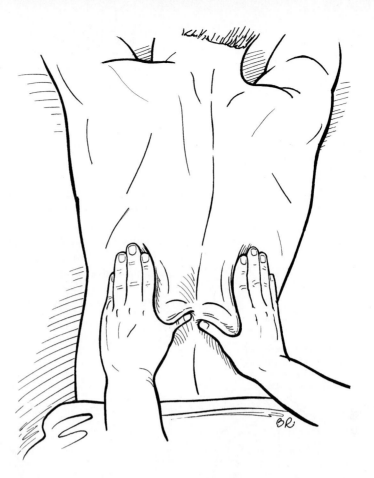

Figure 11.10
Use of petrissage or skin rolling to assess skin and superficial connective tissues by lifting the tissues.

soft gelcaps. The compression of the joint action assists in lymphatic flow. A client with enlarged lymph nodes should be referred to a medical professional for diagnosis.

The sixth level is skeletal muscle. Muscle has a distinct fiber direction that can be felt. This texture feels somewhat like corded fabric or fine rope. Muscle is made of contractile fibers embedded in connective tissue. When the muscle fibers end and the connective tissue continues, the tendon develops. This is called the muscular tendinous junction. It is a good practice activity to locate this area for all surface muscles and as many underlying ones as possible. Almost all muscular dysfunctions, like trigger points or microscaring from minute muscle tears, will be found at the muscular tendinous junction. Most acupressure points, now often classified as motor points, are also in this area.

There are often three or more layers of muscle in an area. Compressing systematically through each layer until the bone is felt is important. The layers usually run cross grain to each other. The best example of this is provided by the abdominal group. Even in the arm and leg, where it seems the muscles all run in the same direction, there is a diagonal crossing and spiraling of the groups.

The seventh level is the tendons. Tendons have a higher concentration of elastin fibers and feel more pliable and less ribbed than muscle. A wide rubber band is a good comparison. Tendons attach muscles to bones. These attachments can be directly on the bone, but it is just as common to find tendons attaching to ligaments, other tendons, and fascial sheaths to provide for indirect attachment to the bone. The important thing to remember is that these attachment areas are made of various types of connective tissue. The difference in the connective tissue is the ratio of collagen, elastin, and water. Under many tendons is a fluid-filled bursa cushion that assists the movement of the bone under the tendon.

The eighth level of palpation is fascial sheaths. Fascial sheaths separate muscles and expand the connective tissue area of bone for muscular attachment. Some run on the surface of the body like the lumbar dorsal fascia, the abdominal fascia, and the iliotibial band. Others run perpendicular to the surface of the body and the bone, such as the linea alba and the nuchal ligament. Still others run horizontal through the body. This occurs at joints, the diaphragm muscle (which is mostly connective tissue), and the pelvic floor. Fascial sheaths separate muscle groups. The larger nerves and blood vessels lie in grooves created by the fascial separations. Careful comparison reveals that the location of the traditional acupuncture meridians corresponds to these nerve and blood vessel tracts, as do the motor points that correspond to the acupuncture points. The layers can be separated by palpating with the fingers. With sufficient pressure, the fingers will tend to fall into these grooves, and then they are able to be followed. These areas need to be resilient but distinct. They serve both a stabilizing and separation purpose (Fig. 11.11).

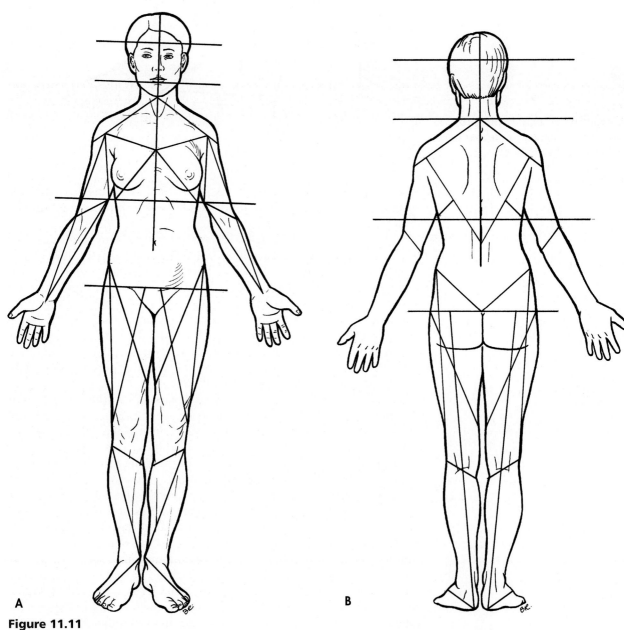

A   B

**Figure 11.11
Fascial planes.**

The ninth level is the ligaments. They are found around joints and are high in collagen and not very stretchy. They feel like small ropes that have a little give to them. Some are flat. Ligaments hold joints together and maintain joint space in synovial joints by keeping the joint apart. Ligaments need to be flexible enough to allow the joint to move, yet stable enough to restrict movement. It is important to be able to recognize a ligament and not mistake it for a tendon.

The tenth level of palpation is the joints. Joints are found where two bones come together. Careful palpation should reveal the space between the synovial joint ends. Most assessment, at the basic massage level, is with active and passive joint movements. An added source of information is to palpate the joint while in motion. The sense should be a stable, supported, resilient, and unrestricted range of motion. See Box 11.2 for a summary of joint function.

With the joint movements, it is important to assess for *end-feel*. End-feel is the perception of the joint at the limit of its range of motion. The end-feel is either soft or hard. In most joints, it should feel soft. This means that the body is unable to move anymore through muscular contraction, but a small additional move by the therapist would still produce some give. A hard end-feel is what the bony stabilization of the elbow feels like on extension. No more active movement is possible, and passive movement would be restricted by bone.

**Box 11.2
JOINT FUNCTION**

For the most part, massage practitioners work with synovial (freely movable) joints. The focus of this text is on the synovial joints. All joints are basically the same. The amount of joint movement depends on the bone structure, supportive elements of the ligaments, and arrangement of the muscles. Almost all joint movement is based on the basic flexion-extension concept. Flexion decreases the angle of a joint, and extension increases the angle of a joint. Circumduction is a combination of flexion-extension movements.

In order for a joint to move, the muscular elements must be functioning properly, and the joint structure including the cartilage must also be functional. Joints are designed to fit together in a specific way. In order for a joint to be able to move, there must be a space between the bone ends. This space must be smooth and lubricated to avoid friction. Anything that interferes with these key elements will interfere with joint function. Balance is another key element in joint function. If the positional receptors in a joint relay information to the central nervous system that indicates that damage to the joint may occur, the motor activity (muscles) will be affected.

The basic configuration of muscles around a joint is a one-joint muscle and a two-joint muscle. One-joint muscles consist of short levers and long levers. Short levers initiate and stabilize movement. They often have the best mechanical advantage in joint movement. They are usually located deep to the long levers. Long levers have the strength to carry out the full range of motion of the joint pattern. They are superficial to the short levers and deep to the two-jointed muscles. Two-joint muscles are muscles that cross two joints and coordinate movement patterns. They are usually the most superficial of the muscles. A noted exception to this is the psoas muscle (Fig. 11.12).

When evaluating joint function, the massage professional is most concerned with pain free, symmetric range of motion. It is difficult to tell if pain on movement is a muscle or tendon problem

continued

Box 11.2
JOINT FUNCTION
(continued)

or a ligament or joint problem. Therapeutic massage can deal with nonspecific soft tissue dysfunction. Joint dysfunction is out of the scope of practice for the massage professional unless specifically supervised by the chiropractor, doctor, or physical therapist.

It is important to be able to distinguish between the muscle and tendon components and the ligament and joint components in a restricted movement pattern.

The following two ways are recommended:

1. Pain on gentle traction is usually a muscle or tendon problem. Pain on gentle compression is usually a problem with the ligament and joint.
2. If active range of motion produces pain and passive range of motion does not, it is usually a muscle or tendon problem. If both passive and active ranges of motion produce pain, then the problem is usually a ligament or joint.

When in doubt, ALWAYS refer suspected joint problems to a medical professional.

When working with joints, it is important to distinguish between the anatomic barrier and the physiologic barrier. The anatomic barrier is the bone contour and soft tissue, especially the ligaments, that serve as the final limit to motion in a joint. Beyond the motion limit, tissue damage occurs. The physiologic barrier is more of a nervous system protective barrier that prevents access to the anatomic barrier where damage to the joint could occur. It is important for the massage therapist to stay within the limits of the physiologic barrier to avoid possible hypermovement of a joint. Therapeutic massage may increase the range of motion of a jointed area by resetting the confines of the physiologic barrier of the joint.

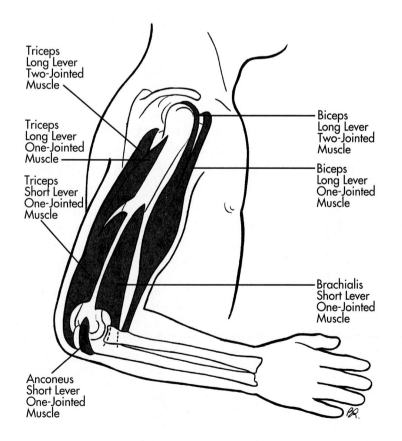

Figure 11.12
One-jointed and two-jointed muscles. Functional short and long lever muscles.

The eleventh level is the bone. There is a firm, but detectable pliability to bone for those who have developed their palpation skills. For the massage practitioner, it is important to be able to palate the bony landmarks that indicate the tendinous attachment points for the muscles and to be able to trace the bone shape.

The twelfth level of palpation is the viscera. The abdomen contains viscera or internal organs of the body. The massage therapist should be able to palpate the distinct firmness of the liver and the large intestine. Although deep massage to the abdomen is not suggested for those trained in basic massage, light to moderate stroking of the abdomen is beneficial for the large intestine. The massage therapist should be able to locate and palpate this organ. It is important for the massage professional to be able to locate and know the layering of the organs in the abdominal cavity. A good anatomy text will help with this information.

The thirteenth level is the body rhythms, which are even pulsations. The three basic rhythms are the respiration, the blood, and the cranial sacral rhythm.

The breath is easy to feel. It should be even and follow good principles of inhalation and exhalation (see Chapter 14). The movement of the blood is felt at the major pulse points. The pulses should be balanced on both sides. The cranial sacral rhythm, sometimes called the primary respiratory mechanism, and related cranial rhythmic impulse is a subtle, but detectable widening and narrowing movement of the cranial bones. A to-and-fro oscillation movement of the sacrum should be noted.[3] Specific training for cranial sacral therapy focuses on this mechanism.

Basic palpation of the breath is done by placing the hands over the ribs and allowing the body to go through three or more cycles as you evaluate the evenness and fullness of the breath. Basic palpation of the movement of the blood is done by placing the finger tips over pulse points on both sides of the body and comparing for evenness (Fig. 11.13). Basic palpation of the cranial sacral rhythm is done by lightly placing the hands on either side of the head and sensing for the widening and narrowing of the skull. Also place a hand over the sacrum and feel for the to-and-fro movement. These sensations normally occur at a rate of ten to fourteen times per minute.[3] The movement of the cranium and the sacrum should feel coordinated and even.

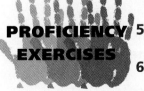

PROFICIENCY EXERCISES

1. **Massage an animal. You will be more likely to feel all of the structures.**
2. **Feel different textures. Then feel the same materials through a sheet, towel, blanket, and foam. See how many you can recognize.**
3. **Have people walk up to you while you are blindfolded. Pay attention to when you sense the people.**
4. **Feel heat radiating off various objects. How far away can you get from the object before you cannot feel the heat?**
5. **Feel appliances or machinery as the motor runs. Pay attention to the vibrations. How far away can you get and still feel the vibration?**
6. **Put a dime in a phone book under two pages. Locate the dime. Keep increasing the number of pages over the dime until you cannot feel it.**
7. **Get two magnets and play with them. Feel for the "force field."**
8. **Using the following list, palpate and observe all of the following on ten clients. Compare with related areas.**
   - **Hot and cold**
   - **Air pressure shifts**
   - **Damp or dry skin**
   - **Goose bumps**
   - **Color**
   - **Hair**

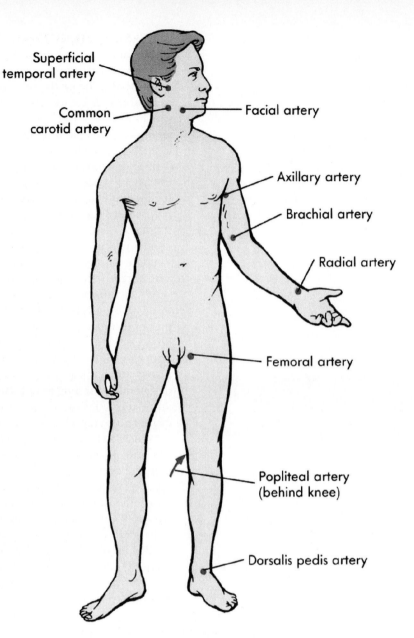

Figure 11.13
Pulse points. Each pulse point is named after the artery with which it is associated. (From Thibodeau/ Patton: The human body in health & disease, St. Louis, 1992, Mosby–Year Book, Inc.)

Superficial temporal artery

Common carotid artery

Facial artery

Axillary artery

Brachial artery

Radial artery

Femoral artery

Popliteal artery (behind knee)

Dorsalis pedis artery

- Nails
- Skin texture
- Skin roughness or smoothness
- Skin and superficial connective tissue connection
- Superficial connective tissue
- Blood vessels
- Pulses
- Lymph nodes
- Skeletal muscle fiber direction
- Muscular tendinous junction
- Motor points
- Muscle layers
- Tendons
- Fascial sheaths
- Ligaments
- Bursa
- Joints
- Joint space
- Joint movement
- Joint movement end-feel
- Bone
- Bony landmarks
- Bone shape
- Viscera
- Cranial sacral rhythms
- Breathing

Muscle Testing Procedures

Muscle testing procedures are used for different purposes. Strength testing seeks to discover if the muscle being tested is responding with sufficient strength to perform the required body functions. Another type of muscle testing seeks to discover if the neurologic interaction of the muscles is working smoothly. The third type of muscle testing is used in applied kinesiology and relies on muscle strength or weakness as an indicator of body function. It is somewhat like a body biofeedback mechanism. The system itself is too complex to cover in this book, but it is important to say that applied kinesiologic muscle testing procedures are a method of assessment and evaluation.

Strength testing determines a muscle's force of contraction. The preferred method is to isolate the muscle or muscle group by positioning the muscle with its attachment points as close together as possible. The muscle or muscle group being tested should be isolated as specifically as possible. Many good kinesiology manuals are on the market and provide instruction on how to specifically isolate a muscle or muscle group. The client holds or maintains the contracted position of the muscle isolation while the therapist slowly and evenly applies a counterpressure to pull the muscle out of its isolated position. The massage therapist needs to use sufficient force to recruit a full response by the muscles but not enough to recruit other muscles. If strength testing is done this way, there is little chance of the therapist injuring the client. As with palpation, it is necessary to compare the muscle test with a similar area, usually the same muscle group on the opposite side.

Another method is to compare the muscle group strength with the antagonist pattern. It is essential to remember that the body is designed so that muscles that are flexors and adductors are about 25 to 30% stronger than extensors and abductors. The body is designed so that flexors and adductors are usually working against gravity to move a joint. The main purpose of extensors and abductors is to balance the flexors and adductors movement and to return the joint to a neutral position. Less strength is required because gravity is assisting the function. Strength testing should reveal that there is a difference in the pattern between flexors and adductors and extensors and abductors in a prime mover/antagonist pattern. These groups should not be equally strong. Flexors and adductors should show more muscle strength than the extensors and abductors. In general, the purpose of strength testing is to determine if the muscle or muscle groups are able to respond with adequate force to a demand without excessive recruitment of other muscles, and if the muscle strength patterns are similar on both sides of the body. It is also important to consider the pattern of muscle interactions that occurs with walking. Remember that gait has a certain pattern for efficient movement.

For example, if the left leg is extended for the heel-strike, then the right arm will also be extended. This results in the flexors of both the arm and leg being activated and the extensors being inhibited. It is common to find a strength imbalance in this gait pattern. If one muscle in the pattern is out of sequence with the others, it could set up hypertonic or hypotonic muscle imbalances. Whenever a muscle is contracting with too much force, it overpowers the antagonist group, which results in inhibited muscle function. The imbalances can be anywhere in the pattern.

Neurologic muscle testing is focused more to the patterns of muscle communication. A small force is used for testing because only the nervous system is activated. An efficient pattern would show that the muscles contract evenly without jerking and without a lot of synergistic (helper muscle) activity. The same isolation of muscle groups is used as in strength testing. The client holds the contraction, and the massage therapist provides moderately light pressure against the muscle. As always, the goal is to locate the muscle interaction pattern. When testing the neuromuscular activity, it is important to notice what the rest of the body does when the muscle group isolated is being tested.

For example, if the neck flexors are tested and the left leg rolls in when the muscles respond to the test, a pattern of interaction has shown itself.

These patterns may be natural, such as the gait reflexes, but often a mixed-up set of signals fires off, which causes the body to respond inappropriately. Inefficient patterns cause some muscles to contract more than is necessary. Muscles may not be able to stop contracting and maintain hypertonicity. Whenever there is a pattern of hypertonicity (too tight muscles), there is a pattern of hypotonicity (weak muscles). These imbalances use energy and contribute to fatigue and pain in the client.

The two basic types of muscles are those that support the body against gravity, called postural muscles, and those that move the body, called phasic muscles (Box 11.3).[1] The two are made of different types of muscle fibers. Postural muscles have a higher percentage of slow- twitch red fibers, which can hold a contraction for a long time before fatiguing. Phasic muscles have a higher percentage of fast-twitch red fibers, which contract quickly but tire easily. There is a difference in how these two types of muscles are tested and what types of dysfunction they develop.

Postural muscles are relatively slow to respond when compared with phasic muscles. They do not display bursts of strength if asked to respond quickly and may cramp. They are the deliberate, slow, steady muscles that require time to respond. If compared with the story about the tortoise and the hare, these muscles are the tortoises. It is common to find inefficient neurologic patterns, hypertonicity, excessive build-up of connective tissue, and trigger points in postural muscles.[1] If posture is not balanced, postural muscles are required to function more like ligaments and bones. When this happens, additional connective tissue develops in the muscle to provide the ability to stabilize the body against gravity. The problem is that the connective tissue freezes the body in the position because, unlike muscle that can contract and lengthen, connective tissue is static tissue.

Box 11.3
MAJOR POSTURAL AND PHASIC MUSCLES

Main Postural Muscles:
Gastrocnemius
Soleus
Adductors
Medial hamstrings
Psoas
Abdominal
Rectus femoris
Tensor fascia lata
Piriformis
Quadratus lumborum
Erector spinae group
Pectorals
Latissimus dorsi
Neck extensors
Trapezius
Scalene
Sternocleidomastoid
Levator scapula

Main Phasic Muscles:
Neck flexors
Deltoid
Biceps
Triceps
Brachioradialis
Quadriceps
Hamstrings
Gluteus maximus
Anterior tibialis

Connective tissue shortening is dealt with mechanically through forms of stretch. Hypertonicity of muscles is dealt with through reflexive lengthening procedures. Postural muscles tend to shorten and be hypertonic when under strain. This information is important when attempting to assess which muscles are hypertonic and, therefore, in need of lengthening and which groups of muscle are apt to develop connective tissue changes and require stretching (see Chapter 10, pg. 281).

Phasic muscles will quickly jump into action when tested, and they will tire out fast. It is more common to find muscular tendinous junction problems in phasic muscles. The four most common problems are microtearing of the muscle fibers at the tendon, inflamed tendons (tendinitis), tendons adhered to the underlying tissue, and bursitis. Phasic muscles will weaken in response to postural muscle shortening. Sometimes the weakened muscles will also shorten. This allows for the same contraction power on the joint. It is important to not confuse this condition with hypertonicity. Phasic muscles can become hypertonic. This almost always results from some sort of repetitive behavior and is a common problem of athletes. The other reason that phasic muscles become hypertonic is in response to a sudden posture change that causes the muscles to assist the postural muscles in maintaining balance. These common, inappropriate muscle patterns often result from an unexpected fall or almost-fall, an auto accident, or other trauma. Basic massage methods discussed in this text can be used to reset and retrain them.

There is no set system for figuring out neuromuscular patterns. They are activated in response to a disruption in balance against gravity, as in a fall. A general pattern can be detected, and then modification for the individual client can be taken from there.

The body is a circular form divided into four basic quadrants: a front, a back, a right side, and a left side. With divisions on the sagittal and frontal planes, the body must be three-dimensionally balanced against the forces of gravity. The body moves and is balanced in the following areas: the atlas, C6 and 7, T12 and L1 (the thoracolumbar junction), L4 and 5 and S1 (the sacral lumbar junction), at the hips, knees, and ankles, with stabilization at the shoulder (Fig. 11.14). If there is a postural distortion in any of the four quadrants or within one of the jointed areas, the entire balance mechanism will need to be adjusted. This happens in a pinball-like effect that jumps front to back and side to side at the movement lines. This is a general guideline to give an idea where to start the work.

Remember from the discussion on joints that there are one-jointed muscles and two-jointed muscles for most joints. Muscles are tested in groups because it is almost impossible to isolate just one muscle. The brain does not process this type of information. It is more important to work with muscles in patterns of flexion and extension, adduction and abduction, or elevation and depression than to be concerned with the function of individual muscles. Each synovial joint's movement pattern is based on the flexion and extension principle. In order to move in gravity, each joint must be stabilized by some sort of diagonal pattern as a counterbalance. Therefore, the entire body is indicated for all movement patterns.

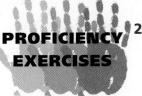

PROFICIENCY EXERCISES

1. **Develop an assessment form using the information in this chapter. Use the form to do a complete assessment of yourself.**
2. **Have three different students do an assessment of you. Include all the postural and phasic muscles listed for both strength and neuromuscular function. Compare the information they gather with what you gathered. Compare assessment forms.**
3. **Do a complete assessment of ten different people.**

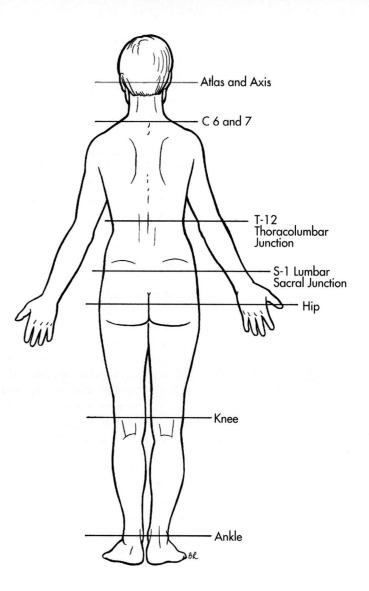

Figure 11.14
Movement segments.

INTERPRETATION OF INFORMATION

SECTION OBJECTIVES

Using the information presented in this section, the student will be able to:

➊ Interpret assessment information for the purpose of designing a basic full-body massage session focused to the specific outcome desired by the client.

➋ Refer clients for care when the assessment information indicates the need for specific diagnosis and treatment.

➌ Choose specific massage approaches to use as intervention methods during the massage session.

Once the information has been gathered, it is time to connect all the pieces to develop the best massage for the individual client. It is easier to learn this way, but with experience, these two segments of assessment and interpretation are woven into one.

When rapport is established, the client will be comfortable and will trust the practitioner enough to let any guard down. The client will communicate a variety of information during the discussion or the massage session. The therapist should listen for repeated phrases such as "It is a real pain in the neck" or "I can hardly stand up to it." The practitioner should not counsel or explain the ramifications of the information, only notice the pattern and keep general clinical notes. Careful attention should be paid to the order of priority in which the client relays the information. If the headache is mentioned first, the knee ache second, and the tight elbow last, then the areas should be dealt with in that order, if possible, in the massage flow.

General Presence

In general, excessive sympathetic activation would be balanced by a relaxing massage, and excessive parasympathetic activation would be balanced by a stimulation massage. But it is not quite that easy. In the discussion of rapport, it was mentioned to work with a client by meeting the current state of the client. This is also very true in deciding whether the general massage approach will be stimulation or relaxation.

If the client is functioning from sympathetic nervous system control, and relaxation methods such as rocking and slow *effleurage* are initially used, the work will often be irritating to the client. By beginning with a more stimulating approach and using such strokes as rapid compression, PNF (proprioceptive neuromuscular facilitation), lengthening, and *tapotement,* the design of the massage fits the physiologic level of the client. Once some of the nervous energy is discharged, the client is ready for the more relaxing methods. The same is true with parasympathetic patterns. If the client is "down" that day, beginning with a stimulation approach may feel like an attack. It is better to begin with the more subtle, relaxation methods and progress slowly into the stimulation approaches.

Gesturing

The general guidelines for gestures listed are not written in stone. Professional experience indicates that those listed in this text are fairly dependable beginning points. Until the student is more experienced with interpreting an individual's body language, the suggestions provided do give some initial direction for the student. People tend to be consistent with their gestures and word phrases within their own internal body language system. However, body language is as individual as the person. Particular gestures or styles of body language cannot be generalized to mean one specific thing. It is the professional's responsibility to understand what a gesture means for the individual. Because of nervous system patterns and basic universal body language connected with survival emotions such as fear, anger, distress, and happiness, some body language is fairly consistent from person to person. But it cannot be assumed that a certain gesture always means the same thing with every person. It takes time and careful observation to decipher an individual body language code. This is done by watching for repetitive body language of a client and by connecting the particular gesture or posture to the mood state or content of the conversation. Eventually the client will repeat the body language patterns enough so that the individual pattern is evident.

Common gestures to watch for are:

- A finger pointing to a specific area could suggest an acupressure or motor point hyperactivity or a joint problem. What the pointing means depends on the area being pointed to.
- If the point is directed to a specific area but then the hand swipes in a certain direction, it may be a trigger point problem.
- If the area is grabbed or pulled or held and moved like it is being stretched, this often indicates muscle or fascial shortening.
- If movement is needed in order to show the area of tightness, then the area may need muscle lengthening combined with proprioceptive facilitation work to prepare for the stretch and reset of neuromuscular patterns.
- If the client moves into a position and then acts as if stuck, it may indicate the need for connective tissue stretching.
- If the client draws lines on his or her body it may indicate nerve entrapment in the fascial planes or grooves.

Posture Assessment

The focus is symmetry. Body areas that are out of alignment can be caused by muscles that pull or do not stabilize, connective tissue shortening or laxity, or, more likely, a combination of these. It is best to follow the lead of the body. It may be hard to tell if one shoulder is too high or the other one is dropped. Instead, the bodyworker should exaggerate the pattern and have the client push or pull out of the stabilizing pressure. Attention should be paid to the pattern where the client uses the most effort when pushing or pulling. This will indicate where to look for further dysfunction. Connective tissue approaches will normalize the twists and pulls from shortened connective tissue.

Asymmetry usually results from hypertonic muscles or shortened connective tissue pulling the body out of alignment. Direct trauma will push joints out of alignment. Weak stabilizing mechanisms, such as overstretched ligaments or inhibited antagonist muscles, contribute to the problem. In these situations, a chiropractor, osteopath, or another trained medical professional skilled in skeletal manipulation is needed. So often a multidisciplinary approach to client care is necessary.

Gait Assessment

When interpreting the information gathered from gait assessment, the focus should be put on those areas that do not move easily when walking and areas that move too much. The areas that do not move are restricted; the areas that move too much are compensating for the inefficient function. By releasing the restrictions through massage and reeducating the reflexes through neuromuscular work and exercise, the gait pattern can be improved. The techniques followed are similar to those for postural corrections. The shortened and restricted areas are softened with massage, then the neuromuscular mechanism is reset with PNF (proprioceptive neuromuscular facilitation) and muscle energy techniques, muscle lengthening, and stretches. Slow lengthening and stretching procedures should be taught to the client. After toning the muscles in weakened areas, the client can be taught strengthening exercises. The therapist must be sure the adaptation methods are built into the context of a complete massage as opposed to spot work on isolated parts of the body. Suggestions could be made to the client to evaluate factors that may contribute to these adaptations, such as posture, foot care, chairs, tables, beds, clothing, shoes, work stations, physical tasks such as shoveling, and other repetitive exercise patterns.

Proper functioning of the sacral iliac joint is an important factor in walking patterns. Because there is no direct muscular component to the sacral iliac joint movement, it is difficult to use any kind of PNF/muscle energy lengthening when working with this joint. The joint is embedded deep in supporting ligaments. To keep the surrounding ligaments pliable, direct and specific connective tissue techniques are indicated, unless the joint is hypermobile. If so, then external bracing is suggested. Sometimes the ligaments will stabilize. Connective tissue tends to thicken with immobility. Stabilization should be interspersed with massage and gentle stretching to ensure that the ligaments remain pliable and do not become adhered to each other. This process takes time. Diagnosis and fitting for external bracing is outside the scope of practice for therapeutic massage and the client would need to be referred to the appropriate professional.

Physical Assessment

Physical assessment becomes part of the massage. In any given massage, about 90% of the touching is assessment, developed as part of *effleurage, petrissage,* or joint movement. Assessment meets tissue but does not override it or encourage it to change. This type of work will generally relax or stimulate the client, depending on the type of stroke used.

The main approach is to help the body regain symmetry. Therefore, when observing gait or posture, areas that seem pulled, twisted, or dropped must be noted. The job of the massage therapist is to use all massage methods to lengthen shortened areas, untwist twisted areas, raise dropped areas, soften hard areas, firm soft areas, warm cold areas, and cool hot areas.

The assessment procedures help find these areas. Palpation is the comparison of smaller areas of the body in relationship to each other. When applying the techniques, a general rule is to honor what the body is doing. This can be done by creating a slight exaggeration of the asymmetric pattern found and then by slowly encouraging the body to shift to a more symmetric pattern.

For example, a client has a long left leg with an externally rotated foot. As part of the massage, a good approach would be to stretch the long leg further and rotate the foot even more. Then the corrective pattern can be encouraged by having the client pull and rotate the leg in the opposite direction against stabilizing pressure. As the client finishes this move, the lengthening and the stretch should be continued in the same direction as the client's pulling force. All the shortened areas should then be massaged, and the overstretched areas toned.

The method just described works well for neuromuscular problems. It is not as effective for altering connective tissue dysfunction but does prepare the body for connective tissue work. If the areas of contracted and shortened connective tissue were stretched without this preparation, the body may respond with protective spasms. Working with connective tissue often requires slow, sustained stretching that puts a sufficient pull into the connective tissue and specific application of friction massage manipulations.

Hot areas could be caused by inflammation, muscle spasm, hyperactivity, or increased surface circulation. Cold areas are often areas of decreased blood flow, increased connective tissue formation, or muscle flaccidity. The focus is to cool down the hot areas. One method is to use ice (see section on hydrotherapy in Chapter 13). Another way is to reduce the muscle spasm and encourage more efficient blood flow in the surrounding areas. The cold areas may have heat applied to them. Stimulation massage techniques tone muscles to increase muscle activity. Connective tissue approaches will soften connective tissue and help to restore space around the capillaries and release histamine, a vasodilator.

Skin

Skin should be contained, resilient, elastic, and even, with rich coloring. There should not be tinges of blue, yellow, or red to the skin. Blue coloration suggests lack of oxygen, yellow coloration indicates liver problems such as jaundice, and redness suggests fever, alcohol intake, trauma, or inflammation. Color changes are most noticeable in the lips, around the eyes, and under the nails. Bruises are to be noted and avoided. If a client displays any hot redness or red streaking, he or she should be referred to a doctor immediately. This is especially important in the lower leg because of the possibility of deep vein thrombosis (blood clot). The skin should be watched carefully for changes in any moles or lumps. As massage therapists, we often spend more time touching and observing a person's skin than anyone else, including the person. If we keep a keen eye to changes and refer clients to doctors early, many skin problems can be treated before they become serious.

Depending on the area, the skin may be thick or thin. The skin of the face is thinner than the skin of the lower back. The skin in a particular area, however, should be similar. Over areas of dysfunction, the skin loses its resilience and elasticity. It is important to know visceral referred areas to the skin. If changes occur to the skin in these areas, refer the client to a doctor (see Chapter 4, pg. 97).

The skin is a blood reservoir. At any given time it can hold 10% of available blood in the body. The connective tissue in the skin needs to be soft to allow for the capillary system to expand to hold the blood. Histamine is released from mast cells found in the connective tissue of the superficial fascial layer, and it dilates the blood vessels. Histamine is also responsible for the client's reported sense of "warming and itching" felt in an area that has been massaged.

Damp areas on the skin show that the nervous system is activated in that area. This small amount of perspiration is part of a sympathetic activation called a facilitated segment. Surface stroking, with enough pressure to drag, will elicit a red response over the areas that are hyperactive. Deeper palpation will usually show a tender response. The small erector pili muscles attached to each hair are also under sympathetic autonomic nervous system control. Light fingertip stroking will produce goose bumps over areas of hyperactivity.

Methods of palpation that lift the skin, such as *petrissage* and skin rolling, will give much information. Depending on the area of the body and the concentration of underlying connective tissue, the skin should lift and roll easily. Loosening these areas is very beneficial and can be done by being more deliberate and slow with the methods to allow for a shift in the tissues. A constant drag should be kept on the tissues because both the skin and superficial connective tissue are being affected.

Hair and Nails

The hair and nails are part of the integumentary system and can reflect health conditions. The hair should be resilient and secure; hair loss should not be excessive when massaging the scalp. The nails should be smooth. Vertical ridges can indicate nutritional difficulties whereas horizontal ridges can be signs of stress caused by changes in circulation that would affect nail growth. Clubbed nails may also indicate circulation problems. The skin around the nails should be soft and free of hangnails. During times of stress, the epithelial tissues are affected first. Hangnails, split skin around the lips and nails, mouth sores, hair loss, dry scaly skin, or excessively oily skin are all signs of prolonged stress or other pathology. Only a physician is able to tell the difference. Refer to the contraindications in Appendix A for more information.

Pulses and Lymph Nodes

Pulses should be compared by feeling for a strong, even, full-pumping action on both sides of the body. If differences are perceived, a referral to the doctor is needed. Sometimes the differences in the pulses can be attributed to soft tissue restricting the artery, which will be determined by the physician. Enlarged lymph nodes may indicate local or systemic infection or more serious conditions. The client should be referred immediately.

Skeletal Muscle

Skeletal muscle is assessed for both texture and function. It should be firm and pliable. Soft, spongy muscle or hard, dense muscle indicates connective tissue dysfunction. Muscle atrophy makes the muscle feel smaller than normal. Hypertrophy makes the muscle feel larger that normal. Application of the appropriate techniques can normalize the connective tissue component of the muscle. Excessively strong or weak muscles can be caused by problems with the neuromuscular control or from imbalanced work or exercise demand. Weak muscle can be a result of wasting (atrophy) of the muscle fibers.

Tendons

Tendons should feel elastic and mobile. If a tendon has been torn, it may get stuck to the underlying bone during the healing process. Some tendons, like the tendons of the fingers and toes, are in a sheath and must be able to glide. If they cannot glide, inflammation builds, and the result is called tendinitis. Overuse can also cause inflammation. Inflammation signals the formation of connective tissue, which can interfere with the movements or adhere the tendons to surrounding tissue. Frictioning techniques help these conditions.

An important area is the muscular-tendinous junction where the nerve usually enters the muscle. As pointed out earlier, motor points (acupressure points) will cause a muscle contraction with a small stimulus, somewhat like a pilot light for a gas stove. Disrupted sensory signals at the motor point cause all kinds of problems, including trigger points and referred pain, hypersensitive acupressure points, and restrictive movement patterns caused by the increase in the physiologic barrier. The condition that develops depends on heredity, activity level, and general health of the individual. It would be nice to give suggestions on how to proceed, but in this case, careful assessment of the entire pattern, the skills to "make it up as you go," and good general massage addressing all tissue components, are the best recommendations.

Fascial Sheaths

Fascial sheaths should be pliable, but they are stabilizers and therefore may be more dense than tendons in some areas. Problems arise if the tissues these sheaths separate or stabilize become stuck to the fascial sheath. Myofascial and cranial sacral approaches are best suited to dealing with fascial sheaths. This type of bodywork is not usually included in basic massage training. Mechanical work such as slow sustained stretching and methods that pull and drag on the tissue are used to soften the sheaths. Because it is often uncomfortable, the work should not be done unless the client is committed to regular appointments until the area is normalized. This may take from six months to one year. Chronic conditions almost always show dysfunction with the connective tissue and fascial sheaths. Any techniques discussed as connective tissue approaches will work, as long as the practitioner goes slowly and follows the tissue pattern. It is imperative that the massage therapist does not override the tissue or force the tissue into a corrective pattern. Instead, the tissue must be untangled or unwound. Highly developed assessment and palpation skills are a must for working specifically with connective tissue. General massage methods that are slowed down and gently pull the tissue are the best recommendations until more specific training is obtained. If there is going to be an emotional component to the client's pattern, it will often surface when dealing specifically with the connective tissues. It seems that emotional chemicals and residue from addictions and toxicity are stored in this tissue. Because of this, the effects of connective tissue work are widespread. Water is an important element of connective tissue. In order for connective tissue to stay soft, the client must rehydrate the body by drinking a minimum of the eight eight-ounce glasses of clean pure water recommend by nutritionists and doctors.

Fascial separations between muscles create pathways for the nerves and blood vessels. When palpated, these pathways feel like grooves running between muscles. If these areas become narrow or restricted, blood vessels may be constricted and nerves impinged. A slow specific stripping *effleurage* along these pathways can be beneficial. The nerves run in these fascial pathways, and the nerve trunks correlate with the traditional meridian system. Therefore, most meridian and acupressure work takes place along these fascial grooves.

Ligaments

Dealing specifically with ligaments, joints, and bone is out of the scope of practice of basic massage therapy as presented in this text. With additional education, such as found in Ontario and British Columbia, Canada, massage applications are beneficial for ligaments, joints, and bones. All of these tissues and structures are helped by general massage applications because of increased circulation, unrestricted soft tissue, and normalized neuromuscular patterns. Massage can greatly affect the physiologic barrier. Joints may be traumatized, and the surrounding tissue becomes "scared," almost saying, "This joint will never get in that position again." When this happens, all the proprioceptive mechanisms reset to limit the range of motion. Massage and appropriate muscle lengthening and general stretching, combined with muscle energy or PNF (proprioceptive neuromuscular facilitation) techniques and self help, can affect ligaments, joint function, and bone health. These tissues are relatively slow to regenerate, and it takes time to notice prolonged improvement.

Abdomen

Refer the client to the doctor if any hard, rigid, stiff, or tense areas in the abdomen are noticed. Close attention must be paid to the viscerally referred pain areas (see Chapter 4, pg. 97). If tissue changes are noticed, the practitioner must refer the client to the doctor. The skin will often be tighter in these spots and should be stretched by the massage therapist. There is some indication that normalizing the skin over these areas does have a positive effect on the organ function. If nothing else, circulation is increased and peristalsis (intestinal movement) is encouraged. By carefully following the recommendations for colon massage (see Chapter 10, pg. 234), repetitive stroking in the proper directions stimulates smooth muscle contraction and can improve elimination problems and intestinal gas. An understanding practitioner is prepared for the results and will offer the restroom to the client.

Body Rhythms

The body rhythms must be assessed before and after the massage. An improvement in stability, rate, and evenness will be noticed after the massage. Improved breathing function helps the entire body. If hyperventilation is a problem and the person is prone to anxiety, work must be done to soften and normalize the upper body and breathing mechanism. The muscular mechanism for the inhalation and exhalation of air is designed like a simple bellows system and depends on unrestricted movement of the musculoskeletal components of the thorax. The muscles of respiration include scalenes, intercostals, anterior serratus, diaphragm, abdominals, and pelvic floor muscles. Because of the whole-body interplay between muscle groups in all actions, it is not uncommon to find tight lower leg and foot muscles interfering with breathing. A person can try this alone by contracting the lower legs and feet and taking a deep breath. Breathing is a whole-body function. Disruption of function in any of these muscle groups will inhibit full and easy breathing. For additional information see Chapter 14. Slow lengthening and stretching and the breathing retraining pattern found in Chapter 14, pg. 385 should be taught to the client. It can also be suggested that the client not wear restrictive clothing nor hold in the stomach. General relaxation massage and stress reduction methods seem to help the most.

Muscular Imbalance

Muscle imbalance, discovered through muscle testing procedures, indicates how the body is compensating for imbalances. Muscle testing can also locate main problems. Usually the dysfunctional group of muscles being tested causes all the other body compensation patterns to activate and exaggerate, but there is no set system. The massage professional must become a detective, looking for clues to unwind the pattern. By concentrating on symmetry of function, the body will work out the details. A major problem is hypertonic muscles. If these muscles can be relaxed and lengthened and stretched, the rest of the pattern takes care of itself. If the extensors and abductors are stronger than the flexors and adductors, there is a major body imbalance and postural distortion will result. Similarly, if the extensors and abductors are too weak to balance the other movement patterns, the body curls into itself, and nothing works properly.

If shortened postural muscles are found, they need to be lengthened and then stretched. This takes time and uses all the bodyworker's skills. Because of the fiber configuration of the muscle tissue, techniques will need to have sufficient intensity and be applied long enough to allow the muscle to respond.

If shortened and weak phasic muscles are located, they will first have to be lengthened and stretched. Eventually, strengthening techniques and exercises will be needed.

If the hypertonic phasic muscle pattern is from repetitive use, the muscles will need to be fatigued with muscle energy or PNF (proprioceptive neuromuscular facilitation) techniques and then lengthened. Hypertonic muscles will often increase in size (hypertrophy). The client will need to reduce activity of the muscle group until balance is restored, which usually takes about four weeks. Muscle tissue that has undergone hypertrophy will begin to return to normal if it is not used for the activity during that time. Athletes will often display this pattern and will very likely be resistant to complete inactivity. Reduced activity level and a more balanced exercise program combined with flexibility training is beneficial.

Reassessment

Once the massage is complete, it is a good idea to do a quick reassessment to see what changes the body has made. This can be quickly done by targeting a few major areas that were the core focus of the massage. The reassessment process helps the client to integrate the body changes. The before and after awareness is a reinforcing factor for the benefits of massage. The entire process of massage is an assessment, an intervention for adaptation, and then a reassessment to see if the approach was beneficial. This takes practice. During the learning process, assessment and reassessment can feel choppy. The skilled massage professional will learn by practice to flow between these three steps of assessment, intervention/adaptation, and reassessment during the context of the massage session, providing a sense of continuity and fluidity to the massage session.

PROFICIENCY EXERCISE
• **Design and do ten massage sessions following the assessment guidelines in this chapter.**

SUMMARY

Massage is a whole-body system. Assessment skills are the basis for developing intuition by learning to pay attention and becoming skilled in the interpretation of the assessment results. With practice and experience, these skills become second nature. The trained massage professional modifies intensity and method to best fit the client's needs. Massage routines are not done. The methods look and are simple, but applied with the right intensity and in the right location, the body recognizes the stimulation and can respond. This learning is continuous. The clients never stop teaching the therapist. The more reliable the assessment information, the more likely the interpretation of it will be accurate. The more accurate the interpretation, the more specific the application of massage methods. The detective work and skills required to assist the client in figuring out each individual pattern prevents massage from becoming boring. Massage and bodywork techniques are relatively basic. Soft tissue can be pushed, pulled, shaken, stretched, or pounded, regardless of the bodywork system. The only variables are the location of the application, the intensity, and the duration.

After completing one thousand massage sessions, the massage professional begins to own the information learned in school. After five thousand massage sessions, the massage professional has enough experience to begin to trust the process of massage. After giving ten thousand massages, the massage therapist allows the massage to happen. A master of massage has learned to respect the client and to follow the lead of the client. This take years of practice.

The bottom line is this. The client knows his or her body best. It is the job of the practitioner to understand what the client says verbally, visually, through body language, in the tissues, and the movement patterns. Each person's body language is unique. It takes time to learn it. Only by listening, observing, and touching will the patterns begin to show, and then the solutions can be found for the individual. The therapist should not hesitate to ask for help and should refer when the problem is bigger than the professional skills determined by scope of practice for massage therapy. By joining into the team approach with other health professionals, massage in some form, can be an important part of the client's solution.

Practice must be continued because it allows the massage professional's skills to increase. The student will be surprised at how perceptive and sensitive the body actually is once we learn to pay attention. We must also learn not to be attached to the client's outcome by gauging personal or professional success or failure to the progress noted by the client.

Robert Fulghum tells a story about hiccups that epitomizes massage. "The reason most cures work, at some time on some people, is that hiccups usually last from between seven and sixty-three hicks before stopping of their own accord. What ever you do to pass the time while the episode runs its course seems to qualify as a cure, so the more entertaining the cure is, the better . . . The hiccupper will be treated with great solicitation while in the throes of these miniconvulsions, and the shaman who has come up with the winning cure will be looked upon with the respect. . . .[2] When massage intervention does provide for more efficient function for the client, the massage professional needs to be mindful of not being a "Shaman" but instead focus on educating the client about the body's responses so that the client begins to experience personal empowerment and recognizes the body's own healing potential.

1. Why is it important to understand massage methods as opposed to doing a massage routine?
2. What is always the first manipulation of a massage?
3. Explain the concept of "broth of the massage."
4. What is the goal of the general massage?
5. Why are there a million ways to do a massage?
6. How does the massage therapist determine what kind of massage to give?
7. Why does the massage practitioner do an assessment?
8. What is assessment?
9. What are SOAP notes?
10. What or who is the most important source of information during the assessment process?
11. What is rapport?
12. Is observation only limited to vision? Why?
13. What is considered when observing the general presence of the client?
14. What information can be gathered by watching a person's gestures?
15. What is the importance of patterns?
16. What is the importance of open-ended questions?
17. Why is it important to repeat what the client has told you?
18. When explaining something to someone, what kind of words are used?
19. What interferes with listening ability?
20. At the beginning of the physical assessment, what question is important to ask?
21. What are the three factors that influence posture, and which one is easiest to affect?
22. What other factors influence posture?
23. What is the fundamental determining factor in posture?
24. What is the essence of mechanical balance?
25. What is required to stand?
26. What is the "screw home" mechanism of the knee?
27. What do shoes with high heels do?
28. What are the two main stances used in standing?
29. Why is an understanding of this information important for the massage therapist's body mechanics?
30. What is the position of the client during assessment of the standing position?
31. What is the importance of bony landmarks in the assessment process?
32. Why assess for efficient gait patterns?
33. What is the importance of the sacral iliac joint during walking?
34. What are the two main factors to look for during the assessment of gait?
35. What are the most common reasons for dysfunctional walking patterns?
36. Why is full-body massage beneficial for efficient gait patterns?
37. What is palpation?
38. Why is the hand such an effective assessment tool?

39. How does the brain interpret sensory information?
40. Why is self massage less effective?
41. Are palpation skills limited to the hand?
42. Why is it important to trust first impressions during palpation?
43. Why can we feel something that does not touch us?
44. What is intuition?
45. What type of information is gathered with near touch or palpation that does not actually touch the body?
46. What types of things are noticed when palpating the skin?
47. What does the superficial connective tissue layer feel like?
48. Where are the superficial blood and lymph vessels located?
49. Why refer client's with enlarged lymph nodes to the doctor?
50. How can you tell if you are feeling skeletal muscle?
51. What is the importance of the muscular tendinous junction?
52. Do tendons only attach muscle to bone?
53. What is the function of fascial sheaths?
54. Why is it important for the massage therapist to be able to palpate and recognize a ligament?
55. What is joint end-feel?
56. What should a joint feel like?
57. What is the basic premise that all joint function is based on?
58. What is the basic configuration of muscles around a joint?
59. What would pull the alignment of a joint out of its anatomic position?
60. Why is it important to differentiate between joint and soft tissue dysfunction?
61. Explain why you palpate bone.
62. What are the important things to look for when palpating the abdomen?
63. What are body rhythms?
64. What are the three basic types of muscle testing?
65. What is the difference between strength testing and neurologic muscle testing?
66. When evaluating muscles both for strength and for neurologic function, what is the importance of the pattern?
67. What are the two basic types of muscles?
68. Typically, how do muscle imbalances set up patterns?
69. When is the information from the assessment interpreted?
70. What are some key elements to designing the massage?
71. What is the purpose of the design of the massage?
72. How does the massage therapist decide what method to use?
73. What is the importance of reassessment?
74. How does the quote from Robert Fulghum on page 320 pertain to massage?

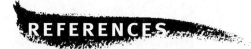

REFERENCES

1. Chaitow L: Soft tissue manipulation, Rochester, Vermont, 1988, Healing Arts Press.
2. Fulghum R: Uh-oh, New York, 1991, Villard Books.
3. Greenman PE: Principles of manual medicine, Baltimore, 1989, Williams and Wilkins.
4. Lehmkuhl LD and Smith LK: Brunnstrom's clinical kinesiology, ed 4, Philadelphia, 1983, FA Davis Company.
5. Norkin CC and Levangie PK: Joint structure and function: a comprehensive analysis, ed 2, Philadelphia, 1992, FA Davis Company.

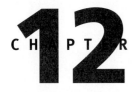

CHAPTER 12

SPECIAL POPULATIONS

After completing this chapter, the student will be able to do the following:

❶ Develop a massage environment to best serve individuals with special needs.

❷ Demonstrate the communication skills important when working with a client who has special needs.

❸ Gather data about additional training and information about massage for those with special needs.

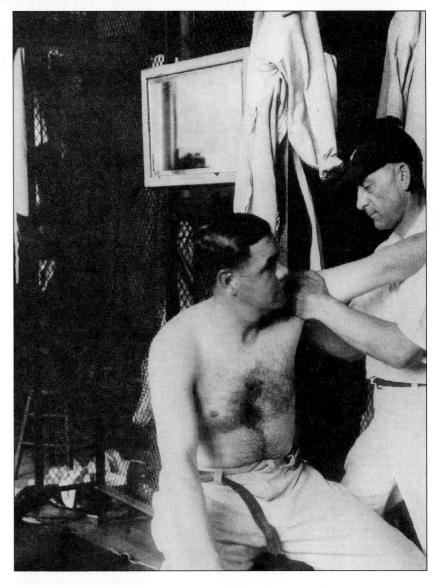

Babe Ruth receiving an arm massage by a coach before a game. (Bettmann Archive)

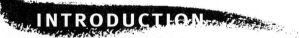
INTRODUCTION

In this chapter we examine ways in which the massage professional can respect and help those who need additional consideration. The intent is to help the massage professional focus the benefits of general massage on clients with specific needs. What is offered in each section is a general description of the special situation, the application for wellness massage, and directions for obtaining further training and information.

The following special populations or circumstances are considered:

Abuse
Athletes
Children
Chronically ill
Terminally ill
Elderly
Pregnant women
Infants
Physically challenged
- Amputation
- Burns
- Hearing impairments
- Mobility impairments
- Size (height and weight)
- Speech impairments
- Visual impairments

Psychologically challenged
- Addictions
- Chemical imbalances in the brain
- Developmental disabilities
- Learning disabilities
- Mood disorders

As each special situation is explored, it is important always to see the individual as a person first, and the special need as only a secondary consideration. There are no visually impaired, hearing impaired, or abused people, but there are people who have visual or hearing impairments, or who have been abused. Basic massage skills are sufficient to serve all people in order to facilitate general health enhancement and increase well-being. Rehabilitative massage will require additional education. The basic skills presented in this textbook seldom change. Effleurage for someone with special needs is still effleurage. The difference will be in who is receiving the effleurage and how it is done.

It is the massage professional's responsibility to learn as much as possible about the situation with which the client is dealing. If the work is with a tennis player, the therapist should learn about tennis. If the work is with survivors of abuse, then the therapist should learn about abuse. The scope of these studies is beyond the context of this textbook. The best way to obtain information about special needs is to ask the client directly. Each situation is different.

We all need help at times. For most of us; however, the condition requiring assistance is limited or short-lived. Those with disabilities or special needs live with the challenge *every day*. Life may be harder and the person may be experiencing more stress. Massage can be a wonderful way to reduce this stress and promote well-being.

ABUSE

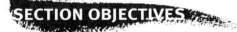

SECTION OBJECTIVES

Using the information presented in this section, the student will be able to do the following:

1. Define abuse.
2. Explain state-dependent memory.
3. Recognize dissociation.
4. List the elements needed in additional training to work specifically with abuse issues.
5. Respond resourcefully if a client responds emotionally during a massage.

The following are words synonymous with abuse: exploit, misuse, prostitute, batter, mishandle, mistreat, molest, ravish, violate, harass, condemn, persecute, torment, belittle, ridicule, insult, offend, neglect, ignore, berate, criticize, defile, desecrate, dishonor, perversion, attack, and reject. Words with the opposite meaning include honor, respect, consider, regard, protect, defend, preserve, praise, value, safeguard, shelter, sustain, support, tolerate, appreciate, approve, recognize, understand, accept, and unharmed.

When people are abused, whatever the form of abuse, they must learn to survive, as best they can, at the time of the abuse. These survival mechanisms take many forms, such as dissociation, hypervigilance, aggressive behavior, learning to "disappear," low self-esteem, withdrawal. These patterns may generalize into many life situations. If the abuse happens to a young child, the victim's coping mechanisms develop around a twisted reality. The younger the child, the more difficult survival will be, and possibly the more magnified the survival mechanisms that develop.

People want to think of abuse as physical or sexual torture. It is safer to consider the acts of the "monster" or "sociopath" than to recognize the subtler abuses that we have all experienced. Most abusers are members of our families (including siblings) and friends. Mixed signals can be very devastating; those who have experienced both abuse and support from the same person have difficulty with trust and esteem. Guilt is common and secrecy the norm. Subtler forms of mistreatment, especially emotional abuse, are also frequent. The effects of the abuse should not be judged on the intensity of it. A child or adult who has been deceived has had trust violated and personal power taken away just as the person who has been raped. Abuse removes a person's self-empowerment, no matter what the means. The severity of the results depends on the frequency of the situation, whether someone was able to validate our worth and help us cope at the time, and our inner resources. The older we are, the more inner resources we have.

Sexual and physical abuse attacks the very form of the person, and the physical body remembers in some way. The technical term for this is *state-dependent memory*. This type of memory is encoded in the brain in a manner that includes the position, emotion, chemicals, nervous system activation, and all other combined physiology affecting the internal functions of a person at the time the experience happened. Later, when the physical and emotional states change, the memory may be vague or forgotten. State-dependent memory functions in all life experiences. When someone gets ready to hit a baseball or drive a car, that person will assume the appropriate position, and the body will remember. During trauma, this mechanism locks in all the factors that coincide with the experience. In the future, this repressed memory may be triggered by any one of the sensations and physiology involved in the state-dependent memory. The sense of smell often triggers a memory. When working with massage, the pressure, location of the touch, and the position or movement of the client may trigger a memory.

From birth to about age three years, the myelination of nerves and development of the nervous system are still occurring. During this time, memories are transient, spotty, and may be stored in the memory centers in scattered ways. During the first year of life, the senses of touch, sound, smell, taste, and vision are functioning and in some ways are more keen than in the adult. What is not keenly developed is the processing, storage, and retrieval of all this information. Abuse is particularly devastating during this critical time of learning about the world and dependence on a caregiver to meet not only basic needs (e.g., food, clothes) but also the need for connection, bonding, and love. Physical, sexual, and emotional abuses at this time are remembered by the body, but are not always understood, coped with, or remembered in detail. The adult who experienced abuse during his or her formative years may have difficulty sorting it all out in adulthood. The memories may be spotty, in pieces, or it is possible that only one of the sensations such as smell, touch, or position was encoded in the memory. It is important not to discount this memory pattern simply because all the pieces do not fit together to form a whole picture. It may be affirming to know that all the pieces do not have to fit together to have enough information to resolve and integrate past experiences, and to develop more resourceful behavior for the present and future.

Sexual abuse that occurs in the older child is often laden with mixed signals, role confusion, and secrecy. Role confusion occurs when the child takes on the duties or family function of one of the parents. Because the child is older, memories may be clear, or because of state-dependent memory patterns, clouded or shut off and separated. The perpetrator may develop a relationship with the child and then use the child to meet the adult's or older adolescent's sexual needs. Again, feelings, emotions, roles, coping styles and behavior all shift somehow to put the abuse into a form that can be survived.

Physical abuse (e.g., beatings, neglect) and emotional abuse (e.g., criticism, unrealistic expectations) will demand survival as well. How many times have we been expected to do something that we did not have the skill, physical ability, or knowledge to accomplish and were belittled after trying our very best? This type of abuse riddles holes into the self-esteem.

Some life experiences that may affect a person in a manner similar to abuse are illness, medical procedures, hospitalization, accidents, or other trauma. The success of the individual's coping skills will depend on the type of support received during and soon after the traumatic event, as well as the dynamics surrounding the situation. A child who attempts to hide the pain during a medical procedure in order not to upset his or her parents has been denied full emotional and physical expression in the situation. If the medical staff does not explain the procedure, or the child is too young to understand, this too may become a difficult situation to integrate into a person's life experiences. If a parent or support person is physically separated from or emotionally unavailable for a child or adult during a critical time, this can also have an effect.

Abuse of an adult, such as spouse beating, and abuse of the elderly also need to be considered. Typically, the adult feels powerless in the situation, and may feel as if the abuse is deserved. If the elderly are also mentally impaired, such as with Alzheimer's disease, they may become childlike in their reasoning and survival mechanisms.

The touch of the massage therapist may remind the body of the abuse. It is possible that as the body remembers, it can somehow resolve and integrate the experience. Often, the client does not remember the details, or recall who, what, where, when, and how. Instead, a vague uneasiness or dissociation (detachment, discontentedness, separation, isolation) develops. One mechanism for surviving physical, sexual, and emotional abuse is to "leave the body," to not feel, or to believe that the abuse is happening to someone else. There are many types of dissociative coping mechanisms that are valuable in times of emergency and survival. If the pattern of dissociation becomes repetitive and generalized, one of the results is that we are unable to feel. One way to relearn feelings and appropriate touch is through both receiving and giving massage.

The massage professional should be aware when a client dissociates during a massage. It is not our job to change the dissociative pattern by reminding the client to remain aware of his or her body, unless specifically requested by the client. More specialized training is required to deal effectively with all the ramifications of a shift in coping style. This frequently includes professional counseling. The massage practitioner should never remove a coping mechanism for a client or imply guilt for using it when it still serves a purpose. It takes time to learn to cope differently. Most of the time people dissociate in order to avoid feeling pain. The timing and situation must be right to be able to focus the energy necessary to feel again. The process must happen gently, at the client's pace, and must never be hurried. The client leads, and the therapist follows that lead. As this happens, the practitioner can begin to recognize the pattern of the dissociation, and what massage techniques or positions are being used that seem to trigger the pattern. With this information, the therapist can alter his or her approach to the massage, providing the opportunity for the client to stay with the body more easily.

If the therapist notices, for example, that every time the left knee is bent a client's body becomes unresponsive, the eyes distance, or breathing shifts, then it is best to work with the knee in a different position. The client can also move into the position instead of being moved, which is more empowering for him or her. Over time, it will be easier to notice these little steps which will reacquaint the client with his or her body.

Some people who have been abused will self-abuse, which can take many forms including a destructive lifestyle, addictive processes, and self-inflicted trauma. The massage professional may notice bruises, cuts, burns, or other injuries on the client's body. Professionally, these areas need to be brought to the client's attention and noted in the client's records. By acknowledging an injured area to a person who self-abuses, the client may feel guilty or ashamed, tell a cover story, or ignore the question. It may seem hard to understand, but self-abuse may be calming for the person. During self-abuse, endorphins and other chemicals are released. The mechanisms of counterirritation and hyperstimulation analgesia come into play.

Occasionally, a client will demand or request very deep massage when the soft tissue condition does not indicate the need for this type of invasive work. It may be possible that self-abuse mechanisms are involved in this situation. It is important not to become involved in a situation that perpetuates an abuse pattern. The therapist needs to trust intuition, and should not force the person to face the situation. If the therapist is uncomfortable, the client must be told of the discomfort.

The decision to deal actively with an abusive history requires commitment and time by the client. Professional help and support groups are often needed. There are those who do not want to recover their memories of abuse. This is a valid response for these clients. The practitioner must not suggest that a client was abused or that the client needs to deal with his or her situation. Our job is to honor, respect, consider, regard, protect, defend, preserve, praise, value, safeguard, shelter, sustain, support, tolerate, appreciate, approve, recognize, understand, accept, and to never harm.

Boundaries are very important (see Chapter 2, pg. 30). Review the importance of respect for personal boundaries.

Listening and believing what the body and the client say is significant. Referral is important. When someone is actively exploring personal abuse and its results, it is important that the therapist does not take on the client's problems (counter-transference). The client may personalize (transference) the nurturing touch being received, and may want to involve the therapist in the experience. Working with those who have been physically or sexually abused is rewarding work, but it can be very difficult. Before serving clients with abusive histories, more training is necessary. The actual techniques of massage are no different, but an understanding of coping mechanisms and somatic (body) memories requires additional study. Bodywork in some form may be a valuable tool for those wishing to resolve these issues while for others it is not the best choice.

There is a difference between the re-enactment of abuse and an integration process that may result from the physical triggers produced by massage. Re-enactment does not necessarily provide the awareness and understanding necessary to integrate the physical response and feelings into the client's experience in an empowering way. Instead, with re-enactment the client repeats an abusive pattern and feels disempowered and lost. The massage professional needs to be aware of the potential for causing possible harm to the client from deliberately triggering a re-enactment response. Without the additional and necessary support of qualified counselors and other support personnel to provide for an integration process, the re-enactment is undesirable.

If a client should respond during the massage by crying, shaking, panicking, becoming agitated or fearful, or through another emotional pattern, it is important for the massage professional to be still and let the person experience the emotion. In most instances, it is best to continue to massage the area in the same way as triggered the response, to slow it down, and to allow the body to integrate the information. The client should be asked no questions other than, "Do you want me to continue?" The practitioner should be calm and accepting of the response, and should never try to encourage or stop the response. It is important not to interfere with the person's experience by interjecting suggestions. If needed, tissues should be provided in an unobtrusive way. It is important for the therapist to stay connected with the client, but distanced from the client's experience. The emotional experience belongs to the client, not to the practitioner, who works as a support in a quiet, simple way. When the emotional response dissipates, the massage can be continued. If the client asks what happened, a simple explanation based on state-dependent memory is sufficient. If the client seems unsettled and needs additional coping help, he or she should be referred to a qualified counselor.

Confidence, respect, and trust are necessary in order to provide the type of massage that will enhance the well-being of those who have been or are being abused. Always remembering that confidentiality is a sacred trust, the therapist does not talk about clients or any experience with clients.

PROFICIENCY EXERCISES

1. **Find and read three books that deal with abuse.**
2. **Visit a "safe house" or shelter for abused women and talk with the volunteers who work there.**
3. **Contact the child protection agency in your community and obtain information on how to recognize child abuse and how to report suspected cases.**
4. **Write about three times that you felt abused, and three times when you feel you have abused someone.**

ATHLETES

SECTION OBJECTIVES

Using the information presented in this section, the student will be able to do the following:

❶ List the experts in care and training for athletes.

❷ Explain the concept of event sport massage.

❸ List the components necessary for additional sports massage training.

Athletes are people who participate in sports either as amateurs or professionals. Athletes require precise use of their physical bodies. The athlete trains the nervous system and muscles to perform in a specific way. Often the activity involves the repetitive use of one group of muscles more than others, which could result in hypertrophy, changes in strength patterns, additional connective tissue formation, and compensation patterns in the rest of the body. These factors contribute to the soft tissue difficulties that often develop in athletes. Massage can be very beneficial for athletes if the professional performing the massage understands the biomechanics required in the sport. If not, massage could impair the optimum function of the athletic performance. Because of the physical activity, an athlete may be more prone to injury. All injuries must be referred for evaluation.

The experts for athletes are the sports medicine doctor, physical therapist, athletic trainer, exercise physiologist, and sports psychologist. It is especially important for competing athletes to work under the direction of these professionals. The psychological state of an athlete is critical to his or her performance. With athletes, the competition often is won in the mind.

The athlete is dependent on the effects of training and the resulting neurologic response for quick and precise function. It is easy for a massage therapist to disorganize the neurologic responses if the patterns required for efficient function in the sport are not understood. This is temporary, however, and unless the athlete is going to compete within twenty-four hours it is not significant. If the massage is given just before competition, however, the results could be devastating. Any type of massage before a competition must be given carefully.

If a massage professional plans to work with an athlete, it is important that he or she know the person and become part of the training experience. The therapist should learn about the sport, what is required of the athlete's body and mind, how to best use massage to enhance performance, and how to support the body in compensating patterns.

If a massage professional is doing promotional work at sports massage events, working with many unfamiliar athletes, it is best to do post-event massage. This way, the effects of any neurologic disorganization caused by the massage are not significant. No connective tissue work, intense stretching, trigger points, or other invasive work should be done with an athlete at a sporting event. The massage should be superficial, supportive, and focused more toward circulation enhancement. That is the reason that an experienced massage professional who is familiar with the sport is in charge at the sporting event. All of the massage therapists participating follow a routine. If this "team spirit" is also adopted by the massage therapists, each person will do essentially the same routine consistently throughout the event. Each member of a sports massage team represents the entire profession. The attitude should be one of helpfulness and concern, and therapeutic opinions must be avoided.

Promotional massages are usually given at events for amateur athletes. The massages are offered as a public service to provide educational information about massage. This type of public, promotional environment is one area where following a sport massage routine is important. The massage lasts about fifteen minutes and is quick-paced. Lubricants may not be used because of the risk of allergic reaction, staining an athlete's uniform, or other unforseen happenings. It is important to watch for any swelling that could be a sign of sprains, strains, or compression fractures, and to refer the athlete to the medical tent for immediate evaluation. It is also important to watch for thermoregulatory disruption or hypo- and hyperthermia and refer immediately.

Pre-Event Massage

Pre-event, warm-up massage is a stimulating, superficial, fast-paced, rhythmic massage lasting ten to fifteen minutes. The emphasis is on the muscles used in the sporting event, and the goal is for the athlete to feel that his or her body is perfect physically. Avoid uncomfortable techniques. The warm-up massage is given in addition to the physical warm-up; it is not a substitute. Use this style of massage from three days before the event until just before the event. Massage techniques that require recovery time or are painful are strictly contraindicated. Focus on circulation enhancement, and be very careful of overworking any area. Sports pre-event massage should be general, nonspecific, light, and warming. Avoid friction or deep, heavy strokes. Massage should be pain-free!

Inter-Competition Massage

Inter-competition massage, given during breaks in the event, concentrates on muscles that are being used or are about to be used. The techniques are short, light, and relaxing.

Post-Event Massage

Post-event, warm-down massage can reduce muscle tension, minimize swelling and soreness, encourage relaxation, and reduce recuperation time. The massage techniques can spread muscle fibers to minimize fascial adhesions and encourage circulation. Be aware of possible sprains, strains, and blisters. Use ice for inflammation and areas of microtrauma.

In athletes, regular massage allows the body to function with less restriction and accelerates recovery time. Many specialized training programs for sports massage are offered. If the massage professional intends to work with athletes, additional training must be pursued. Such training should include the physiologic and psychologic functions of an athlete, overuse and repetitive use syndromes, biomechanics of specific sports, use of cryotherapy, ice massage, and other hydrotherapy methods, injury repair and rehabilitation, exposure and education about training regimens, and education by exercise physiologists, athletic trainers, and sports psychologists.

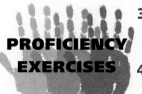

PROFICIENCY EXERCISES

1. **Look through professional journals and send for information about three advanced sports massage training sessions.**
2. **Contact a university with a sports team and speak with the athletic trainer to discover ways in which massage might be used to enhance athletic performance.**
3. **Contact a local exercise club or physical therapy department and talk with the exercise physiologist about how massage could enhance the work being done.**
4. **Volunteer to work at a sponsored sports massage event held by your school or local professional massage organization.**
5. **With your classmates, organize a sports massage event for a local sporting function.**
6. **Obtain a catalog from a university that offers degrees in athletic training or exercise physiology. List the classes required to earn these degrees.**

CHILDREN

SECTION OBJECTIVES

Using the information presented in this section, the student will be able to do the following:

❶ Apply general massage methods to ease growing pains.

❷ Train family members in massage techniques for use at home.

Providing massage services for children is not much different than for adults. For the purposes of this textbook, "children" are people ranging in age from three to eighteen years. From three to puberty the physical growth is mostly in height. At adolescence, not only is there an accelerated growth in height from the influence of the increased hormone levels, and there is sexual maturation taking place as well. Both physical and emotional growing pains are common. The physical type of growing pains occurs because the long bones grow more rapidly than the muscle tissue. There is a pulling on the periosteum or connective tissue bone covering. This is a very pain-sensitive structure. Massage can help by gently stretching the muscles and connective tissue, providing symptomatic relief of pain through the effects of counterirritation, hyperstimulation analgesia, gait control, and endorphin release.

Children love physical contact. It is interesting to note that the horsing around and wrestling of kids looks a lot like massage. Because children and adolescents may have shorter attention spans than adults, a thirty-minute massage is usually sufficient.

Adolescents live in a body that is changing every second. Hormone fluctuations are constant, and moods swing in response. Growth is accelerated and natural sleep-wake patterns are often disrupted. It is not uncommon for a teenager to be up all night and want to sleep all day. Massage may help an adolescent become more comfortable with this ever-changing body. It certainly will help with the growing pains. Use special caution when working with adolescent boys. The reflexive sexual erection response is sensitive, and almost anything can trigger an erection. The therapist should be sensitive to this by not using a smooth sheet over the groin area when working with male adolescents. Instead, keep the sheet bunched in this area to disguise any physical response to the massage.

It is also important that the practitioner never work with children and adolescents without parental or guardian supervision. The massage time can be used to teach the parent or guardian some massage methods to use to help the child, and to teach the child some massage methods for use on the parent. Massage provides for a structured approach to safe touch. Perhaps massage can help families stay connected during good times, as well as during difficult times (Fig. 12.1).

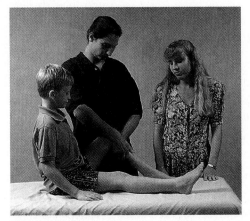

Figure 12.1
Child receiving a massage with parent or guardian present.

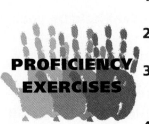

PROFICIENCY EXERCISES

1. **Give massages to three children of various ages. Make sure the parent or guardian is supervising.**
2. **Develop a one-page handout with five massage techniques that families can share.**
3. **Teach the five massage methods to three different families. After each session, write a one-page description about what you learned from the experience.**
4. **In a group session, share one of the learning experiences above with your classmates.**

CHRONIC ILLNESS

Using the information presented in this section, the student will be able to do the following:

1 Obtain a basic understanding of the etiology of chronic illness.

2 Explain the difference between acute illness and chronic illness.

3 Develop realistic expectations for working with people who have chronic illnesses.

Chronic illness is defined as a disease, injury, or syndrome showing little change or slow progression. Dealing with chronic illness is difficult for the person who has it, for the doctor, and for the massage therapist. In many situations not much can be done except to make the day-to-day living with the illness more tolerable. Healing is an option in some situations, but even the healing is a long process, and requires work, commitment, and support. The dynamics of family relationships, work, and emotional and coping skills play an important role in the etiology of a chronic illness. It affects every aspect of a person's life and the lives of those around him or her. An entire family's dynamic and functioning pattern may be set up around a chronically ill family member. Shifting illness patterns may be difficult. Entire relationship dynamics may change if the chronically ill individual improves. Personal and professional responsibilities of the client that have been able to be avoided due to the illness will have to be addressed if chronic conditions improve. The dynamics required to support chronic illness patterns reach far beyond the physiology of the disease, and professional counseling may be required.

Acute illness and injury are relatively easy to deal with, since there are measurable results in healing. This is the realm of the medical professional. Working with chronic illness does not often produce measurable results. More commonly there is a slow deterioration and at best a stabilization. Because of this, working with chronic illness does not fit easily into the current medical system, which is geared mostly toward acute and trauma care.

The massage professional who wishes to work with the chronically ill needs to have realistic expectations. Instead of developing a massage approach to bring about a cure in the illness, which is out of the scope of massage practice, the focus should be on helping the client feel better for a little while. Although this can get very frustrating for the therapist, we can see that our work has value if we remember that we may be the only ones who will provide this type of care, that not getting worse is an improvement, that some people need their illness to survive, and that massage helps them not to suffer so much in the illness pattern.

Long-term debilitating diseases like Parkinson's disease, multiple sclerosis, lupus, rheumatoid arthritis, fibromyalgia, chronic fatigue syndrome, asymptomatic human immunodeficiency virus infection, acquired immune deficiency syndrome, and disk problems resulting in back pain respond well to the short-term relief of symptoms provided by massage. Massage can also reduce general stress levels by helping the individual to cope better with his or her condition. If the person is having a bad day, the massage should not be overdone. It may be better to give massages more often for shorter periods of time. Chronic illness runs an uneven cycle with good and bad periods. During good days, the person may overexert and deplete an already weakened energy source. The immune system may be compromised, making the person with a chronic illness more susceptible to infection like colds and flu.

One of the methods used to rehabilitate the chronically ill are hardening programs. *Hardiness* is the physical and mental ability to withstand external stressors. Those with chronic illnesses often reduce activity levels, isolate themselves, and become less hardy. Massage, hydrotherapy, specially designed hardening programs, and exercises are ways of increasing a person's hardiness.

People with chronic illnesses are usually under the care of a physician and may be taking medications. It is important to work closely with the medical professionals involved to understand the effects of the various medications. Because massage does influence the physiology, there can be an interplay with the medication. Additional training is often required just to understand chronic illness patterns, the effects of the medication involved, and the skill necessary to work in conjunction with these professionals. As with athletes, if work is to be done with someone who has a chronic illness, the massage therapist should understand as much as possible about the illness. By using this information and consulting with the doctor and other health care professionals involved with the client, the effects of massage can be integrated into a comprehensive treatment plan to help the client achieve the highest quality of life possible.

Mind/body approaches, behavior modification, relaxation techniques, spiritual healing, and other types of interventions and alternatives are helpful to those with chronic illnesses. All these approaches tend to empower the client, rallying the powerful internal resources that humans have. It is important not to discount a method that a person may use for self-help. The only caution about alternative interventions is that some of the people offering these services do not have the highest good of the client as their priority. Instead they prey on the misery of the chronically ill. These people usually offer cures, charge a lot for the sessions, require frequent sessions, and try to convince people with chronic illness that their way is the only way, making the client dependent on them. This type of behavior is unethical.

A resourceful goal for working with people with chronic illnesses is helping a client rediscover the fact that each person is in charge of his or her own life, and the illness is not. The illness may have been allowed to take over the person's life and personal power. "Healing" may be the act of taking back self control of life, not getting rid of the disease. The benefits of massage may provide enough relief for clients to be able to find the necessary inner resources to constructively deal with the effects of chronic illness, increasing the quality of their lives and the lives of those around them. *Author's Note: I speak from personal experience and continue to learn from an endocrine condition and a compressed disk in my lower back.*

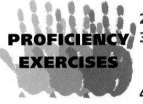

PROFICIENCY EXERCISES

1. **Contact the local support groups for those with chronic illness and request any information these groups may have.**
2. **Choose one chronic illness and investigate it thoroughly.**
3. **Develop an educational brochure explaining how massage can be beneficial as a part of coping with the chronic illness you have investigated.**
4. **Share the brochures with fellow students.**
5. **Volunteer to do a presentation for a support group for the chronic illness for which you developed the brochure.**

THE ELDERLY

Using the information presented in this section, the student will be able to do the following:

❶ **Provide a rationale for the benefits of massage for the elderly.**

The age range for the elderly is seventy years and above. There are some sixty-year-olds who have the problems of the aged and some eighty-five-year-olds with a physiology better than some sixty-year-olds. Because of this, it may be well to consider physiologic instead of chronologic age in those over sixty.

In the industrialized societies, the fastest growing segments of the population are those over eighty. People in their advanced years can benefit greatly from massage. Although the methods of massage are no different, the elderly do present specific situations. Muscle tissue has decreased and been replaced by fat and connective tissue. Bones are not as flexible and are more prone to breaking. Joints are worn and osteoarthritis is common. Skin is thinner and circulation is not as efficient. Medications may be prescribed to control blood pressure and other conditions. People who are elderly are not sick; the aging process is normal.

The body tends to collapse a bit during aging. The spaces provided for the nerves are reduced and bones and soft tissue structures may put pressure on the nerves, resulting in sciatica and thoracic outlet syndrome. Feet hurt because the intricate joint structure of the foot has broken down. Circulation to the extremities is reduced, often resulting in a burning pain. These conditions are not life-threatening, but they surely can cause someone to be miserable. If only temporarily, massage can help ease the discomfort from these conditions.

Many elderly are alone; their spouses have passed away and their families are busy with their own lives. We all need to be touched. If a person is not physically and emotionally stimulated, neurologic function begins to deteriorate. The interaction with a massage therapist provides both physical and emotional stimulation for the elderly. Because they are often alone and on a limited income, the massage therapist should consider not only the fees charged, but also the amount of time spent with the elderly client. Many of the elderly will want to talk. This social interaction may be just as important as the physical interaction of the massage. If the massage professional listens attentively, much can be learned from the elderly, who have many years of experience to share. The time should be given willingly. However, professional boundaries need to be maintained. When the massage practitioner tells an elderly person how much time can be spent, most will respect the time limitations.

If a person does not have functioning cognitive skills, as in cases of dementia caused either by the aging process or by drugs taken for other conditions, he or she will be unable to give informed consent for the massage. The guardian, doctor, or other health care professional will need to intervene to give the necessary permission to provide massage.

As in the previous discussions, if work is to be done with the elderly, then more training may be needed to learn about their special needs. Usually, a general massage session and an attentive caring spirit are sufficient for interacting professionally with the elderly (Fig. 12.2).

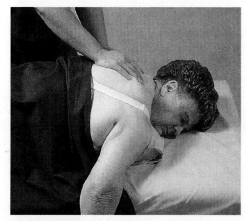

Figure 12.2
Elderly client receiving massage. Note placement of support due to kyphosis.

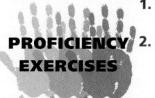

PROFICIENCY EXERCISES

1. Volunteer to give massage and teach classes at the local senior citizen center for at least four weeks or a total of thirty-two hours.
2. Contact a local nursing home and ask if there is a resident who has few visitors and would appreciate the volunteer services of a massage therapist. Commit to a minimum of two massages per month for six months.

INFANTS

SECTION OBJECTIVES

Using the information in this section, the student will be able to do the following:

① Explain the importance of the first year of life for an infant.

Most authorities classify infants as those from birth to eighteen months of age. This textbook expands this period to three years of age since infants are still developing neurologically until that time. Compared with other mammals, human infants are born about halfway through the gestation period. This is so the head is still small enough to pass through the birth canal. Otherwise, babies would stay in the womb at least another year. The womb is a much safer place to be unless the pregnant mother uses tobacco, drugs, alcohol, or other chemicals that cross the placental barrier, or if the pregnant mother does not provide adequate nutrition and care for herself and her baby.

2 Explain the importance of organized sensory stimulation for infants.

3 Teach parents to massage their babies.

4 Understand the importance of a confident touch when working with infants.

For the human infant, protection, nutrition, connection, bonding, stimulation, and soothing acceptance are critical. Unlike insects or fish, which hatch impersonally from deserted eggs, human infants are born with a need for sociability along with the more basic need for food, shelter, etc. Most cultures massage their infants. Although this practice has been almost lost in the westernized world, it is being revived. Research by Dr. Tiffany Fields and her associates shows that premature infants who have been massaged fare much better than those who have not. Massage provides an organized approach to sensory stimulation, which is important for infants. Part of their growth is being able to sort and organize sensory stimulation.

Physiologically, the infant's growth pattern is not completed until three years of age. By twelve months of age (when a child would just be born if our heads were not so big), the infant is able to independently move from place to place, but is still utterly dependent on the protection of a parental person or group. Two-year-olds are still babies. Three-year-olds are quite different in both function and body form. By the time a child can control bladder and bowel functions reliably (about age three), cognitive functions are better able to be organized. Now is the time to work on learning the meaning of "no," picking up toys, and sharing. This infant is ready to pass into childhood.

Understanding the limitations of these walking infants is important. How many two-year-olds have been spanked for not sharing toys or putting toys away, when physically and developmentally they are incapable of understanding the concept? Lots of hurts happen at this age. Expectations from parents are often too high, resulting in frustration on the parts of both the parents and the child. These "wonderful and challenging" twos are a great time to take time out and give a massage. If the child is approached appropriately, this experience can be calming for both the parent and the child.

When working with any person, the massage professional needs to meet the person where he or she is at the moment. This is even more important when working with infants. A fussy baby and a two-year-old in a tantrum are caught up in their physiology. It takes time for both the nervous and endocrine systems to calm down. The crying may be a way to burn off the internal agitation that has built up throughout the day when verbal skills are not sufficient to express the problem. If the parent or the massage practitioner expects the infant to settle into the massage immediately, he or she may be disappointed. Relaxing takes time. Repetitive long strokes and rhythmic movement of the limbs can start the soothing. Even lateral (on the side) stimulation is calming. Swaddling provides this type of consistent, even pressure that reduces neural activity. If the baby stiffens with the massage, the tactile stimulation may be too intense. The nervous systems of infants are very sensitive. Confining the massage to the feet or rhythmic rocking may be preferable to stroking. When just the right combination of methods is found, the infant will respond to the touch.

Infants cannot give informed consent so parents must provide this permission. It is appropriate to teach parents to massage their own babies. Massage may be especially helpful for those parents who have trouble bonding.

Other than in a hospital-type setting, developing a clientele of infants is not very likely. But teaching infant massage can be an exciting career addition. There are classes available that instruct therapists on how to teach infant massage. The skills a beginner has are usually sufficient to work with well-baby care. Consideration must be given to a shorter massage time (between fifteen and thirty minutes), to the smaller, still developing anatomy, and to the needs of the parents as they learn to communicate, through touch, with their babies. A confident touch is important;

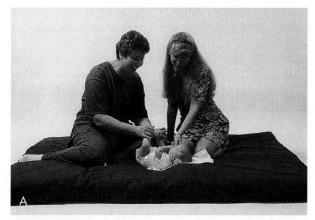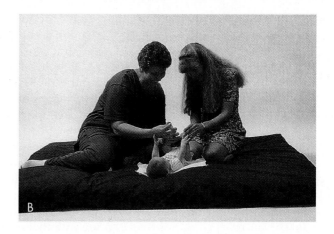

Figure 12.3
Parent being taught infant massage by massage therapist.

babies will detect nervousness immediately. To them this is not a "safe" touch. The baby will not respond and may even try to withdraw. The parents may feel rejected by the infant. Learning massage is a way for parents to become confident with their touch (Fig. 12.3).

Infants born of drugs and alcohol-addicted mothers have a nervous system that is especially challenged. Research is currently being done to see if the gentle, organized, tactile approaches of massage can help these special little babies. The initial findings are promising. Babies, especially babies of drug-addicted mothers, are sometimes abandoned. Hospitals will place these infants in what is called a border nursery. A hospital may be open to the volunteer efforts of a massage therapist, which would provide a great learning experience for both the massage professional and the hospital staff.

Remember, each baby is different. "Listen" to these little bodies, structure the massage to best meet those needs, and the baby will respond with a purity that fills your heart.

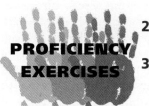

PROFICIENCY EXERCISES

1. **Using professional journals, investigate resources for learning more about infant massage.**
2. **Volunteer at a border nursery in the local hospital for a minimum of thirty-two hours.**
3. **Contact the Lamaze birth classes, LaLache League, or other organizations that provide support for new parents and volunteer to give a presentation about massage.**
4. **Locate a litter of puppies or kittens and massage these "babies."**

PHYSICALLY CHALLENGED

SECTION OBJECTIVES

Using the information presented in this section, the student will be able to do the following:

❶ Communicate more effectively with people who have a physical disability.

According to McGladrey and Pullen's assessment of the Americans with Disabilities Act, a *physical disability* or *impairment* is any physiologic disorder, condition, cosmetic disfigurement, or anatomic loss affecting one or more of the following body systems: neurologic, musculoskeletal, special sense organ, respiratory (including speech organs), cardiovascular, reproductive, digestive, genitourinary, hemic and lymphatic, skin, and endocrine. Extremes in size and extensive burns may also be considered physical impairments.[1]

People with physical impairments can benefit from massage for all the same reasons as any other individual. The client's body may develop a compensation for the disability. For instance, a person in a wheelchair

2 Adjust the massage environment to better support those with physical disabilities.

3 Become aware of subtle discrimination.

could experience increased neck and shoulder tension from moving the chair. In addition, dealing with a physical impairment daily can make routine functions more stressful.

People who are not physically challenged may be uncomfortable around those who are. This discomfort comes from not knowing what to do or say, from being afraid of the disabled, or from various other reasons. It is common to put the disability first instead of the person. When the disability is first in the therapist's mind, then the person is not. Ignorance is a huge factor. Over-compensation and patronization by the nondisabled person makes normal communication difficult. The massage professional is responsible for professional behavior and the ability to communicate effectively with all clients, including with those who have disabilities. Not knowing how is not an excuse. The best source of information is the person with the impairment. Ask your client to explain his or her limitations, what assistance, if any, might be needed, and how that assistance should be given if requested.

The following are some guidelines that may help the therapist deal with these special clients. The person with a disability should be treated the same as anyone else. The right of individuals to choose the kind of help they need must be respected. The practitioner should use good judgment when deciding whether to ask if assistance is needed, and then wait until the person accepts the offer before providing assistance. The client can give the best directions on how to proceed.

For example, if assistance is offered, it may be best to say, "If you need any assistance, I am glad to help. Tell me what you need." If the offer is declined, no offense should be taken. If the person is abrupt, it may be that this question has been asked many times already, and not in such a pleasant and respectful manner. All remarks need to be directed to the individual, and not to a friend who is nearby. This behavior is very degrading, and occurs when the therapist is more comfortable with the able-bodied companion and therefore finds it easier to address him or her.

When assisting a client with a visual impairment, the therapist should never push or pull on the person. Instead, if guiding is necessary, the therapist should stand just in front and a bit to the left of the client, who can then touch the therapist's right elbow when following. Useful directions should also be given to a person with a visual impairment. If asked where something is, the therapist should not point and say "over there." Instead, terms such as left, right, about ten steps, and so on, are much easier to follow. It is not necessary to talk louder to a person with a visual impairment since they usually can hear just fine. The conversation should begin with the therapist addressing the client by name, so that he or she is aware of being spoken to. The therapist should then state his or her name, never touching until the person is aware of the therapist's presence in the room.

If a person with a visual impairment places anything, it should not be moved. If a door is opened, the direction of the opening (toward or away from the person) and the location of the hinges (left or right) should be explained. It is best to let the client open the door to be better oriented to its position. Most people with visual impairments have some type of sight. Comparatively few people have no vision at all.

If a service dog is harnessed and working, be it a guide dog for someone with a visual impairment or any other support service, the therapist must not pet, feed, or in any other way interact with the dog. This distracts the dog and makes the job difficult. It must become very tiresome for a person with a service dog to be stopped repeatedly and asked if someone can pet the dog (Fig. 12.4).

It may be difficult to understand a person with a speech problem. The therapist should ask the person to repeat anything that was unclear until it

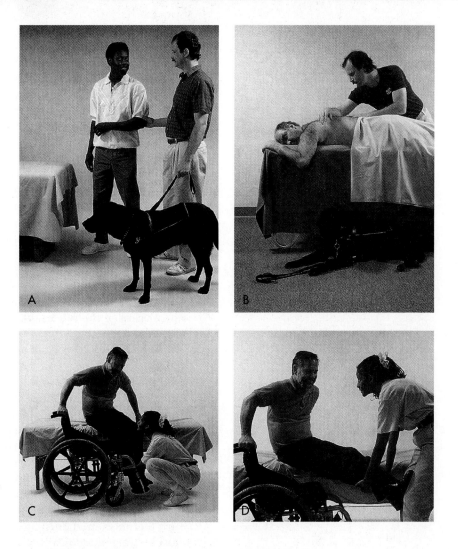

Figure 12.4
A, The sighted individual provides sighted guiding by offering elbow and concise verbal instruction. B, Guide dog is trained to lay quietly by the massage table. C, Transfer from chair to massage table. D, A low table providing for a lateral transfer is best.

is understood, and should then repeat it so the person can give additional clarification as needed. If the therapist cannot understand what is being said, the client should be told.

In order to gain the attention of a client with a hearing impairment, the therapist should tap him or her on the shoulder or wave a hand. If there is no interpreter, all talking should be done using a normal tone and rhythm of speech. When a person can lip read, it is important that the therapist stay facing the person and not cover his or her own mouth when talking. A normal tone of voice and speed should be used unless the therapist talks quickly, in which case the speed should be slowed down a bit. If necessary, a note pad can be used to write down communication.

Hearing aids amplify sound; they do not make sound clearer. Reducing background noise will help the hearing impaired to hear better. Therefore, it may be wise to ask before using any music during the massage session. Getting too close to a hearing aid may make it squeal, so care must be taken when massaging the ears.

When speaking to a client in a wheelchair or talking to a person who is small, it is best to do so from eye level. This would obviously require the massage therapist to sit down. There are many types and reasons for paralysis. Just because someone is paralyzed does not mean that he or she has no feeling in a particular area. Just because someone is in a wheelchair does not mean that he or she is paralyzed.

A wheelchair must never be pushed unless permission is given by the person in the chair. This same person will give directions as to how to push the wheelchair over inaccessible curbs or stairs. When transferring a client from chair to massage table, he or she can give the best directions on how to proceed. It may be that a transfer to a mat on the floor is easier to accomplish and the massage should be given there. The most efficient transfer is a lateral transfer to a table that is the same height as the wheelchair. This will entail a shift in body mechanics by the massage therapist to a lower table.

When giving a massage to a person with paralysis, the client should do the guiding since normal feedback mechanisms are not functioning. Those clients with catheters or other equipment must instruct the therapist as to how the items are to be handled. In most cases, the catheter can be ignored. If a client has an amputation, and a prosthesis is used, the client may or may not want it removed during the massage. Permission must be granted to massage the stump. If the client is comfortable with this, massage is especially beneficial if a prosthesis is used. Although there is no scientific validation, professional experience has shown that massage strokes carried the full length of the amputated limb seem to feel good to the client.

If the client is short, a stool may be needed to help reach the massage table, clothing hangers, or bathroom fixtures. A very large person may not trust the massage table and will be more comfortable on a floor mat. Ask the client what is preferable. If the therapist is nervous about doing the massage on the massage table, the client must be told (disclosure) since the nervousness of the therapist will affect the quality of the massage.

People who have been burned may have an assortment of challenges ranging from mobility impairment to disfigurement. As burns heal, scaring replaces functioning epithelial tissue. All of the functions of the skin, including excretion, sensation, and protection are compromised. Scar tissue tends to contract and pull, which can make the area of the healed burn feel shortened or tight. Severe contractures sometimes develop and must be treated medically. The approaches of myofascial release, cranialsacral therapy, and other connective tissue techniques will work to soften and gently stretch connective tissue. Massage of this type may somewhat reduce the effect of this shrinkage. Those seeking to serve a client who has been burned will need additional training in these methods.

All massage facilities must be barrier-free. A therapist must never assume to know, understand, or anticipate a client's need. *It is important to ask!* A good therapist will not try to pretend that the disability is not there, but will respond professionally. The disability affects only a small part of the whole person. Once the client has provided the necessary information and education about his or her disability, the therapist should then ignore the impairment. Focus conversations to discuss other aspects in the client's life.

PROFICIENCY EXERCISES

1. **Contact your local building department and speak with the person in charge of the barrier-free code requirements. Find out what the requirements are and why each requirement exists.**
2. **Obtain and read the Americans With Disabilities Act from the United States Government.**
3. **Spend a twenty-four hour period "disabled". Rent a wheelchair, tie one arm down, blindfold yourself, use ear plugs, or do not speak. When you remove the "disability," remember that a person with a disability wakes up the next morning and it is still there.**

PSYCHOLOGICALLY CHALLENGED

Using the information presented in this section, the student will be able to do the following:

❶ Comprehend the importance of verifying informed consent when working with those with a psychological disability.

❷ Structure a massage to support other psychological interventions.

McGladrey and Pullen[1] cite that in the Americans With Disability Act, a *mental impairment* is defined as any mental or psychological disorder, such as mental retardation (developmental disabilities), organic brain syndrome, emotional or mental illness, and specific learning disabilities.

We will consider addictions, brain chemical imbalances, developmental and learning disabilities, anxiety, depression and other mood disorders, and eating disorders. Again, the actual massage is really not different. What is important is who is receiving the massage.

Informed consent is a big concern with those who are influenced by drugs (both prescribed and not), internal chemicals, internal imbalances, as well as developmental disabilities. Special care must be given to ensure that the client is able to provide informed consent. When in doubt, the massage should not be given.

Massage for those with developmental disabilities has the same effect as for everyone else. Care needs to be taken to communicate at the level of the client, but not below functioning level. Adults with developmental disabilities are not children and should not be treated as such. Developmentally disabled people may become frustrated and anxious during a day of challenges. Life is harder for them. Massage is soothing, calming, and beneficial if it is accepted by the client. Not everyone likes to be touched. This needs to be respected.

Those withdrawing from chemical and alcohol addictions may find that massage helps to reduce stress levels. The type of chemical the person is addicted to will determine the types of stressful experiences incurred. The therapist listens to the client and helps decide if the massage could calm an anxious client or give a boost to a depressed client. Heavy connective tissue massage should be avoided during withdrawal periods. Toxins released from this type of massage may overtax an already burdened detoxification system.

Massage affects the brain chemicals by encouraging the release of serotonin and the endorphins, which alter mood. Certain types of mental disabilities are based on an imbalance in the brain chemicals. Hyperactivity, attention deficit disorder, bipolar (manic depressive) disorder, schizophrenia, seasonal affective disorder, and clinical depression are just a few brain chemical disorders. Medication is importation in helping those with brain chemical imbalances. The massage professional should never make the client feel guilty for taking medication or suggest that medication is not necessary. Medication must be monitored carefully, with the smallest effective dose given to avoid side effects. Massage cannot replace medication, but the client receiving regular massage may be able to reduce the dose and duration of its use in some situations. It is very important to work with the client's doctor, and to carefully chart the response of the client to the massage.

Massage has a strong normalizing effect on the autonomic nervous system. Mood disorders such as depression, anxiety, and panic interplay in a combination of autonomic nervous system functions and hormone neurotransmitters, neuropeptides, and other brain chemicals. General stress reduction massage may take the edge off the mood through the influence of massage on the autonomic nervous system. The type of massage given can be adjusted to be a little more stimulating or a little more relaxing. The key is to begin where the person is at the time of the massage. Someone who is anxious may initially resist long slow strokes and instead do better with a more active strategy for the massage that incorporates active joint movement, post-isometric relaxation, lengthening and stretching, rapid compression, and gradually shifts into a calming, rocking, long slow stroke massage. The person who is a little depressed may not initially want to join in with an active participation massage. Instead, the work might begin with rocking, long slow strokes, and end with stimulating active joint movement, rapid compression, and tapotement.

Eating disorders involve mood disorders, physiologic responses to food, and control issues. They are complicated situations that usually require professional help. The job of the massage therapist is to be aware and to refer. Any substantial weight loss must be referred to a physician. Those with anorexia nervosa lose a great deal of weight. It is more difficult to recognize bulimia, which involves binge eating and purging by vomiting and laxatives. The teeth and gums become affected by the stomach acids and the massage professional may notice this. Referring should be done because of symptoms, and not from the therapist attempting to diagnose the disorder.

Difficulties with sensory processing that occurs in some learning disorders may be helped with the organized systematic sensory stimulation of massage. Having a learning difficulty is stressful. *Author's Note: I have dyslexia as well as an inner ear dysfunction that makes eye/hand coordination difficult. Thank goodness for computers, spell checkers, and editors.* Life is more difficult when dealing with any special situation. Stress makes the learning difficulty worse. Self-esteem is hard to maintain when the person has been made to feel stupid in school for not being able to write, spell, or read. People with learning disabilities are not stupid, they just need to learn differently. Massage helps to reduce stress.

Those wishing to work with clients with mental impairments will need additional training to be able to understand the physiology and psychology of the various disorders and challenges their clients face. This type of work should be supervised closely by a psychologist or psychiatrist.

At times we are all challenged psychologically. It is important to understand how our minds work, and the interaction between the mind/body connection. Results of research are becoming available that show the connection between the mind, the body, and health. The sincere student of massage will seriously consider taking some psychology courses at a community college or other educational resource and keeping up to date on the new findings. Massage will have a very important place in mind/body medicine and therapies.

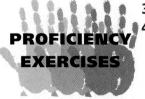

PROFICIENCY EXERCISES

1. **Contact a drug rehabilitation counselor and discuss the stages of drug withdrawal and rehabilitation.**
2. **Check out Alcoholics Anonymous or other twelve-step programs and ask to sit in on a minimum of three meetings to learn about addictions.**
3. **Volunteer to work at a Special Olympics event.**
4. **Each student in the class chooses one type of brain chemical disorder, mood disorder, eating disorder, or learning disorder. Research it and write a five-page paper on the subject. Include one page devoted to the implications for massage intervention. Include all resources in a works-cited page. Combine all of the papers into a resource book and provide a copy for each classmate.**
5. **For a minimum of six months, collect one article per month on mind/body medicine from a professional medical or research journal. At least one article should focus on body therapies.**

PREGNANCY

SECTION OBJECTIVES

Using the information presented in this section, the student will be able to do the following:

❶ Explain the importance of prenatal care.

❷ Describe the three basic stages of pregnancy.

❸ Design a general massage session to meet the needs of a pregnant woman.

❹ Teach a support person basic massage methods to use during labor.

Good, early prenatal care is very important for pregnant women. The massage professional must have permission from the doctor or licensed midwife to work with a woman during this time. Pregnancy is not an illness; it is a natural event. Prenatal care is needed to make sure that proper nutrition is provided to the mother, that the pregnancy is progressing normally, and to catch any potential problems early. If a woman is planning to become pregnant, it is useful for her to build her health up for about six months. This means eliminating all alcohol, drugs, and nicotine, normalizing her weight, developing a moderate exercise program, and eating a nutritious diet. These activities prepare the best environment for the baby to grow. Smoking, alcohol, and drug use is very dangerous to the unborn child.

A woman who is pregnant is undergoing extensive physical and emotional changes. Pregnancy is divided into three distinct segments—the first, second, and third trimesters. During the first three months (first trimester), the woman's body is adjusting to huge hormonal changes that are likely to cause mood swings. The most common complaint is morning sickness or nausea, which results from the physical body adjusting to the growing baby. This is also a very vulnerable time for the developing baby. Massage given at this time is general wellness massage, which may help to level out the mother's physiologic responses. Positioning is not a concern because the abdomen has not yet started to expand. Deep work on the abdomen is avoided, while surface stroking may be pleasurable.

The second trimester usually brings a leveling of the hormones, and the woman feels better. During this time she may start to show and feel the first movements of the baby. If the pregnancy is a choice, this is a joyful time. If not, the physical evidence of the growing baby may cause additional stress for the mother. Toward the end of the second trimester, the connective tissue begins to soften to allow the pelvis to spread. The joints seem to become sloppy. Overstretching must be avoided. Alternate positioning for side-lying or support for the abdomen is important. (Fig. 12.5) As in the first trimester, deep work on the abdomen must be avoided.

During the last trimester, the weight of the growing baby, the postural shifts, and the movement of the internal organs may cause discomfort for the pregnant woman. Because many of the internal organs are pushed up

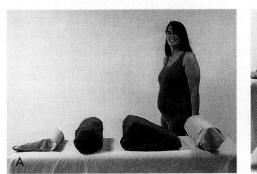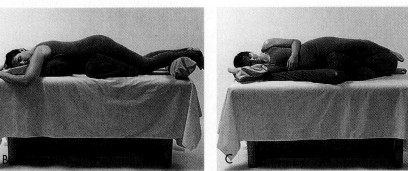

Figure 12.5
A, Placement of supports for massaging a pregnant woman. Positioning for B, prone and C, sidelying.

and back, the diaphragm does not work as efficiently. The mother will use her neck and shoulder muscles to breathe, possibly causing discomfort or thoracic outlet symptoms. Massage offers temporary relief. About two weeks before birth (in the first pregnancy), the baby will turn head down and drop into the birth canal. This provides more space for the diaphragm to work and breathing becomes easier, but pressure on the bladder causes frequent urination. Lymph vessels may be impinged so that the legs and feet swell. Edema or fluid accumulation could be a symptom of more serious complications, and the client should be referred to a doctor immediately. The low back may ache from the postural shift. The breasts have enlarged in preparation for lactation. A woman may not feel very attractive at this point. Massage is gentle and assists circulation. If a comfortable position cannot be found, the client is allowed to change positions often and to use the rest room as needed. General massage may help the woman to feel better for a little while.

It may be appropriate to teach the woman's support person some massage techniques. Massage of the lower back and stroking of the abdomen may provide comfort and distraction during labor. Massaging the feet is often helpful. Massage can relax the body and divert the attention of the nervous system, thereby providing distraction during early labor. Labor proceeds easier and faster if the woman is relaxed and works with her body. Massage given by the support person helps him or her feel useful and involved with the pregnancy and birthing process. During a phase of labor called transition, it is not uncommon for the woman to not want to be touched. Transition occurs just before the second stage of labor, with the actual movement of the baby down the birth canal. The contractions at this time are very hard and have not yet been replaced by the urge to push. After delivery, massage may help the woman's body return to normal, reduce the stress from taking care of a new baby, and give the client some time to take care of herself.

Unless there are specific circumstances or complications, massage for pregnant women should be a wellness personal service massage. Do not massage vigorously or extremely deep, overstretch, or massage the abdomen other than superficial stroking. Make sure the woman's doctor or midwife has given permission for her to receive massage. Watch for edema, varicose veins, and severe mood swings. After the birth, postpartum depression can get very serious for some women. Refer these conditions immediately to the client's doctor.

There are times when pregnancy is not joyous, as in an unwanted pregnancy. The therapist must not try to convince the woman that she really does want the baby or try to change her mood. She needs to be supported with caring quiet touch.

Interrupted pregnancies are also difficult. Whether spontaneous abortion in the first three months, induced abortion, or miscarriage, an interrupted pregnancy is a strain on a woman's body and emotional well-being. If a client has had an interrupted pregnancy, watch for emotional changes at what would have been the projected time of birth. Extra caring and support are helpful.

Giving a general massage to a woman who is pregnant can be a very rewarding experience, allowing the massage professional to watch the miracle of life develop.

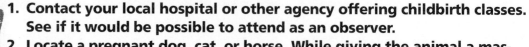

PROFICIENCY EXERCISES

1. **Contact your local hospital or other agency offering childbirth classes. See if it would be possible to attend as an observer.**
2. **Locate a pregnant dog, cat, or horse. While giving the animal a massage gently palpate the abdomen.**

3. **Volunteer to massage a woman weekly for her entire pregnancy and for four weeks after the birth.**
4. **At local childbirth classes, volunteer to teach a class on foot massage to the support people.**

TERMINAL ILLNESS

SECTION OBJECTIVES

Using the information presented in this section, the student will be able to do the following:

❶ Obtain additional information about the dying process.

❷ Explain the importance of comfort measures.

In cases in which there is nothing more that can be done to prolong life, the focus of care is more on comfort measures. The experts in this situation of terminal illness are the dedicated hospice nurses and staff who treat death with dignity. It has been said that the staff of hospices are midwives to the dying.

In order for the massage therapist to work successfully with those dealing with a terminal illness, the therapist must be aware of his or her personal feelings about death. It is strongly encouraged that every massage professional who wishes to work with clients during this very important, challenging, and special time become hospice volunteers and take the training that hospice offers.

No one knows when a person is going to die. However, two very powerful psychological forces influence living and dying—hope and the will to live. Attitudes about death vary. Adults may have more fears about death than children do. They fear pain, suffering, dying alone, the invasion of privacy, loneliness, and separation from family and loved ones. They worry about who will care for and support those left behind. Elderly persons usually have fewer fears than younger adults. They may be more accepting that death will occur, and have had more experience with dying and death. Many have lost family members and friends. Some welcome death as freedom from pain, suffering, and disability.

Dr. Elizabeth Kubler-Ross has written about death and her works have much to offer. Bernie Siegal's books are also excellent. Massage professionals interested in working with the terminally ill would benefit from reading their works.

Massage has much to offer in comfort measures. Being bedridden and immobile is painful. Massage can distract the sensory perception and provide temporary comfort measures. It provides continued human contact, and can give caregivers something useful, rewarding, and positive to do for their loved one who is dying.

Massage can become an important stress reduction method and a means of support for family members and caregivers. Caring for someone who is terminally ill can be very stressful. This support person may need to receive massage if for no other reason than to have someone take care of him or her for an hour.

The massage professional should be an integral part of the team working together to make this time of passage as gentle as possible. This means that once the decision to work with someone who is terminally ill is made, it is important to stay until the client dies (if possible). Abandonment at this time is very painful. The therapist will likely grow to care for the person, to cry when death comes, and to mourn and grieve. The therapist will probably miss the client, and may grow from the experience.

As always, it remains the choice of the client about what is wanted and to give informed consent. The client who is dying needs to retain as much personal empowerment as possible. It should not be discouraging if all that is done during a massage session is to stroke a client's hands. At this time especially it is crucial to "listen."

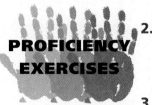

PROFICIENCY EXERCISES

1. Plan your funeral. List all plans and details regarding these final arrangements.
2. Talk with an attorney about living wills. Write a few paragraphs regarding how you wish to be taken care of when it is your time to die. How much intervention do you want? Do you want to die in a hospital or at home? When do you want hospice services?
3. Volunteer to provide massage for hospice staff. Spend a minimum of thirty-two hours.

Respect is important in any interaction with another person. In all situations remember to see and address the needs of the person first and then to accommodate the individual's special needs by offering assistance and following the directions provided by the person.

The massage therapist who desires to focus his or her professional skills to best meet the specific needs of a person will continue to seek out training and information pertinent to the therapeutic needs of each client. Often the knowledge base required becomes too extensive and it becomes necessary to specialize. When this is the situation, such as when a massage professional obtains additional training for sports massage, the information is built on the fundamentals of massage and the additional training is focused on the application of the massage fundamentals for the special situation. It is the wise professional who recognizes when less intervention is more appropriate. It requires much learning, great skill, and patiently-developed empathy to therapeutically hold someone's hand.

REVIEW QUESTIONS

1. What is the single most important factor for effective communication with those who have special needs?
2. What special massage skills are needed to work with those with special needs?
3. What is the best source of information about any special situation?
4. What is a generalized definition of abuse?
5. What importance is state-dependent memory in working with those who may have an abuse history?
6. What responses might the massage practitioner receive when pointing out a area of injury to a client who self-abuses?
7. How should a massage practitioner respond if a client experiences an emotional response during the massage?
8. Why is massage beneficial for athletes?
9. When working with athletes, what factors are important?
10. What type of massage is provided at sports events?
11. What adjustment to a massage session may need to be made when working with children?
12. Why do children like massage?
13. What is a major benefit of massage for children and adolescents?
14. Why is it important to teach parents and children some basic massage methods to share with each other?
15. Who gives informed consent for massage for those under the age of eighteen?
16. What is a realistic goal for the massage professional when working with those who have a chronic illness?
17. What is the importance of hardiness and how does massage encourage it?
18. Why is close supervision by the doctor or other health professional important when working with those who have a chronic illness?
19. What can the massage therapist learn from working with the elderly?
20. What special physical conditions are common for the elderly to experience?
21. Are there special skills required for working with the elderly?
22. What is the unique physiologic state of an infant?
23. Why is massage beneficial for infants?
24. Who is the best person to massage a baby?
25. What key elements are important when massaging an infant?
26. What are important things to remember when working with clients who have a physical disability?
27. When working with those who have an emotional or developmental disability, what important factor must the massage therapist consider?

28. How can massage be beneficial in situations of withdrawal from addictions, learning disabilities, and developmental disabilities?

29. Are there special massage skills required when working with pregnant women? Explain.

30. What part can teaching massage to the expectant father or other support person play?

31. What can providing massage for someone who is dying teach us?

32. What is the best source for information about working with the dying?

33. What can massage offer to someone who is dying?

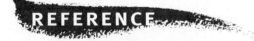

REFERENCE

1. McGladrey and Pullen. *The Americans With Disabilities Act* (Rev.) New York, 1994, Panel Publishers.

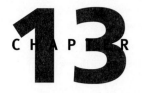

BASIC THERAPEUTIC
APPROACHES

OBJECTIVES

After completing this chapter, the student will be able to do the following:

1 Integrate a variety of therapeutic interventions into a general wellness massage.

2 Understand the physiologic mechanisms through which the therapeutic methods work.

3 Consider a direction of interest for further study.

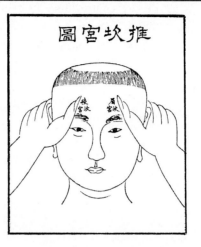

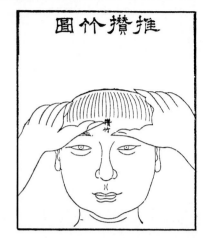

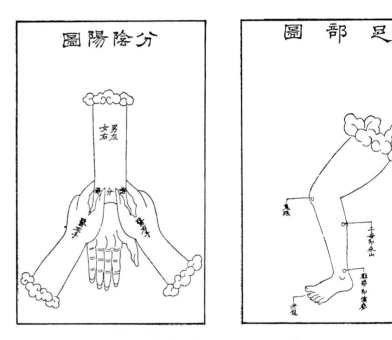

Four Chinese charts giving instructions for acupressure stimulation of acupuncture points. Today, these points are used for the relief of eye strain and myopia in children and for prevention and relief of nausea and vomiting. (Courtesy of New York Public Library)

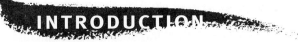

This chapter is called "Basic Therapeutic Approaches" for a reason. This chapter and the next on "Wellness Education" point the way for additional training for the massage professional. As you practice the various methods presented, pay attention to those areas where there is particular interest and talent. This information can help direct you to specific avenues for continuing education. Both of these chapters provide a general overview and simplified application of many different methods. Each topic is a specific study. The information contained in this chapter is not sufficient training to be able to purposefully and intelligently understand and use these methods for anything other than a general enhancement of the skills you have already developed. However, with a commitment to further education, the methods mentioned can add efficiency, effectiveness, and enthusiasm for what therapeutic massage has to offer for wellness, prevention, rehabilitation, and client-directed healing.

The purpose of this textbook is to train the massage professional to use massage methods intelligently in a way to promote health and well-being. There are times when the client may present the massage professional with minor problems that can be helped though the use of the techniques offered in this chapter. These same methods can be used for rehabilitative massage. In order for the massage professional to use the methods in a more specific way, additional training is needed, especially pathophysiology, medical terminology, and charting. It is important for the massage professional to confer with the medical team when dealing with clients who are undergoing medical intervention (e.g., medications, physical therapy, psychotherapy, chiropractic therapy, etc.). The massage should be integrated into the entire treatment protocol. Supervision by a licensed medical professional can help to ensure that all the methods used for a particular client are monitored and evaluated for effectiveness.

Healthy people can benefit from stimulation of the normalizing effects from the approaches of hydrotherapy, connective tissue, lymphatic and blood circulation, trigger point, acupressure, and reflexology work. These methods, when integrated into the massage methods already used, can add one more dimension to the effectiveness of the massage.

HYDROTHERAPY

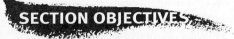

Using the information presented in this section, the student will be able to do the following:

❶ Explain the general effects of hot and cold water applications.

Hydrotherapy is a separate and distinct form of therapy that combines well with massage. Water can be used in many different ways depending on the health needs and condition of the client and the facilities available for therapy.

Water is a near-perfect natural body balancer and is necessary for life. It comprises the largest percentage of our body weight. A universal solvent, it is a perfect detoxifier for our bodies. It is available in many forms, all of which are therapeutically beneficial. Water can relax or stimulate, anesthetize, and reduce or increase circulation. It works naturally, is non-allergenic, tissue-tolerant, inexpensive, and readily available.

② Incorporate simple hydrotherapy methods into the therapy setting.

③ Suggest easy self-help techniques for clients using basic hydrotherapy.

Water therapy is as old as the human race. One of the first recorded mentions of the use of water as medicine involves the temples of the Greek god of medicine, Asclepius. At the temples, bathing and massage were part of the treatment for the sick. Hippocrates used water as a beverage in reducing fever and for treating many diseases. He also stressed the value of using various types of baths, each with a different temperature, as a therapeutic tool to combat illness. Later, the ancient Roman physicians Galen and Celsus also recommended specific baths as an integral part of their remedies. Almost every warm-climate civilization has at some point in its history used baths for therapeutic reasons.[1]

Water's three forms (liquid, steam, and ice) allow for use in a variety of temperatures. As a liquid, water can be pressurized and used as a relaxing massage shower or as a whirlpool for muscle and joint therapy. As steam, it provides relaxation and cleansing in a steam bath or humidity in a winter home, or acts as a breathing aid to a congested child or senior. As heat, it can increase circulation, and as ice, reduce it. When warm, it can increase body temperature; when cool, reduce or increase it. As ice, it is an effective anesthetic and can minimize edema. It is an antiseptic when boiling or as steam. In a flotation tank or soaking bath, it can reduce stress. Water can be used internally by drinking it, or by forcing streams of water into orifices, as in an enema, douche, bidet, or nose or ear bath. Water can be used externally as full or partial baths, or showers, in compresses, packs, hot water bottles, frozen ice bandages, or wrapped ice, and as steam in several different ways.

The effects of water are primarily reflexive and focused to the autonomic nervous system. The addition of heat energy or dissipation of heat from tissues could be classified as mechanical in its effect. In general, cold stimulates sympathetic responses and warm activates parasympathetic responses. There are differences with short- and long-term applications of hot or cold. For the most part, short cold applications stimulate and increase circulation. Long cold applications depress and decrease circulation. Short applications of heat depress and deplete tone, while long hot applications result in a combined depressant and stimulant reaction.

Skillful use of hydrotherapy methods requires long-term study. The advanced-level massage therapist should be well trained in hydrotherapy. These methods have very powerful physiologic effects and have been used for centuries as part of the healing process. Before the development of depressant and stimulant drugs, hot, warm, and cold applications were used to stimulate the autonomic nervous system. Cold shock was used instead of electric shock to treat depression. Warm baths of long duration were used to calm anxious persons. Herbal additives to water have also been used for centuries to enhance the effects of hydrotherapy.

The information presented in this section is only meant to be an introduction to hydrotherapy and basic techniques that can be used by the massage practitioner or taught as self-help to clients. Although many massage therapy facilities do not have access to hydrotherapy equipment, simple hot and cold compresses can be used. A warm foot bath is easy to incorporate into a massage and will serve the double purpose of relaxing the client and freshening "stale" feet before the massage. A bag of frozen peas makes a great cold pack since it will mold to almost any area. Hot water bottles can be safer to use than heating pads. They will naturally cool down before they could burn someone. Water frozen in a paper cup with a stick in it makes an effective massage tool, especially when using ice as a counter-stimulant to assist in lengthening and stretching procedures. Clean, pure drinking water should be available for both the client and the therapist.

Rules of Hydrotherapy

Hydrotherapy has a powerful effect on the body. The following rules, taken from the Ontario, Canada curriculum guidelines for massage therapy, need to be followed when using hydrotherapy in the massage setting:

1. Always take a thorough case history to check for possible contraindications. Contraindications include various circulatory and kidney problems as well as skin conditions.
2. Always adapt the method to the individual and not vice versa. The procedures given for time length, temperatures used, and other variables should be used as guidelines and not absolutes.
3. Have the client go to the bathroom before treatment begins.
4. Stay with the client during treatment or have some way for the client to contact you, such as by using a bell.
5. Explain the complete treatment to the client beforehand so he or she knows what to expect and what is expected.
6. Make sure the room is draft-free, clean, and quiet. All equipment should be sanitary and in good working condition. Each client should have clean towels and sheets.
7. Keep the client from becoming chilled during or after the treatment.
8. When using cold temperatures, the water should be as cold as possible, within the tolerance of the client. A 10° difference is the minimum needed to create stimulation and change in the circulation.
9. Warm temperatures should be as warm as necessary and within the client's tolerance. Too hot a temperature can be debilitating.
10. More is *not* better. It is not always more effective to use greater extremes in temperature or greater lengths of time. The aim is to achieve a positive change, and too much can overtax, damage, or set back the condition.
11. Ask pertinent questions during the treatment, including questions about comfort level and thirst, but keep talking to a minimum to allow the client to relax.
12. Check the client's pulse before, during, and after treatments as required, especially with prolonged hot treatments. The pulse should stay fairly even.
13. Watch for discomfort and/or negative reactions to the treatment.
14. Stop the treatment if a negative reaction occurs.
15. Generally, short cold treatments are followed by active exercise. Both prolonged cold and hot treatments are followed by bed rest and then exercise.
16. Apply cold compresses to the head with both hot treatments and prolonged cold treatments.
17. Never give a cold treatment to a cold body. Always warm the body first. The easiest method for this is a warm foot bath.

Use Box 13.1 as a guide when classifying water temperatures for treatments.

Box 13.1 HOW TO CLASSIFY WATER TEMPERATURE		
	Very cold	32° to 56°
	Cold	56° to 65°
	Cool	65° to 92°
	Neutral	92° to 98°
	Warm to Hot	98° to 104°
	Very Hot	104° and above

Types of Water Application for Health Purposes

The types of water application used for health purposes include the following:

1. Local heat: Apply heat to a specific area of the body such as a joint, the chest, throat, shoulders, or spine. Use hot, moist compress or a hot water bottle.
2. Local cold: Apply cold to a specific area of the body. Use cold compress, ice bag, ice pack, ice hat, or frozen bandage.
3. Tonic friction: Water sponging and washing combined with some form of friction, from either the hand or a rough wash cloth, produces a tonic effect in the body. Use cold friction massage or a cold sponge rub.
4. Sponging: Use alcohol, water, or witch hazel applied with a sponge to wash the body.
5. Baths: The body is immersed in cold, hot, or tepid water. Use foot, sitz, full, or herb baths. Any part of the body may be partially bathed, as in an arm, eye, or finger bath. A whirlpool is a bath in which the water is moving under pressure.
6. Compresses and packs: Compresses and packs are folded cotton, flannel, or gauze soaked in water or liquid medications or herbs. A pack covers a larger area than a compress.
7. Showers: Several kinds of water streams can be directed against the body. Alternate streams can also be directed against the body, or large quantities of water can be poured from a height.
8. Shampoo: When soap and water are used together on one or all parts of the body, it creates a shampoo. Use to cleanse hair, or after sauna or steam room.
9. Steam: A vaporizer can cleanse the upper respiratory system, and a steam room or sauna increases body perspiration and releases many stored toxins. Cold steam, as from a humidifier, moistens dry rooms in winter and is important in preventing colds and sinus headaches.
10. Sauna (dry heat): An intense but tolerably heated room. Take a tepid or cold shower after a sauna.

Mechanical Effects

Different pressures of water can exert a powerful mechanical effect on the nerve and blood supply of the skin. Techniques that are used include a friction rub with a sponge or wet mitten, and pressurized streams of hot and cold water directed at various part of the body (Box 13.2).

R.I.C.E. First Aid

Everyone should understand basic first aid. The R.I.C.E. application of hydrotherapy is appropriate for most soft tissue injuries, especially sprains or strains. Always refer serious injuries to a medical doctor.

R—rest
I—ice
C—compression
E—elevation

R.I.C.E. decreases recovery time by decreasing the secondary injury to tissue caused by the inflammatory response, since there is less total damage and thus less to be repaired. By decreasing pain and muscle spasm there is a more normal range of motion and muscular strength. The client can therefore return to activity much quicker, reducing other complications set up by the injury.

Rest allows the injured area(s) or the entire body to best use regenerative energy to heal. *Ice* decreases metabolism, resulting in lessened secondary injury due to swelling from primary injury. Ice does not affect the

Box 13.2
HEAT, COLD, AND ICE APPLICATIONS

Effects of Heat
- Increased circulation
- Increased metabolism
- Increased inflammation
- Decreased pain
- Decreased muscle spasm
- Decreased tissue stiffness

As a sedative, water is a very efficient, nontoxic, calming substance. It soothes the body and promotes sleep.

Techniques: Use hot and warm baths to quiet and relax the entire body, salt baths, neutral showers to relax certain areas, or damp sheet packs.

For elimination, the skin is the largest organ, and simple immersion in a long hot bath, sauna, or steam room can stimulate the excretion of toxins from the body through the skin. Inducing perspiration is useful in treating acute diseases and many chronic health problems.

Techniques: Use hot baths, epsom salt or common salt baths, hot packs, dry blanket packs, hot herbal drinks.

As an antispasmodic, water effectively reduces cramps and muscle spasm.

Techniques: Use hot compresses (depending on the problem), herbal teas, or abdominal compresses.

Effects of Cold
- Increased stimulation
- Increased circulation
- Decreased inflammation
- Decreased pain
- Increased muscle tone
- Increased tissue stiffness

Water not only restores the body's normal circulation and temperature, but intelligent water treatment, especially with cold water, can also act to restore and increase muscle strength and increase the body's resistance to disease. Cold water boosts vigor, adds energy and tone, and aids in digestion.

Techniques: Use cold water treading (standing or walking in cold water), whirlpool baths, cold sprays, alternate hot and cold contrast baths, showers or compresses, salt rubs, apple cider vinegar baths, and partial packs.

For injuries, the application of an ice pack will control the flow of blood and reduce tissue swelling.

Technique: Use an ice bag, plus compression and elevation.

As an anesthetic, water can dull the sense of pain or sensation. *Technique:* Use ice to chill the tissue.

For minor burns, water, particularly cold and ice water, has been rediscovered as a primary healing agent.

Technique: Use ice water immersion or saline water immersion.

To reduce fever, water is nature's best cooling agent. Unlike drugs, which usually only diminish internal heat, water both lowers and removes heat by conduction.

continued

Box 13.2
HEAT, COLD, AND ICE APPLICATIONS
(continued)

Effects of Ice
- Decreased circulation
- Decreased metabolism
- Decreased inflammation
- Decreased pain
- Decreased muscle spasm
- Increased stiffness

Application Type
- Ice packs
- Ice immersion (ice water)
- Ice massage
- Cold whirlpool
- Chemical cold packs
- Cold gel packs (caution)

Contraindications
1. Vasospastic disease (spasm of blood vessels)
2. Cold hypersensitivity
   - Skin = itching, sweating
   - Respiratory = hoarseness, sneezing, chest pain
   - Gastrointestinal = abdominal pain, diarrhea, vomiting
   - Eyes = puffiness of eyelids
   - General = headache, discomfort, uneasiness
3. Cardiac disorder
4. Compromised local circulation

Precautions
1. Do not use frozen gel packs directly on skin.
2. Do not use cryotherapy applications for longer than 30 minutes continuously.
3. Do not do exercises that cause pain following cold applications.
4. Do not use cryotherapy for treating persons with certain rheumatoid conditions, or for those who are paralyzed or have coronary artery disease.

Ice is a primary therapy for strains, sprains, contusions, hematomas, and fractures. It has a numbing, anesthetic effect and helps control internal hemorrhage by reducing circulation to, and metabolic processes within, the area.

original injury but does keep body processes from making the injury worse. *Compression* acts to increase pressure outside the vasculature. This will help control edema formation by promoting reabsorption of fluids. *Elevation* reduces blood and fluid flow to injured areas.

A wrapped ice bag is the most effective initial therapy for many injuries, especially sports injuries. An ice bag held to the injury site with an elastic bandage is ideal because the resulting compression reinforces the physiologic action of the application. An ice bath or ice massage is also effective.

To avoid frostbite, place a layer of fabric between the ice and the skin. Ice therapy varies with the injury and its severity. Most injuries respond within twenty-four to forty-eight hours. Ice bag compression should be used for twenty minutes, twice a day, or for shorter applications, four times a day. Apply ice periodically, not continuously. Between ice applications, rub the body part briskly with the hand. When heat is ineffective for muscle spasms, use ice. Often a sciatica attack that does not respond to moist heat will respond to one or two frozen bandages.

Be sure the injury has been evaluated by a physician. Apply ice to the injured area by immersion in ice water (ice bath), massage with ice cubes or pops, an ice bag, or ice packs.

Ice application continues through four sensations (over a ten- to fifteen minute time period): appreciation of cold (pain), warming, ache or throbbing, and skin anesthesia (numbness).

The effects of alternating hot and cold include constriction and dilation of vessels, and decreased congestion. Techniques include hot and cold compresses, ice bags, warm or hot baths, hot packs, whirlpool baths, and hot and warm or alternate hot and cold showers. Do not use heat on a fresh injury; it increases the blood flow and inflammation, and therefore tissue swelling.

PROFICIENCY EXERCISE

• **Visit a whirlpool, sauna, and steam room. Hotels may have this equipment available. Use the equipment and pay attention to how you feel.**

LYMPH BLOOD AND CIRCULATION ENHANCEMENT

SECTION OBJECTIVES

Using the information presented in this section, the student will be able to do the following:

❶ Explain the general effects of lymphatic and circulation enhancement massage.

❷ Incorporate the principles of lymphatic and circulation massage into the general massage session.

One of the most documented benefits of massage is stimulation of the lymphatics and circulation. A style used for lymphatic drainage is manual lymph drainage, which was developed by Vodder. There are many variations and styles of massage that are used to stimulate lymphatic and blood circulation. When the massage is focused to specifically stimulate the lymphatic or circulatory system, a special type of massage is performed. Because an entire body system is being stimulated, the approach is called *systemic massage*. In this section we discuss the important physiology and methods of focusing the massage to accomplish lymph and blood circulation enhancement.

Lymphatic Drainage

Lymph drain is a specific therapeutic method. Specialized training is required to use it well. All massage stimulates the circulation and lymph movement, but structuring a massage to focus on this system is a particular therapeutic intervention. When an individual body system is focused, and the effects of the massage concentrated to a certain response, it is not uncommon for the client to feel the effects of the methods more than with general or local massage. When working with lymph and the precise movement of lymph, the client may feel listless, fatigued, or achy for forty-eight hours after the massage. Some have described this feeling as a massage "hangover." The physiologic effects of toxin overload are similar to an alcohol hangover. Anything other than a general approach presented in this text is likely to be outside the scope of practice for personal service wellness massage. The information presented here should provide enough background information for the massage professional to refer to another more appropriate professional should special circulation work be needed.

The lymph system permeates the entire tissue structure of the body in a one-way drainage network of vessels, ducts, nodes, lacteals, and lymphoid organs such as the spleen. It is helpful to visualize roots on a plant to get an idea of the extensive lymph network. Tiny lymph vessels, known as *lymph capillaries*, are distributed throughout the body, except in the eyes, brain, and spinal cord. The lymph fluid is collected in the capillaries somewhat like water is drawn up into the plant roots. There are major lymph plexus on the soles of the feet and the palms of the hands. It is pos-

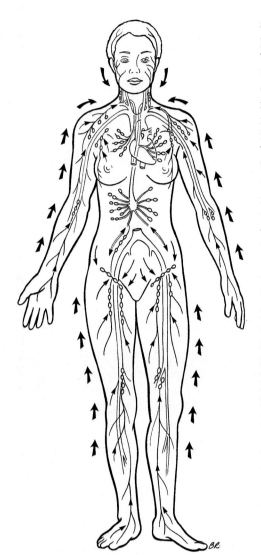

Figure 13.1
Direction of strokes for facilitating lymphatic flow.

sible that the rhythmic pumping of walking and grasping facilitates lymphatic flow. The tubes merge into one another until major channels and vessels are formed. These vessels run from the distal parts of the body toward the heart, usually along veins and arteries. Lymph nodes are enlarged portions of the lymph vessels that generally cluster at the joints for assistance in pumping when the joint moves. These nodes filter the fluid and produce lymphocytes. All of the body's lymph vessels converge into two main channels: the thoracic duct and the right lymphatic duct. Vessels from the entire left side of the body and from the right side of the body below the chest converge into the thoracic duct, which in turn empties into the left subclavian vein situated beneath the left clavicle. The right lymphatic duct collects lymph from the vessels on the right side of the head, neck, upper chest, and right arm. It empties into the subclavian vein beneath the right clavicle. Waste products are then carried by the bloodstream to the spleen, intestines, and kidneys for detoxification.

The lymph system is a specialized component of the circulatory system, responsible for waste disposal and immune response. Lymph and blood are very similar except lymph does not have red blood cells and platelets, has a slightly higher protein content, and carries bacteria and other debris. Lymph is the interstitial (around the cell) fluid. It moves from the interstitial space into the lymph capillaries through a pressure mechanism exerted by respiration, the compression of muscles, and the pull of the skin and fascia during movement. This action is especially prominent at the plexus in the hands and feet. It does not take much pressure to move the fluid. The pressure provided by massage mimics the compressive forces of movement and respiration.

Simple muscle tension puts pressure on the lymph vessels and may block them and interfere with efficient drainage. Massage can normalize muscle tone. As the muscles relax, the lymph vessels open. The methods of lymphatic massage are fairly simple, but lymph massage, when indicated, is a very powerful technique with body wide responses. Lymphatic massage stimulates the flow of lymph mechanically with very light pressure on the surface of the skin tracing the lymphatic routes. Rhythmic gentle passive joint movement reproduces the body's normal means of pumping lymph. The client helps the process by deep slow breathing, which stimulates lymph flow. When possible, position the area being massaged above the heart so that gravity can also assist the lymph flow.

The massage consists of a combination of short, light, pumping, effleurage strokes followed by long surface effleurage strokes. The direction is toward the drainage points (following the arrow on the diagram in Fig. 13.1). The focus of the pressure is on the dermis just below the surface layer of skin and the layer of tissue just beneath the skin and above the muscles. This is the superficial fascial layer. It does not take much pressure to contact the area. Too much pressure presses capillaries closed and nullifies any effect. With lymphatic massage, light pressure is indicated.

Designing a massage for the healthy client that provides a more specific focus to the lymphatics is appropriate.

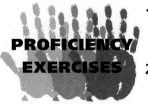

PROFICIENCY EXERCISES

1. Fill a long balloon with water. Leave an air bubble in it. Use short effleurage strokes to move the bubble. Notice the level of pressure that moves the bubble most effectively.
2. Design a lymphatic self-massage. Incorporate deep breathing and compression action at the joints, palms, and soles of the feet.

Circulatory Massage

Circulatory massage is focused specifically to stimulate the efficient flow of blood through the body. As with lymph massage, specific application for an impaired circulation disease process is out of the scope of practice for the massage professional trained in wellness personal service massage. Those clients who are not sick can still benefit greatly from increased efficiency in the circulatory system. This type of massage tends to normalize blood pressure, tone the cardiovascular system, and undo the ill effects of occasional stress. It is an excellent massage approach to use with athletes and after exercise. Circulatory massage also supports the inactive client by increasing the blood movement mechanically, but it in no way replaces exercise. Both circulatory and lymphatic massage are very beneficial for the client who is unable to walk or exercise aerobically, whatever the reason.

The circulatory system is a closed system that is composed of a series of connected tubes and a pump. The heart pump provides pressure for blood to move out through the body in the arteries and eventually to the small capillaries where the actual oxygen and nutrient exchange happens. The blood then returns to the heart via the veins. Venous blood is not under pressure from the heart; it relies on the muscle compression against the veins to change the interior venous pressure. As in the lymphatic system, backflow of blood is prevented by a valve system.

Veins and arteries are different. Massage to encourage blood flow to the tissues (arterial circulation) and then back to the heart (venous circulation) is different. Because of the valve system of the veins and lymph vessels, any deep stroking over these vessels, from proximal to distal (from the heart out), is contraindicated. There is small chance of breaking down the valves. However, compression, which does not slide like effleurage or stripping, is appropriate for stimulating arterial circulation. Compression is applied over the main arteries beginning close to the heart (proximal), and systematically moves distally to the tips of the fingers or toes. The manipulations are applied over the arteries and pump at a rhythm of approximately sixty beats per minute or with the client's resting heart rate. Compressive force changes the internal pressure in the arteries and encourages the movement of blood (Fig. 13.2).

The next step is to assist venous return flow. This resembles the lymphatic massage in that a combination of short and long effleurage strokes is used with movement. The difference is that lymphatic massage is done over the entire body and the movements are passive. With venous return flow, the effleurage strokes move distally to proximally (from the fingers and toes to the heart) over the major veins. The short effleurage stroke is about three inches long and moves the blood from valve to valve. Long effleurage strokes carry the blood through the entire vein. Passive and active joint movements help venous circulation. Placing the limb or other area above the heart brings in the gravity assistance (Fig. 13.3).

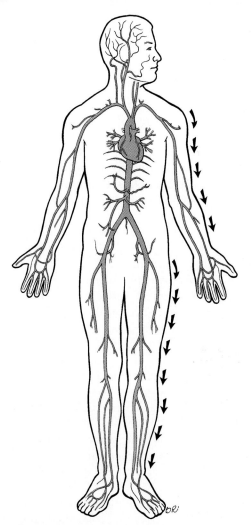

Figure 13.2
Direction of compression over arteries to increase arterial flow.

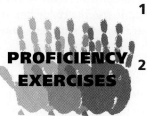

PROFICIENCY EXERCISES

1. Hook a hose up to a faucet and barely turn on the water. This simulates the heart pump. Use compression to facilitate the movement of "circulation" of the water in the hose.
2. Obtain a three-foot piece of clear soft plastic tubing. As if sucking on a straw, draw up a small amount of water into the tubing. Massage the water to the other end of the tube. This is similar to venous return massage.

REFLEXOLOGY

SECTION OBJECTIVES

Using the information presented in this section, the student will be able to do the following:

❶ Explain the physiologic benefits of foot and hand massage.

❷ Incorporate the principles of reflexology into the general massage session.

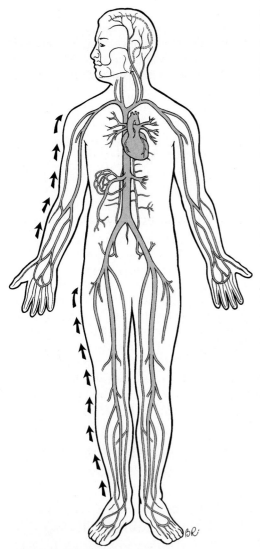

Figure 13.3
Direction of effleurage strokes to facilitate venous flow.

In the bodywork community, *reflexology* is taken to mean the stimulation of areas beneath the skin to improve the function of the whole body or of specific body areas that are away from the site of the stimulation. Eunice Ingham has been given credit for formalizing the system, which is based on the theory that certain points in the foot and hand will affect other body organs and areas. Foot reflexology is the most popular. However, the whole body, including the hands, head, ears, and torso, has reflex points. As Dr. Leon Chaitow put it, "If you consider all of the reflexology points, acupuncture points, neurolymphatic points, motor points and other reflex points, the body is a point."

Another approach to reflexology is referred to as zone therapy. It is postulated that there are ten zones running though the body. Reflex points for stimulation can be located within the zones.

Reflexology applies the stimulus/reflex principle to healing the body. The foot has been mapped to show what areas to contact to affect what areas of the body. All of the charts vary somewhat. Typically, the large toe represents the head and the junction of the large toe to the foot represents the neck. The next toes represent the eyes, ears, and sinuses. The waist is about midway on the arch of the foot with various organs above and below the line. The reflex points for the spine are along the medial longitudinal arch. It is thought that this stimulus/response reflex is conducted through neural pathways in the body that activate the body's electrical and biochemical activities (Fig. 13.4).

The medical definition of reflexology is "the study of reflexes." *Reflexotherapy* is the treatment by manipulation or other means applied to an area away from the disorder. In physiologic terms a reflex is an involuntary response to a stimulus.

This discussion of reflexology attempts to explain why foot and hand massage is beneficial though standard physiology and avoids the issue of whether there are actual corresponding points on the foot relating directly to other body areas. An explanation based on standard anatomy and physiology is better suited to the format of this textbook and may be better accepted by the public.

The foot is a very complex structure. The ankle and foot consist of 34 joints, with many joint and reflex patterns (Box. 13.3). There is extensive nerve distribution to the feet and hands. The position of the foot sends considerable postural information from the joint kinesthetic receptors through the central nervous system. The sensory and motor centers of the brain devote a large area to the foot and hand.

It seems logical to assume that stimulation of the feet would activate the responses of the gait control mechanism and hyperstimulation analgesia. Body wide effects are the result. This fact alone is sufficient to explain the benefits of foot and hand massage. There are many nerve endings on the feet and hands that correlate with acupressure points, which, when stimulated, trigger the release of endorphins and other endogenous chemicals. In addition, major plexuses for the lymph system are located in the hands and feet. Compressive forces in this area would stimulate lymphatic movement.

An excellent way to massage the foot is to systematically apply pressure and movement to the entire foot and ankle complex. This pressure will stimulate the circulation, nerves, and reflexes. Moving all of the joints stimulates large-diameter nerve fibers and joint kinesthetic receptors, initiating hyperstimulation analgesia. The result is a shift in proprioceptive and postural reflexes. The sheer volume of sensory information

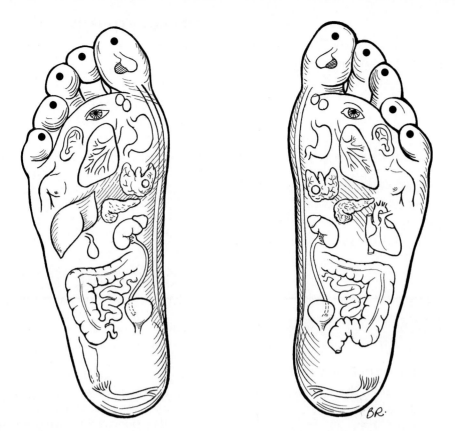

Figure 13.4
A generalized reflexology chart.

flooding the central nervous system must have some significant effects within the body.

Foot massage is usually boundary-safe. Most people will accept foot or hand massage when the idea of removing the clothing is objectionable. Hand and foot massage is likely to be the most effective form of self-

Box 13.3
REFLEXES ASSOCIATED WITH THE FOOT

Achilles tendon reflex: Plantar flexion/extension of the foot resulting from the contraction of calf muscles following a sharp blow to the Achilles tendon. Similar to the knee jerk reflex.

Extensor thrust: A quick and brief extension of a limb upon application of pressure to the plantar surface.

Flexor withdrawal: Flexion of the lower extremity when the foot receives a painful stimulus.

Mendel-Bekhterev: Plantar flexion of the toes in response to percussion of the dorsum of the foot.

Postural reflex: Any reflex that is concerned with maintenance of posture.

Rossolimos reflex: Plantar flexion of the second to fifth toes in response to percussion of the plantar surface of the toes.

Proprioceptive: Reflex initiated by movement of the body to maintain the position of the moved part. Any reflex initiated by stimulation of a proprioceptor.

massage. The hand and the foot have similar motor cortex distribution patterns. The stimulation of the hands while doing the massage does not override the sensations to the feet being massaged. The hands are massaged while they massage the feet.

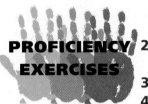

PROFICIENCY EXERCISES

1. **Exchange foot massage with another student or visit a professional reflexologist. Receive a foot massage and compare the effects with those of a full-body massage.**
2. **Using a skeletal model, move each of the joints of the foot. Then move each of the joints of your foot.**
3. **Teach foot massage to three people.**
4. **Massage your feet daily for fifteen minutes for a period of two weeks and take notice of the effects.**

CONNECTIVE TISSUE APPROACHES

SECTION OBJECTIVES

Using the information presented in this section, the student will be able to do the following:

❶ Modify existing massage methods to address more specifically the connective tissue.

❷ Explain the principles of deep transverse friction massage.

There are several basic connective tissue dysfunctions that can develop. Connective tissue may shorten, lose fluidity, and adhere causing binding, pulling, and restricted movement. Another common problem is overstretched connective tissue at the joint, resulting in laxity and destabilization of the joint, setting the stage for protective muscle spasms causing a reduction in joint space.

The basic connective tissue approach consists of mechanically softening the tissue through pressure, pulling, movement, and stretch on the tissues, which allows them to rehydrate and remold. The process is similar to softening jello by warming it. If you want connective tissue to stay soft, water must be added. This is one reason why it is important for the client to drink water.

The stretching, pulling, or pressure on the connective tissue is a little different from that of neuromuscular methods. Neuromuscular work usually flows in the direction of the fibers to affect the proprioceptive mechanism and creates a quick response. Connective tissue approaches are slow and sustained, usually against or across the fibers. Connective tissue stretching is elongated or telescoped at the point of the barrier.[6] It is important to induce a small inflammatory process in the dysfunctional area. This process initiates the reorganization of tissue.[5] Connective tissue work extends from the very subtle, light work of cranial-sacral and fascial release concepts, to the very mechanical deep transverse frictioning of Cyriax.

The most specific localized example of connective tissue work is Dr. James Cyriax's cross-fiber frictioning concept. This method is effective, especially around joints where the tendons and ligaments become bound. According to Cyriax,

> "During treatment by deep friction, great precision in sitting (positioning) of the patient and of the physiotherapist's hand is essential; throughout the session she keeps her mind on her finger-tip. This type of work involves her in much more concentration and care than most of her other work. There is nothing routine about it; each patient and each lesion must be assessed and given expert and individual attention."[4]

Although mastery of this type of deep transverse friction is beyond the scope of this textbook, it is a very valuable form of rehabilitative massage and any massage practitioner working in a medical setting should be trained in the methods. Specific anatomic knowledge is required for the precision of which Dr. Cyriax speaks. The frictioning can last as long as fifteen minutes. In effect, a controlled re-injury of the tissue occurs, which introduces a small amount of inflammation and traumatic hyperemia to the area. The result is the restructuring of the connective tissue, increased circulation to the area, and temporary analgesia.[4] Proper rehabilitation is essential to produce a mobile scar upon rehealing of the tissue. According to Cyriax,

> "Thus, deep transverse frictions restore mobility to muscle in the same way as manipulation frees a joint. Indeed, the action of deep transverse friction may be summed up as affording a mobilization that passive stretching or active exercises cannot achieve. After the friction has restored a full range of painless broadening to the muscle belly, this added mobility must be maintained. To this end, the patient should perform a series of active contractions with the joint placed in a position that fully relaxes the affected muscle i.e., the position that allows the greatest broadening. Strong resisted movement should be avoided until the scar has consolidated itself; otherwise, started too soon they tend to strain the healing breach again."[4]

Cyriax further teaches that when massage is given to a muscle, tendon, ligament, or joint capsule, the following principles must be observed:

1. The right spot must be found.
2. The therapist's fingers and the client's skin must move as one. Care must be taken to not cause a blister and the client must understand the that deep friction massage to a tender point can be painful.
3. The friction must be given across the fibers composing the affected structure.
4. The friction must be given with sufficient sweep. Pressure only accesses the tender area; it does not replace the friction. Circular friction is not recommended. Only a back and forth friction is effective.
5. The friction must reach deeply enough. If it does not reach the lesion, it is of no value.
6. The client must be placed in a suitable position that ensures the appropriate degree of tension or relaxation of the tissues to be frictioned.
7. Muscles must be kept relaxed while being frictioned. Since the connective tissue of the muscle is affected, the massage must penetrate into the muscle and not stay on the surface.
8. Tendons with a sheath must be kept taut during friction massage.

Proper rehabilitation after the massage is essential for the friction massage to be effective. The frictioned area needs to be contracted painlessly without putting any strain on the frictioned tissue. This is done by fixing the joint in a position in which the muscle is relaxed and then having the client contract the muscle as far as it will go. This is sometimes called a *broadening contraction* (Fig. 13.5).

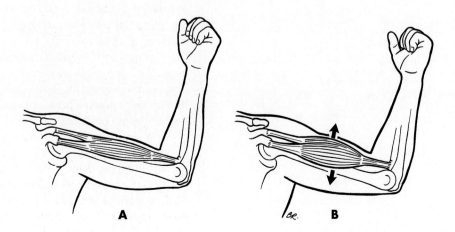

Figure 13.5
Broadening contraction.
A, Beginning point.
B, Contract muscle by flexing the joint.

A   B

Using Cyriax's principles, this textbook introduces a modified version of these methods, which can be incorporated into a general massage session to be used for small areas of adhered tissue. It is true that the modified version of deep transverse friction will not have the same effects on an area of adhesion, but the ability to move the tissue in a transverse way may keep the development of adhesions in check when a person develops minor muscle tears from overstretching or minor muscle pulls. To accommodate the lack of precise location of all of the anatomic structures, the friction suggested will be done over a broader area for a shorter time.

- Locate the area to be frictioned.
- Place the muscle in a relaxed position.
- Provide friction as described in Chapter 10, pg. 258.

Cyriax asserts that the essential component of a transverse friction massage is that it applies concentrated therapeutic movement over only a very small area. The key element is that friction moves the tissue against its grain. Additional training will be required for more specific frictioning methods.

Other forms of connective tissue massage exist. They consist typically of some form of stretching of the connective tissue and are described next.

Professional experience suggests that the longer the problem has existed, the more mechanical the techniques that will be required initially. Mechanical techniques include all gliding, kneading, skin rolling, and compression styles of bodywork as long as the contact elongates and drags or pulls on the tissue for sustained periods of time. The connective tissue responds relatively slowly, sometimes taking sixty seconds or longer. Conversely, neuromuscular techniques usually elicit a response in fifteen to thirty seconds.

Although connective tissue generally orients itself vertically in the body, there are also three or four transverse planes (depending on which resource you use). Adhesions result when connective tissue attempts to stabilize itself by attaching to surrounding tissue. Stabilizing formations can orient in any direction. The intent of connective tissue massage is either to soften the ground matrix, or to introduce small amounts of inflammation, which triggers connective tissue restructuring.[5] Another of the body's responses to inflammation is the generation of injury potentials. In acupuncture, the insertion of a needle into a muscle generates a burst of electrical discharges, which can cause a shortened or hypertonic muscle to relax instantly or within minutes. Injured tissue also yields a current known as the *current of injury*. First detected by Galvani in 1797, this current can encourage healing processes for days until the miniature wound heals.[5]

It is often futile to try to figure out connective tissue patterns. The more subtle connective tissue approaches rely on the skilled development of following tissue movement. This is simple once the student stops thinking about the process and begins to experience it. Pulling, stretching, and frictioning techniques do not require such finesse. The important point is that the pressure actually moves the tissue, puts tension into it, elongates it, and holds it long enough for energy to build and soften it. The development of connective tissue patterns is highly individualized and systems that follow a precise protocol and sequence are often less effective in dealing with these complex patterns.

It is possible that the normalization of connective tissue will allow the joint to function appropriately; however, this process may become problematic. The purpose of the connective tissue is to stabilize; and it may do so while the joint remains out of alignment. Dr. Gurevich, a Russian physician, explained the pattern of degeneration as usually beginning with dystonia or disruption of tone. (Sometimes a direct trauma to a joint could

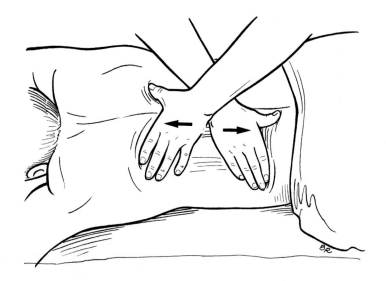

Figure 13.6
Light compressive force is applied, molding hand to the skin. The hands are then separated without adding additional compressive force providing for a fascial stretch.

cause it to misalign, as opposed to increased or decreased muscle tone pulling joints out of alignment.) Bones are designed to fit at the joint in a specific way. When this fit is disrupted, the next step is a protective muscle spasm, followed by connective tissue reorganization to stabilize the area. Areas of disruption in joint play or joint alignment eventually will include a connective tissue component in the dysfunction. Gurevich teaches that the treatment sequence is first massage, then mobilization (movement of jointed areas within comfortable range of motion), and finally joint manipulation. Massage and mobilization are within the scope of a bodywork practice, while joint manipulation is not. The services of a chiropractor, osteopath, or other professional trained in joint manipulation are desirable for those problems that require direct manipulation to the joint.

A fascial restriction involves an area larger than a small localized spot. It is palpated as a barrier or an area of immobility within the tissue. It is worked initially using routine massage techniques. If the area does not release, the pressure must be more specific.

The tissue is stabilized with one hand. With the fingers of the other hand, the tissue is pulled in the direction of the restriction. The heel of the hand or the arm can be used to separate the tissue. Twist and release petrissage and compression applied in the direction of the restriction can also release these fascial barriers (Fig. 13.6).

This style of bodywork is often called *soft tissue manipulation* or *myofascial release.* The procedures described are only a part of these systems and additional training is required to learn these valuable methods in detail. Cranial sacral therapy, which is a subtle connective tissue approach reaching many structures deep with in the body, is a valuable technique to perfect. John Barnes Myofascial Release Seminars and Upledger Institute CranioSacral Therapy Seminars have been a major source of information for this section.

PROFICIENCY EXERCISES

1. Make some gelatin using only half the required water. Let it set. Massage it into liquid form. Pay attention to the type of massage you use.
2. Get some plastic wrap and twist and wad it into a ball. Smooth it out. What methods did you need to use?
3. Take the same plastic wrap and pull it. Take out all the slack and telescope and elongate the tissue. What did you have to do to accomplish the stretch?

TRIGGER POINT THERAPY

SECTION OBJECTIVES

Using the information presented in this section, the student will be able to do the following:

1 Describe a trigger point.

2 Locate a trigger point.

3 Use two methods to massage a trigger point.

Dr. Janet Travell has done extensive research and is considered the foremost authority in myofascial pain involving trigger points.[7] Dr. Leon Chaitow has integrated much additional information about trigger point therapy.[2] These two experts are the resource for the information in this section about trigger point therapy.

There is some confusion about the synonymous use of the two terms neuromuscular therapy and trigger point therapy. *Neuromuscular therapy* is the umbrella encompassing a variety of treatment approaches, one of which is trigger point therapy. *Trigger point therapy* is one of many techniques found to be useful in the treatment of myofascial problems. As with most of the methods discussed in this chapter, additional training will be required by the therapist to be efficient and purposeful with the use of trigger point methods. In general wellness massage it is not uncommon to encounter a mild trigger point that is dealt with effectively by using the methods discussed here.

A *trigger point* is an area of local nerve facilitation of a muscle and is aggravated by stress of any sort affecting the body or the mind of the individual. Trigger points are small areas of hypertonicity within muscles. If these areas are located near motor nerve points, there may be referred pain caused by nerve stimulation. The area of the trigger point is often the motor point where nerve stimulation initiates a contraction in a small sensitive bundle of muscle fibers that, in turn, activates the entire muscle.[5] Any of the more than 400 muscles can develop trigger points. Accompanying the development of the trigger points will be the characteristic referred pain pattern and restriction of motion that is associated with myofascial pain.

All of the basic neuromuscular techniques, including the muscle energy techniques of postisometric relaxation, reciprocal inhibition, isokinetic contraction, strain/counterstrain, positional release, and isolytic contraction, will deal effectively with trigger points *if* the hypertonic area within a muscle is hyperstimulated and then lengthened and the connective tissue in the area softened and stretched. Neuromuscular methods and stretch are explained in Chapter 10. Direct pressure, dry needling (acupuncture), spray and stretch, or ice massage are suggested for trigger areas by Dr. Janet Travell and other professionals in the field. Direct manipulation of proprioceptors by pushing or pulling on a muscle belly or attachments is also very effective (Fig. 13.7).

With classic trigger points, the referred pain pattern can be traced to its site of origin. The distribution of the referred trigger point pain does not usually follow an entire distribution of a peripheral nerve or dermatomal segment.[7]

It is often difficult to decide if the tender spot is really a trigger point, a point of fascial adhesion requiring friction, or a motor point (acupressure point). The massage therapist will usually find trigger points during palpation or general massage using both light and deep palpation consisting of gliding strokes (Box. 13.4). Dr. Chaitow recommends that gliding strokes should cover a region of two to three inches at a time.

Both Dr. Travell and Dr. Chaitow agree that some pain is elicited during assessment and treatment, but they both recognize that the *pain elicited during treatment should be well within the client's comfort zone.* The muscle must be relaxed in order to be examined effectively. If the pressure is too great, severe local pain may overwhelm the referred pain sensation, making accurate evaluation impossible. Trigger points that are so active that referred pain is already being produced have no need for exaggerated pressure. Only those muscles that can actually be treated at the same visit

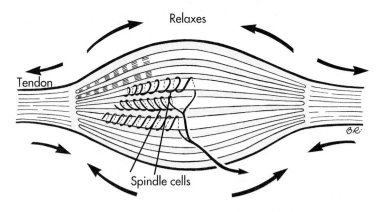

Figure 13.7
Direct manipulation of proprioceptors.

should be examined. Palpating for trigger points can irritate their referred pain activity, so only areas intended for treatment should be palpated. Trigger point therapy is not to be done for extended periods of time. Due to the nature of the syndrome and the irritation involved, fifteen minutes is a sufficient amount of time to spend on trigger points. There will be occasions when thirty minutes of therapy can be tolerated.

Treating Trigger Points Directly

Once a trigger point has been identified, the massage therapist will make use of a pressure technique or direct manipulation method and stretch to eliminate the point (Fig. 13.8). Direct manipulation is the least invasive and gentlest method. It is worth trying before the more intense pressure techniques.

Direct manipulation methods consist of pushing together at the belly of a muscle to affect spindle cells, and pushing on tendons to affect ten-

---

Box 13.4
PALPATING FOR TRIGGER POINTS

In performing **light palpation,** the therapist may notice these responses:

Skin changes: The skin may feel tense with resistance to gliding strokes. The skin may be slightly damp due to perspiration on the skin from sympathetic facilitation, and the hand will stick or drag on the skin.

Temperature changes: The temperature in a local area increases in acute dysfunction but decreases in ischemia, which is an indication of more fibrotic changes within the tissues.

Edema: Edema is an impression of fullness and congestion within the tissues. In instances of chronic dysfunction, edema is replaced gradually with fibrotic (connective tissue) changes.

Deep palpation: During this phase, the therapist is establishing contact with the deeper fibers of the soft tissues and exploring them for:
• Immobility
• Tenderness
• Edema
• Deep muscle tension
• Fibrotic changes
• Interosseous changes

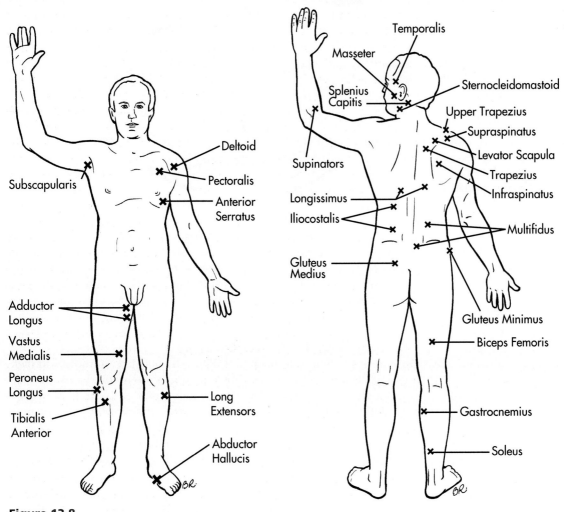

Figure 13.8
A & B, Common trigger points.

don receptors. If the belly of the muscle is pressed together and the desired effect is not given, then the next step should be to separate the tissue from the middle of the muscle belly toward the tendons. The local area must be lengthened. This lengthening is performed either directly on the tissues or through movement of a joint (see Fig. 13.7).

If the trigger point still remains after this is done, then pressure techniques should be tried. The pressure may take the form of *direct pressure,* in which the trigger point is pressed by the therapist against an underlying hard structure (bone), or *pinching pressure,* when no bony tissue lies underneath, as in the "squeezing" of the sternocleidomastoid muscle.

This process can end the hyperirritability by mechanical disruption of the sensory nerve endings mediating the trigger point activity. When using the direct pressure technique, the therapist must hold the compression long enough to stimulate the spindle cells.[7]

It is important that the pressure technique be done properly. Dr. Travell has pointed out that referred pain is usually sensed by the client within ten seconds of applied digital pressure. It is therefore inefficient to hold pressure for longer than ten seconds when trying to locate the trigger. Once the trigger has been located, the *time of applied pressure* will be different than the time used to locate the trigger. Dr. Chaitow recommends a procedure of gradually intensifying pressure, building up to eight seconds, then repeating the process for up to thirty seconds or as long as two minutes, ending when the client reports the referred pain has stopped and/or the therapist feels a "release" in the trigger point tissue.

Sufficient duration is determined by the fiber construction of the muscle. Muscles can be made up of red or white fibers, which can be of the slow or fast twitch variety. The type of fiber a muscle is comprised of is determined by whether the muscle functions as a postural endurance muscle or a phasic movement muscle and the demands exerted by the client's lifestyle. It is easier to fatigue a phasic muscle then an endurance muscle. Once the muscle is fatigued, there is a period of recovery when the fibers will not contract and the muscle can be stretched effectively.

Dr. Chaitow also recommends variable pressure rather than constantly held pressure from beginning to end to avoid further irritation to the trigger area. Students should not misunderstand this idea of variable pressure. It is not a "bouncing" in and out of the tissue but rather a carefully changing pressure for a specific purpose. The pressure used reflects the therapist's sensitivity to what is happening as the tissue responds; the therapist will apply more pressure as the tissue shows it is relaxing and will accept more pressure. When the massage therapist senses that the tissues are becoming tense, pressure is decreased. As an alternative, deep cross-fiber friction over the trigger can be effective, followed by lengthening and stretching. This method is beneficial if the massage therapist suspects that the connective tissue around the trigger point has become immobile.

Dr. Travell recommends that after treating with pressure methods, the practitioner should again stimulate circulation to the local area with circular friction, petrissage, and/or vibratory massage techniques. Localized treatment of the muscle should always end with lengthening and stretching, whether passive or active, of the affected muscle. Both Dr. Travell and Dr. Chaitow agree that gradual gentle lengthening to reset the normal resting length of the neuromuscular mechanism of a muscle and stretching to elongate shortened connective tissue of the treated (involved) muscle must follow therapy for the results to be complete and to be maintained. Incomplete restoration of the full length of the muscle means incomplete relief of pain. Failure to stretch will result in the eventual return of original symptoms. Muscle energy approaches are more effective than passive stretching in achieving the proper response (see Chapter 10). This enables the muscle to "learn" that it can now return to a fuller resting length and more complete range of motion.

Following treatment of a trigger point, the target (referred) area should be searched to uncover and deal with satellite or embryonic triggers. Immediately following treatment, moist heat (hot towel) over the region is soothing and useful. The area will require rest for a few days, avoiding all stressful activity.[3]

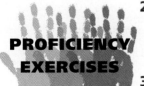
PROFICIENCY EXERCISES

1. **Place a dry pea under a half-inch piece of foam. Locate the pea with light and deep palpation.**
2. **Tie a slip knot in a large rubber band. Apply direct pressure or pinch pressure to the knot. Does the trigger point "go away?" Now pull the ends of the rubber band to stretch the trigger point. What happens to the knot now?**
3. **Use light palpation to locate an area of suspected trigger point activity. Once an area is found, use deep palpation to find the exact area of the trigger point. Then use the methods described in this section to normalize the area.**

ACUPRESSURE

SECTION OBJECTIVES

Using the information presented in this section, the student will be able to do the following:

❶ Explain the basic physiology of acupressure points and the effects of acupressure.

❷ Locate an acupressure point.

❸ Use simple methods to stimulate acupressure points.

Acupuncture, one branch of Chinese medicine, has been proven to be effective for the treatment of many diseases and dysfunctions. The exact origin of acupuncture is unknown. Although it remains a mystery in some respects, science is close to proving the phenomenon. Whatever the physiologic factors that underlie acupuncture, the beneficial changes that occur clearly are a sound basis for acupressure treatment. *Acupuncture* can be defined as the stimulation of certain points with needles inserted along the meridians (channels) and "AhShi" (trigger) points outside the meridians. The purpose of acupuncture is to prevent and modify the perception of pain (analgesia) or normalized physiologic functions.

Acupressure is a modified version of acupuncture that substitutes pressure for needle insertion. The effects of acupressure are not as dramatic as those of acupuncture but are still effective, especially if repeated often with the pressure held long enough. There are 1000 acupuncture points in the human body, most of which are located on twelve paired and two unpaired meridians. According to Chinese theory, the meridians are internally associated with organs and externally associated with the surface of the head, trunk, and extremities. Meridians seem to be energy flows from nerve tracks in the tissue and are located in the fascial grooves.[8]

The Yin and Yang of It

The oriental perspective considers body functions in terms of balance between opposing forces. These opposites are actually a portion of a continuum. A circle is a good example: no matter where you stand on a circle you can look across and see the other side. In this idea of duality, we often forget that a circle is one concept; it is broken into sections only through the limitation of our perceptions.

Yin and yang are representations of the above concept. Yin and yang functions are complimentary pieces of the whole (Fig. 13.9). When functioning equally and in harmony, the natural balance of health exists in all areas of the body, mind, and spirit. Conversely, if part of the continuum becomes out of sync with the rest, stress is put on the entire circle.

The body is physiologically a closed system. There cannot be a "too much" without a "not enough" someplace. Just as muscles work in pairs and facilitate and inhibit each other, so do meridians. The pairing of meridians is called *yin/yang.*

Yin meridians are associated with the parasympathetic autonomic nervous system responses and functions of the solid organs essential to life (e.g., the heart). The energy is considered "female" or of a negative charge. (Terminology and metaphor tend to become confused with the terms "female" and "negative." All they mean is that the functions draw energy in and restore or reproduce.) Yin meridians are located on the inside soft areas of the body and flow from the feet up (arms are lifted into the air).

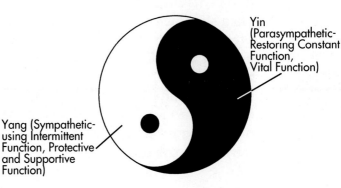

Figure 13.9
Yin/parasympathetic and Yang/sympathetic.

Yin
(Parasympathetic-Restoring Constant Function, Vital Function)

Yang (Sympathetic-using Intermittent Function, Protective and Supportive Function)

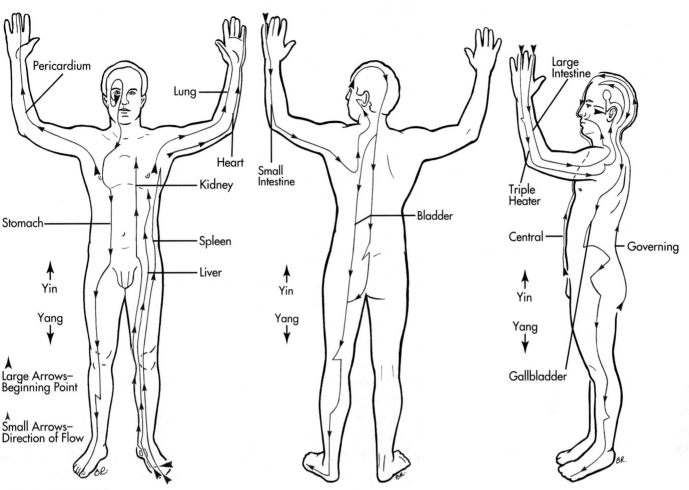

Figure 13.10
**A–C, Typical location of meridi-
ans. Meridians tend to follow
nerves. (see, Fig. 6.3 pg 133.)**

Yang meridians (Fig. 13.10) are associated with the sympathetic autonomic nervous system responses and hollow organs whose functions are
supportive to life, but not essential (e.g., the stomach). The energy is considered "male" and a "positive" charge. (Again, in terms of metaphor
these terms mean that the energy is expended in short bursts as necessary
and moves out from the body). Oriental philosophy teaches that there
must be a balance between the forces of yin and yang in order for health
to exist. This balance changes according to the weather, the seasons and
other rhythms of nature.

Acupressure points usually lie in a fascial division between muscles and
near origins and insertions. The point will feel like a small hole and pressure will elicit a nervy feeling. Unlike a trigger point, which may only be
found on one side of the body, acupressure points are bilateral (i.e., located
on both sides of the body). To confirm the location of an acupressure
point, locate the point in the same place on the other side of the body.

To stimulate a hypoactive or "not enough" acupressure point, use a
short vibrating or tapping action. This method would be used if the area is
sluggish or a specific body function needs stimulation. To sedate a hyperactive or "too much" point for pain reduction, elicit the pain response
within the point itself and use a sustained holding pressure until the
painful over-energy dissipates and the body's own pain killers are released
into the blood stream. The pressure techniques are similar to those used
for trigger points, but it is not necessary to lengthen and stretch an acupressure point after treatment. It is often difficult to determine whether
you are dealing with a trigger point or an acupressure point because the
two often overlap. It might be wise to lengthen and stretch the area gently

after the use of direct pressure methods. The process will not interfere with the effect on the acupressure point and without it a trigger point is not treated effectively.

Acupressure and systems such as shiatsu that use the same concepts are complicated methods of healing that take years to perfect. A wise therapist is careful not to overextend his or her abilities when using these techniques, and to commit to further training in the use of these very valuable therapeutic methods.

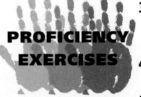

PROFICIENCY EXERCISES

1. Place a piece of grooved paneling or similar board under a piece of half-inch foam. Palpate through the foam for the grooves using both light and deep pressure.
2. Do a massage that incorporates running the hand down each of the meridian grooves in the body. Stop at each hole or point you feel. Compare these points to the location of acupuncture points and motor points.
3. When doing the above massage and locating a point, decide whether the point needs to be stimulated with vibration or tapping, or sedated with sustained direct pressure. How did you decide?
4. Design three original massage sessions that incorporate a principle from each topic covered in this chapter.
5. Exchange massage with three students using one of the massage sessions developed above.
6. While giving ten general massages, make mental notes each time you use one of the methods in this chapter.
7. Using professional journals and massage school catalogs, find a continuing education opportunity for each method discussed in this chapter.

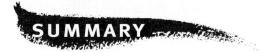

The addition of these methods to the massage professional's skills can provide a more specific focus during the massage. A client could enjoy a relaxing foot bath and sip a cup of hot tea while waiting for the appointment. The client and the massage therapist may drink a glass of pure water together. A cold compress could be placed on the back of the neck, forehead, or other area of the body during the massage. Effleurage could be focused to move lymph and blood in the veins while compression could move down the arteries to stimulate arterial blood flow. Effleurage specifically applied into the grooves of the body may stimulate the meridians. Compression, vibration, or tapping of the acupressure points would normalize body function. Petrissage, stretching, and friction methods, applied slowly and deliberately to drag, pull, and elongate, might soften and normalize the connective tissue. The occasional trigger point might be treated with direct pressure or friction, and with a hot compress applied afterward. An ice pack may sometimes be a better choice after friction to control the amount of inflammation. Every joint in the hands and feet could be moved and attention given to compression on the bottoms of the hands and feet to stimulate lymphatic flow. The client might be instructed in deep breathing to further encourage lymph movement. The body's internal chemicals may be released, thus normalizing body function. It is the intention of the massage interaction for the client to experience a pleasant, relaxed, and alert state in response to the physiologic shifts in the body.

REVIEW QUESTIONS

1. Why is continuing education required to use the methods presented in this chapter effectively?
2. What are the primary effects of hydrotherapy?
3. What are some simple hydrotherapy methods that the massage practitioner can use that do not require special hydrotherapy equipment?
4. What are some important contraindications and precautions for the use of ice?
5. What is systemic massage and what results can be expected from this type of massage?
6. What are the basic procedures for lymphatic massage?
7. What are the basic procedures for circulation massage?
8. What are the physiologic mechanisms that make reflexology a valuable massage approach?
9. What are the recommended methods for foot massage?
10. Why is hand and foot self-massage beneficial?
11. What are connective tissue approaches?
12. What is the intent of connective tissue massage?
13. Why is additional education so important before using connective tissue approaches?
14. What is a trigger point?
15. How are trigger points located?
16. What methods are used to normalize trigger points?
17. After treating a trigger point what types of therapy follow?
18. What is the western terminology for acupressure points, meridians, and yin and yang?
19. What wisdom do the eastern approaches offer for the massage practitioner?
20. Where are acupressure points located?
21. How are acupressure points treated?
22. How can the principles of the therapeutic methods presented in this chapter be integrated into a massage?

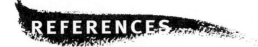

REFERENCES

1. Buchman DD: *The complete book of water therapy: 500 ways to use our oldest natural medicine,* New York, 1979, E.P. Dutton.
2. Chaitow L: *Soft-tissue manipulation,* Vermont, 1988, Healing Arts Press.
3. —Workshop Notes 1988, 1991, 1992, 1993.
4. Cyriax J and Coldham M: *The textbook of orthopaedic medicine treatment by manipulation massage and injection,* vol 2, ed 11, East Sussex, England, 1984, Bailliere Tindall.
5. Gunn C: *Reprints on pain, acupuncture and related subjects,* Seattle, 1992, University of Washington.
6. Kreighbaum E and Barthels KM: *Biomechanics: A qualitative approach for studying human movement,* ed 2, New York, 1985, Macmillan Inc.
7. Travell JG and Simons DG: *Myofascial pain and dysfunction: The trigger point manual.* Baltimore, 1984, Williams and Wilkins.
8. Yao JH: *Acutherapy.* Acutherapy Postgraduate Seminars, 808 Paddock Lane Libertyville, Il 60048:1984.

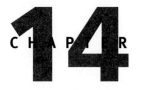

14

W E L L N E S S
EDUCATION

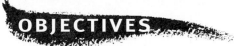

OBJECTIVES

After completing this chapter, the student will be able to do the following:

1 Identify the basic components of a wellness program.

2 Locate resources to develop a wellness program.

3 Develop a personal wellness program.

4 Provide general wellness guidelines to clients.

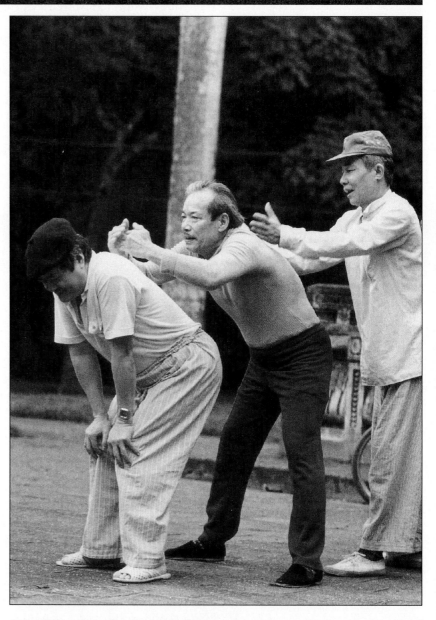

A traditional method of Vietnamese massage applied to the backs of three participants. (Bettmann Archive)

INTRODUCTION

The purpose of this final chapter is to educate the massage professional about the general concepts of wellness. Massage is an important part of any wellness program because it restores body balance and connects us with other human beings. It is necessary for the massage professional to understand all of the other components of "wellness" as well. With this information the professional can explain to his or her clients how massage fits into the whole wellness picture. It is not possible to define a step-by-step process that provides for wellness and spirituality. Each person is an individual and needs to develop a personal plan according to the general concepts of wellness.

We are considered *well* when body, mind, and spirit are in ideal balance. In the words of renowned nutrition scientist, Professor Jeffrey Bland, many people are "vertically ill," that is, not sick enough to lie down, but certainly not well.[1] It does not seem to be just the type of stress involved, but rather the amount of stress that accumulates until the breakdown begins. It will only be a matter of time before physical health, the mind, or life in general will simply fall apart under the accumulation of multiple stressors.

Each individual will need to develop a personal wellness plan. Just as in designing a massage, there is no right or wrong way. Following a few basic guidelines, whatever works is what is best for each person. Massage therapists need to remember that as wonderful as massage is, it addresses only a part of the person. Wellness is about the whole person. The sensitive massage therapist will realize that during a client's search for wellness, the times with the massage therapist, the focused attention, the acceptance, and the "only listening" are as important as the massage methods used.

This chapter examines the basic guidelines necessary for building a wellness program. It provides enough information to give some direction in the development and implementation of a wellness plan. As with massage, often the simpler the program the better it is. We are supposed to be well. Our bodies will recognize the correct process. There may be resistance initially to change, which can come either from our own bodies or coping patterns, or from family and friends. Remember, if our behavior changes, the people around us will have to change as well. Wellness has a domino effect. Making a simple alteration in lifestyle will have a chain reaction through your entire life. Consequently, it is only necessary to commit to a few carefully thought out lifestyle alterations and to be open to letting the rest of the pieces readjust themselves. Resistance comes when the pieces have to adjust. Go slowly and allow the "pieces" (your own body, family, or friends) to complain, but do not give in and quit. Persist with the wellness program and give your body, and your family and friends time to get used to your new lifestyle. Making a change to wellness takes determination. Letting go of behavioral patterns is difficult. It is very hard to do this alone, so relationships with those who are supportive and believe in us, (e.g., support groups or professional therapy) are helpful. The massage professional can be an important support person for the client making wellness changes in his or her life.

STRESS

Stress is our response to any demand on the body or mind to respond, adapt, or alter. It is a state of readiness to survive, requiring hypervigilance from the body and the mind. It is our emotional reaction to stress that may be the difference between positive action and destructive breakdown, especially if many of the stresses seem beyond our control.[1]

An expert on stress, Hans Selye, said, "The ancient Greek philosophers clearly recognized that, with regard to human conduct, the most important, but perhaps also the most difficult thing was 'to know thyself.' It takes great courage even just to attempt this honestly . . . Yet it is well worth the effort and humiliation, because most of our tensions and frustrations stem from compulsive needs to act the role of someone we are not."[4]

Before any wellness program can be developed, a person needs to at least "explore thyself." The next step is to analyze and explore the stresses that we all encounter in our daily lives. The three major elements of stress are the stressor itself, the defensive measures, and the mechanisms for surrender. *Stressors* are any internal perception or external stimuli that demand a change in the body. The *defensive measures* are how our bodies defend against the stressor, e.g., the production of antibodies and white blood cells, or behavioral emotional defenses. There are times when defending is not the best way to deal with stress. It is important and resourceful to know when to quit. Hormonal and nervous stimuli will encourage the body to retreat and ignore stressors. On an emotional level this is sometimes called *denial,* which can be an important method of coping with stress.[4]

It has long been known that mental excitement and physical stressors cause an initial exhilaration, followed by a secondary phase of depression. A law of physics states that for every action there is an opposite and equal reaction. Certain identifiable chemical compounds such as the hormones produced during the acute alarm reaction phase of the general adaptation syndrome (discussed in Chapter 6) possess the property of first keying up for action and then causing a depression. Both effects may be of great protective value to the body. It is necessary to be keyed up for peak accomplishments, but it is equally important to tune down by the secondary phase of depression. This prevents us from carrying on too long at top speed. According to Selye,

> The fact is that a person can be intoxicated with his own stress hormones. I venture to say that this sort of drunkenness has caused much more harm to society than the alcoholic kind. We are on our guard against external toxicants, but hormones are parts of our bodies; it takes more wisdom to recognize and overcome the foe which fights from within. In all our actions throughout the day, we must consciously look for signs of being keyed up too much, and we must learn to stop in time. To watch our critical stress level is just as important as to watch our critical quota of cocktails. More so. Intoxication by stress is sometimes unavoidable and usually insidious. You can quit alcohol and, even if you do take some, at least you can count the glasses; but it is impossible to avoid stress as long as you live, and your conscious thoughts often cannot gauge its alarm signals accurately. Curiously the pituitary is a much better judge of stress than the intellect. Yet, you can learn to recognize the danger signals fairly well if you know what to look for[4] (Box 14.1).

Depending on our conditioning and genetic makeup, we all respond differently to general stress. As a whole, people tend to respond consistently, with one set of signs, in individualized patterns caused by the mal-

Box 14.1
COMMON STRESS RESPONSES

- General irritability, hyperexcitation, or depression
- Pounding of the heart
- Dryness of the throat and mouth
- Impulsive behavior, emotional instability
- Overpowering urge to cry, run, or hide
- Inability to concentrate
- Weakness or dizziness
- Fatigue
- Tension and keyed-up alertness
- Trembling and nervous tics
- Intermittent anxiety
- Tendency to be easily startled
- High-pitched nervous laughter
- Stuttering and other speech difficulties
- Grinding teeth
- Insomnia
- Inability to sit still or physically relax
- Sweating
- Frequent need to urinate
- Diarrhea, indigestion, queasiness, and vomiting
- Migraine and other tension headaches
- Premenstrual tension or missed menstrual cycles
- Pain in the neck or lower back
- Loss of or excessive appetite
- Increased use of chemicals including tobacco, caffeine, alcohol
- Nightmares
- Neurotic behavior
- Psychosis
- Accident prone

The massage professional will recognize that these signs of stress result from fluctuations in the autonomic nervous system and resulting endogenous chemical shifts.

functions of whatever happens to be the most vulnerable part in their physiology. When warning signs appear, it is time to stop, change the activity, and divert the body's attention to something else.[4]

If there is proportionately too much stress on any physical or emotional area of the body, the energy needs to be diverted to a different area. If a person is thinking too much, then he or she should use the larger muscles of the body, (e.g., gardening, taking a brisk walk). If too much exercise is causing stress, balance can be restored by reading a novel, watching a movie, or listening to soft music. If there is too much stress on the body as a whole, rest is required. If we do not rest of our own accord, the body may become ill just so we will lie down for awhile.

WELLNESS COMPONENTS: BODY, MIND, AND SPIRIT

When developing a wellness program, our mental and physical histories are considered. Our sense of self, in relation to others, is also important. If this connection with others is not respected and nurtured, there is a strain on the wholeness of our life. This strain may interfere with our spiritual, emotional, and physical health. People are not designed to be alone, therefore we must be able to communicate effectively with each other. If we do not communicate effectively with others and with ourselves, our energy is confused and our responses inaccurate. Communication is one of the biggest problems for humans because it is so subjective. It is very difficult to be truly objective, and to know this is to know an important part of wellness. Wellness requires responsibiity for our communication.

Wellness training requires an extensive amount of information about diet, exercise, lifestyle, and behavior patterns. It is important to seek out those with experience to provide that information. Do not depend on only one information source. Talk with two, three, or four "experts" and read three or four books on each topic before making decisions about what could be done to benefit or improve upon your wellness. Remember, only a few symptoms combine to create a huge array of illness and disease patterns. Fortunately, a combination of only a few lifestyle changes is required in order to redirect a disease pattern toward a more resourceful and healing pattern.

Today, many of the demands placed on us are outside the design of the body. One such demand is excessive sitting. Our bodies are designed for movement, which is meant to be purposeful and set toward a goal such as gathering food for the day or running for safety. Our bodies still function as if this were the reality, but we do not need to work as hard to gather our food in the grocery store. Exercise and stretching programs are important parts of any wellness program because they replace the activity our body was designed to have. Now we run in place and ride stationary bikes. Exercise has become an essential purpose unto itself. Fitness programs need to be appropriate; it is important to modify exercise systems and stretching programs to fit the individual. There are many resources available to study exercise and stretching programs.

Many of us have been sick, or at the very least "vertically ill." It may take extraordinary effort to turn these situations around. At that point we realize that maybe we should have taken better care of ourselves in the first place. Taking care of ourselves is what wellness and personal service wellness massage is all about. Sometimes an event in life removes some part of us. It could be a body part, a body function, a relationship, a member of our family, or a job. In order to heal, we need to reconstruct that part or learn to live resourcefully without it. Many professionals can help us with specific therapeutic interventions as the wellness program is developed. Doctors, counselors, other health care providers, educators, and religious advisors all have an important part to play in helping us become well again. Ultimately, each of us must do all the work and take responsibility for who, what, and where we are, but it is important to use what help is available. For example, if a person has a large tumor growth, and a surgeon can safely remove it, then the doctor's help will give the body a head start on healing.

There is a balance between intuition and research. In developing a wellness program, it is important to consider these two very important sources of information. If Hippocrates' advice of "do no harm" is followed during the development of a wellness program, and there is balance between what science knows and what we know we need, then the wellness program will be sound. A wellness program needs to change as we change. When a good wellness program is carried out, a person looks forward to getting back to living life to the fullest, and at the appropriate time, dying with dignity.

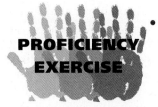

PROFICIENCY EXERCISE

• **Begin to build a library about wellness. Take an inventory of books and magazines you already have. Categorize them and commit to adding one new book at least every three months. Explore your public library and become familiar with what wellness resources it has to offer.**

BODY

Nutrition

Proper nutrition is easy to explain, but people do not always follow recommendations. This is because nutrition involves more than just eating. Eating affects the mood; mood influences feelings; and behavior supports feelings. The whole issue of food therefore becomes an emotional topic.

The basics of balanced nutrition are explained in the Department of Agriculture's new guide to good eating. The original four food group recommendations have been changed to a triangular shape, which suggests a diet high in vegetables, grains, legumes, and fruit. The protein requirement from animal sources has been decreased. Dairy needs are moderate to small. When purchasing any animal products, you might want to locate naturally raised and hormone-free products. Although fat and sugar requirements in the diet are minimal, humans have a strong urge for sweets and fats. It is this instinctive craving for fat and sugar that contributes to most dietary problems. In primitive times these two substances were difficult to find. There had to be a deep instinctual desire to fight the bees for their honey, and the animals for their fat or to gather fatty seeds. Today, these substances are in abundance, but our primitive nature still acts as if we need to store up for a future famine. An ideal diet is low in fats and sugars and moderately low in protein and dairy, with the bulk of the calories coming from complex carbohydrates.

Many people take nutritional supplements, and there are varied opinions on this topic. The only recommendation offered is that the closer a supplement is to a "real food," the better the body will be able to use it. Herbs, which are very powerful substances, should not be used without knowledge of their effects.

Cycles of high and low blood sugar are produced by unbalanced diets, aggravated by improper spacing between meals, and supported by substances such as coffee, tea, alcohol, and cola drinks. These fluids stimulate adrenalin production, which forces sugar to be released into the blood. The body then pushes sugar levels down again with insulin.

Drinking enough pure water is very important to a wellness program. Since our bodies are over 70% water, most diets recommend at least sixty-four ounces of water per day for efficient body function.

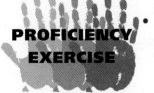

PROFICIENCY EXERCISE

• **Keep a food diary for two days. If your diet is not well balanced, decide what it would take to develop a plan that cuts fat and sugar intake and increases water intake to recommended levels.**

Breathing

Breathing provides us with air—a very essential nutrient. Breathing patterns are a direct link to altering autonomic nervous system patterns, which in turn alter mood, feelings, and behavior. Almost every meditation or relaxation system uses breathing patterns. Other ways to modulate breathing are through singing and chanting. Proper breathing is important, but most of us do not breathe efficiently. For many, the air quality is not very good. The rest of us may be in too big of a hurry to breathe deeply.

Slow, deep breathing takes time. The simple bellows breathing mechanism is a body-wide coordination of muscle contraction and relaxation. A good way to recognize the full body effect of breathing is to do the following activity. Tighten up your feet by gripping the floor with your toes. Take a deep breath and feel what happens. Relax your feet and again notice what happens. Tighten the gluteals and take a deep breath. Then relax the muscles and take another deep breath, again noting what happens. These exercises should demonstrate that breathing involves more muscles than the diaphragm and intercostals.

The shoulders do not move during normal relaxed breathing. The accessory muscles of respiration located in the neck area should only be activated when increased oxygen is required for the fight or flight response. This is the pattern for sympathetic breathing. If the person does not balance the oxygen/carbon dioxide levels through increased activity levels, hyperventilation may occur. Patterns of hyperventilation can perpetuate anxiety states.

If the accessory muscles of respiration, such as the scalenes, sternocleidomastoid, serratus posterior superior, levator scapulae, rhomboids, abdominals, and quadratus lumborum are constantly being activated for breathing when forced inhalation and expiration are not called for, dysfunctional muscle patterns will result. Often, tightness in the quadratus lumborum or shoulder pain is not connected with an inefficient breathing pattern during assessment by the massage professional.

There are three phases of inspiration and two phases of expiration. Quiet inspiration takes place when an individual is resting or sitting quietly. The diaphragm and external intercostals are the prime movers. As deep inspiration occurs, the actions of quiet inspiration are increased. When a person needs more oxygen, she or he breathes harder. Any muscles that can pull the ribs up are called into action. Forced inspiration occurs when an individual is working very hard and needs a great deal of oxygen. Not only are the muscles of quiet and deep inspiration working, but so are muscles that stabilize and/or elevate the shoulder girdle to directly or indirectly elevate the ribs.

Expiration is divided into two phases. Quiet expiration is mostly a passive action. It occurs through relaxation of the external intercostals and the elastic recoil of the thoracic wall and tissue of the lungs and bronchi, with gravity pulling the rib cage down from its elevated position. Essentially no muscle action is occurring. Forced expiration brings in muscles that can pull down the ribs and muscles that can compress the abdomen, forcing the diaphragm upward. Some people may wonder why tightening the feet interferes with breathing. It seems to be a chain reaction between prime mover and antagonist muscle patterns. In order for the abdominals to contract to compress the abdominal cavity, their antagonist patterns have to relax all the way up and down the body[2] (Box 14.2).

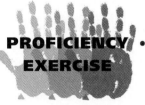

PROFICIENCY EXERCISE
• Develop a "How to breathe" handout to give to clients. Include at least three different breathing patterns.

Exercise and Stretching

The human body is made to wander and gather; it can run when necessary, but was not made to sit all day like many of us do. Exercise replaces the movements lost by inactivity. General recommendations include thirty minutes daily of moderate aerobic activity, which increases the heart and breathing rates. A variety of activities can keep the exercise program from becoming boring. Running, dancing, mowing the yard, and giving massage are examples of aerobic activity. The required activity level varies for each person. Some of us will need vigorous activity like racquetball, while others will fare better with swimming, walking, or gardening.

Muscles and bones need to work against a load or weight to remain healthy, so resistance or weight training of some sort is also needed. Fifteen minutes of resistance weight training three or four times a week is adequate for most people. Carrying groceries is an example of weight lift-

Box 14.2
BREATHING RETRAINING PATTERN

The following breathing retraining sequence should be taught to those who lift their shoulders during quiet and deep inspiration.
Exhale in the following manner first:

1. Tighten toes, buttocks, and abdominals to prepare to compress the abdomen.
2. Lift the chin into the air and relax the shoulders.
3. Slowly exhale through the mouth while tightening the muscles listed above even tighter. Exhale until as much air as possible is expelled without straining.
4. At the bottom of the breath, which is when no further air can be exhaled without strain, stop breathing. (This is different from holding the breath, which requires effort.) It is a resting phase of three to five seconds.
5. Before you begin to inhale, relax all muscles, drop the chin to the chest, and keep the shoulders relaxed.
6. Inhale slowly through the nose until the lungs are comfortably full. This is the top of the breath.
7. Stop breathing for three to five seconds. Repeat the sequence beginning with step one.

The exhalation should take two to four times as long as the inhalation.

There are many additional resources on breathing patterns and the recommendation is to find one that is comfortable and use it regularly.

ing that can be worked into daily activity. The easiest programs build exercise into daily motions in addition to the formal workout.

Slow stretching can replace the bending and reaching that our bodies are designed for. Static positions are very hard on the body because muscles and connective tissue shorten to mold the body to this static position, (e.g., talking on the phone and holding the receiver to the ear with the shoulder). Many types of stretching programs exist. It is important that the stretching be slow, gentle, and sustained. Frequent five-minute stretches and breathing breaks should be built into everyone's day, especially for those who maintain static positions. If this is done, productivity may increase and there may be less fatigue at the end of a busy day.

Any exercise and stretching program must begin slowly. Activity levels can be increased gradually each week. It takes about six weeks for those who are new to movement to reach a level of comfort with the new moves; additional activities may be added more slowly at this point.

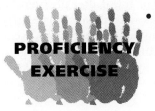

PROFICIENCY EXERCISE

• **Locate an exercise and stretching program taught by a qualified instructor at your local community center, community education, or health club, or purchase an exercise and stretching video. Participate in the program for six weeks, monitoring all movements for correctness and comfort.**

Relaxation

Relaxation methods initiate a parasympathetic response. Muscle tension patterns are habitual. The most successful relaxation methods combine movement, stretching, tensing, and then releasing muscles (progressive relaxation). The heart rate and breathing rate are synchronized while focusing on a quiet or neutral topic, event, or picture. This is called *visualization*. Music can be a beneficial component to add to a relaxation program.

Most meditation and deliberate relaxation processes are built around this pattern. The focus of relaxation is to quiet the physical body, not to create a spiritual experience. Many prayer systems use similar patterns, which are beneficial for relaxation as well. Almost any type of pleasurable, simple, repetitive activity that requires focused attention will induce the relaxation response. Gardening, needlepoint, playing music, watching fish in an aquarium or birds at a bird feeder are all forms of relaxation if there is no need to achieve, compete, or produce results in a specific period. Knitting a sweater for pleasure and having to finish one in a week are two different activities. Relaxation takes time, and when something is urgent, it usually interferes with the ability to relax.

Just as tension patterns are habitual, relaxation can become a habit. Typically, it takes eight to ten weeks of consistent reinforcement to build a habit pattern. Unlike exercise, which can be varied to prevent boredom, a relaxation sequence needs to be the same each time. It is important to use the same location, music, time of day, smells, colors, position, and breathing pattern in the sequence. Any of the components of the relaxation program can soon become triggers to relaxation, creating a continued response. A person should experiment with relaxation methods until the right program is found, then consistently use it every day for at least fifteen minutes. (It takes this long for the physiology to make a shift from an aroused state to a relaxed one.) There are many audiocassette programs available that provide progressive relaxation and self-hypnosis. These cassettes pull together all of the components of a relaxation program. This type of resource can be very useful.

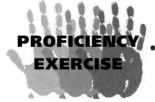

PROFICIENCY EXERCISE

- **Design and carry out a daily fifteen minute relaxation program especially for you.**

Feelings

Feelings are the body's interpretation of emotions. They occur as a response to the effect of hormones, neurotransmitters, and other endogenous chemicals. People use chemical substances like food, nicotine, alcohol, and drugs to create feelings. Behaviors such as creating crisis, eating disorders, accident proneness, hypervigilance, panic, illness, depression, and codependent relationships can be used to change mood and feelings.

Often, if a person's physiology can be changed, his or her feelings can also be changed. The easiest way to change the physiology is to move, as in exercising or breathing. A massage will also change the physiology. This is perhaps why massage feels so good. A wellness plan will alter physiology. Whichever method is chosen, the opposing response will need to be activated in order to restore a balance. For example, if a person is overwrought with thinking, moving around and pulling some weeds in the garden will create a nice balance. If feeling angry, find a way to laugh. If feeling depressed, help someone. If feeling anxious and alone, get a hug or a massage.

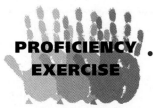

PROFICIENCY EXERCISE

- **Honestly identify two personal behaviors that have a repetitive pattern, one resourceful and one unresourceful.**

MIND

Emotions

Emotions are feelings driven by thoughts and actions that represent the consequences of how we think and what we do. What we think and feel and how we live are all inextricably linked.

The immune system is controlled directly by the mind. The science of psycho-neuro-immunology has clearly established that unresolved emotions and thought patterns of hate, fear, anger, and jealousy reduce the efficiency of the body's defenses.[1]

In 1975, Dr. Robert Adder conditioned rats to dislike sweetened water by injecting them with a chemical to make them feel ill whenever they drank it. After the injections had been stopped for some time, some rats began dying. On investigation, Adder found that the chemical he had used was a suppressor of immune function. The rats had not only become conditioned to feeling ill whenever they drank sweet water, they were also mimicking its other effects and depressing their immune systems. This ability to depress the immune function was proof positive of the nervous system control over the immune system. Many subsequent tests have confirmed this finding in humans. [1]

As humans, we *learn* to be helpless, addictive, and have low self-esteem. We learn to hate. The important point to remember is that if we learned the maladaptive behavior in the first place, we can also learn a more resourceful behavior to use instead.

Emotions can be very powerful. If used resourcefully, they can provide us with the empowerment to reach our goals. Many good things have come from an emotion turned into resourceful behavior. Wellness encompasses a full range of emotion. Some of us pride ourselves on not feeling certain emotions, but if we can experience an emotion in a resourceful way, it is not healthy to deny its expression. For example, if something as powerful as anger is turned inward, it does not lead to positive outcomes. But if expressed resourcefully, to the person or situations involved, then a sense of resolution takes place and we can get on with our lives, free of the anger. The wellness comes from our whole self using the emotion instead of the emotion using us. Used resourcefully, emotions can provide the motivation to achieve wellness; used nonresourcefully, they can make us ill and be destructive to those who share our lives. An adolescent daughter came to her mother one day while the mother was creating a crisis for no apparent reason. The daughter told her mother to "chill out" and left. Sometimes we need someone who loves us in spite of ourselves to put our emotions and resulting behavior into perspective.

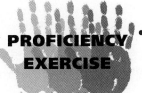

PROFICIENCY EXERCISE

- **List any emotions that gave you the drive to complete this massage therapy program.**

Behavior

Behavior is what we do in response to feelings, to trigger feelings, and occasionally to avoid feelings. Resourceful behavior results in a good feeling and feeling good about what has happened. Unresourceful behavior still results in a good feeling (or we would not do it), but often we feel bad about what happened, and/or others feel bad. Addictive behavior can take many forms. A person who is addicted to food, drugs, alcohol, exercise, pain, crisis, or loss will develop a lifestyle that will both protect and support the substance or behavior of choice. Addictions require a great deal of time and energy. Addictive behavior throws the balance of wellness off course. It takes hard work and lots of support to change an addictive behavior. Sometimes a less damaging addiction is replaced by a more damaging one, and vice versa.[1] A person may alter a food habit by creating an exercise dependency. Whichever is the more damaging addiction needs to be evaluated. These behavior changes are at least steps in the resourceful direction and should not be discouraged. To truly alter behavior the sense of self will need to be evaluated.

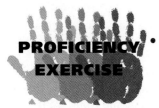

PROFICIENCY EXERCISE

• **List three addictive behaviors. For each, list three alternative behaviors that are less damaging, yet may generate similar feelings.**

Self-Concept

What we think about ourselves and how we talk to ourselves are very important contributors to wellness. Some people do not have a positive self-concept. Most of us want a purpose and a feeling of achievement, success, and self-confidence. This is achievable when we stop comparing ourselves with each other. Instead, wellness involves reaching out to others for support and information. Instead of basing our value on an external standard, people who are well will develop internal standards of self-worth. We need to own both our successes and our mistakes and attempt to correct the mistakes. It is healthy to "clean up our own messes." Putting relationships and mistakes back in order can resolve an issue and allow energy to be used in more beneficial ways. It is also healthy to clean up a mess that someone else may have left in our life. Often the person or situation that made the mess does not, or will not, assume responsibility for it. If we wait for it to be cleaned up, we may have to live with the mess for a long time. Part of wellness is eliminating messes and clutter that we no longer need, no matter who is responsible. As adults, it is also our responsibility to disallow preventable messes. Sometimes we have to be very strong with other people about what we will and will not allow in our space. There are some messes that no one is responsible for, such as natural disasters. It does no good to expect Mother Nature to come clean up the mess.

Everyone is good at something; no one is good at everything. Measure success and self-worth by how good you feel about your accomplishments, instead of by money or fame. Especially with massage, an inner sense of accomplishment is important. Massage is a quiet, unpretentious profession. It does not usually have a lot of public glory. Massage is an important and needed service and its benefits often cannot be objectively measured. As with any type of prevention activity, it is difficult to know what did not happen because someone took preventive measures.

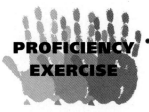

PROFICIENCY EXERCISE

• **Clean up two "messes," one you made in someone else's life and one someone made in your life. Notice how your self-concept blossoms.**

SPIRIT

Coping

Wellness is the ability to live each day and be able to say "a job well done" as we enter sleep with a thankful heart. How we lived that day is the coping part, and sometimes the simplest things can make a difference. One day, when things were going particularly bad in an office, a five-year-old boy walked through. He stopped and said, "Good morning everybody. Have you noticed that the sun is shining today?" It was a better day after that.

Resourceful coping consists of commitment, control, and challenge. Commitment is the ability and willingness to be involved in what is happening around us. Control is characterized by the belief that we can influence events by the way we feel, think, and act. This is internal control, not external control. Internal control involves adjusting ourselves to the situation and looking for ways to respond resourcefully. Those who exert external control attempt to control circumstances and people. It is impossible to control the weather, most circumstances, and most people. Relying on external control is a poor coping mechanism. Those who see change as a challenge cope much better. When there is an expectation of change in life, and resourceful coping mechanisms are available, then most changes can be welcomed as leading to personal development.

Poor stress-coping skills and unresourceful emotions are immune-suppressing and predispose us to infection and poor health. It is the individual's response to the stress that determines the effect of immunity, and not the stress itself.[1] Wellness includes learning more efficient ways to cope with life (through counseling and behavior modification programs if needed). To improve coping skills, pay attention to people who cope well and ask them how they cope. Attending seminars and reading books on effective coping, assertiveness, and development of internal control will provide additional resources. Remember, we learned the coping mechanisms we currently have and we can learn even better ways to cope.

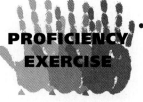

PROFICIENCY EXERCISE

• **Do an inventory of yourself to see what coping mechanisms you possess. List the ones that still work well. Learn a different coping style to replace one coping pattern that does not work as well as the others.**

Faith

Faith is the ability to believe, trust, and know certain things that science cannot prove. Faith is the strength of wellness and involves the expression of that connecting strength each day through faith in ourselves, our partners, our families, and humanity as a whole. Without faith there is little hope of wellness.

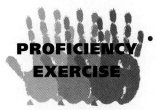

PROFICIENCY EXERCISE

• **Write a poem, story, or song, or draw a picture about your source of faith. This piece of art is just for you, so do not be concerned that anyone else will see it.**

Hope

Hope is the belief, assurance, conviction, and confidence that our future will somehow be OK. It is the belief that the choices we make now will be the most resourceful choices as we create our future. Without hope, there is no sense of continuity. To quote Temple Grandin, an admirable woman who deals daily with autism, "I like to hope that even if there is no personal afterlife, some energy impression is left in the universe . . . I do not want my thoughts to die with me . . ."[3]

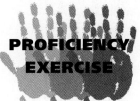

PROFICIENCY EXERCISE

• **Complete this sentence ten different ways: I hope . . .**

Love

Love is the reason why. Love has no concrete explanation. Without love there is no wholeness and without wholeness there is no wellness. This is not romantic love, but is bigger, stronger, more empowering, and mightier. It is quiet, gentle, forgiving, and nonjudgmental. A teenage boy was struggling to put these most important issues into perspective. He came to his mother and said, "I have figured out the meaning of life." Wondering this herself, she asked her son what he had discovered. The son replied, "When I play my music and I feel great and those who listen to me feel great, then I have shared my love, and my power gets bigger and so does theirs. But if I play my music, and only I feel great and those who listen feel bad and weak, then I have taken their power and this is evil. This is the meaning of life." This love celebrates the irrepressible process of life. This is the love of wellness.

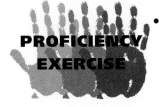

PROFICIENCY EXERCISE

- **During a learning experience, one or two people may emerge who teach us more than we expected to learn. Often the learning has nothing to do with the courses we are studying. This is a love sharing. Go to those who have shared their love with you and say thank you.**

SUMMARY

It will take some time to learn all the information presented in this book. In a year, after some massage experience, reread this textbook. You will be surprised what there is still in it to learn, and you will be impressed with what you now understand. Finishing this textbook and this course of study is an achievement. Be proud of yourself and of all those who helped you in the learning process. Your success now depends on your belief in your own ability. Nothing can stop you if you desire to achieve. Every obstacle is an opportunity to exercise your achievement "muscle." The origin of this muscle is in faith and the insertion is in hope. Its function is love.

Success is the maximum utilization of the abilities you have. If there is a better way to do something, challenge yourself to find it, then share it with others. When in doubt, effleurage! You never fail when you have done your best. All great achievements require time, perseverance, and purpose. Go slowly, evaluate, and adapt to each change, seeing it as an opportunity for growth.

Massage creates space and substitutes one set of signals for another. Hopefully, a more resourceful set of signals frees the energy to reach for our highest potential without restriction. Massage brings an awareness of body, mind, and spirit. Pay attention to the subtleties and quiet messages of life. Let these things teach you. Most importantly, massage touches people, and in turn, we are touched by them.

REFERENCES

1. Chaitow L: *The body/mind purification program,* New York, 1991, Fireside.
2. Lippert L: *Clinical kinesiology for physical therapist assistants,* Portland, 1991.
3. Sacks O: An anthropologist on Mars. *The New Yorker,* Dec. 27, 1993: 106–125.
4. Selye H: *The stress of life,* ed 2, New York, 1978, McGraw-Hill.

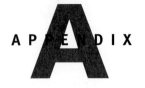

CONTRAINDICATIONS TO
MASSAGE

Because each situation is different, it is difficult to give yes and no recommendations about when to give and when not to give massage. This appendix provides two models for developing guidelines for contraindications and indications for massage. Following are specific conditions, symptoms, indications, and contraindications for massage. Use a medical dictionary for terms with which you are not familiar.

ONTARIO, CANADA GUIDELINES

The following are absolute contraindications (CI) to massage, i.e., massage treatment is not appropriate.

General

1. Advanced kidney failure (very modified treatment may be possible with medical consent)
2. Advanced respiratory failure (very modified treatment may be possible with medical consent)
3. Diabetes with complications such as gangrene, advanced heart or kidney disease, or very high or unstable blood pressure
4. Eclampsia—toxemia in pregnancy
5. Hemophilia
6. Hemorrhage
7. Liver failure (very modified treatment may be possible with medical consent)
8. Pneumonia in acute stages
9. Post–cerebrovascular accident (CVA)—(stroke), condition not yet stabilized
10. Postmyocardial infarction (MI)—(heart attack), condition not yet stabilized
11. Severe atherosclerosis
12. Severe (if unstable) hypertension
13. Shock, all types
14. Significant fever (101° F, 38.3° C)
15. Some acute conditions requiring first aid or medical attention
    anaphylaxis
    appendicitis
    CVA
    diabetic coma, insulin shock
    epileptic seizure
    MI
    pneumothorax, atelectasis
    severe asthma attack, status asthmaticus
    syncope (fainting)
16. Some highly metastatic cancers not judged to be terminal
17. Systemic contagious/infectious condition

Local (Regional)

1. Acute flare-up of inflammatory arthritis (e.g., rheumatoid arthritis, systemic lupus erythematosus, ankylosing spondylitis, Reiter's syndrome)—may be general CI, depending on case
2. Acute neuritis
3. Aneurysms deemed life-threatening, e.g., of abdominal aorta (may be general CI, depending on location)
4. Condition of sepsis
5. Ectopic pregnancy
6. Esophageal varicosities (varices)
7. Frostbite
8. Local contagious condition
9. Local irritable skin condition
10. Malignancy, especially if judged unstable
11. Open wound or sore
12. Phlebitis, phlebothrombosis, arteritis (may be a general CI if located in a major circulatory channel)
13. Recent burn
14. Temporal arteritis
15. Twenty-four to forty-eight hours post anti-inflammatory infection (target tissue and immediate vicinity)
16. Undiagnosed lump

The following conditions require an awareness of the possibility of adverse effects of massage therapy. Substantial treatment adaptation may be appropriate. Medical consultation is frequently needed.

General

1. Any condition of spasticity or rigidity
2. Asthma
3. Cancer, including finding appropriate relationships to other treatments being given
4. Chronic congestive heart failure
5. Chronic kidney disease
6. Client taking anti-inflammatories, muscle relaxants, anticoagulants, analgesics, or any other medications that alter sensation, muscle tone, standard reflex reactions, cardiovascular function, kidney or liver function, or personality
7. Client is immunosuppressed
8. Coma (may be absolute CI depending on cause)
9. Diagnosed atherosclerosis
10. Drug withdrawal
11. Emphysema
12. Epilepsy
13. Hypertension
14. Inflammatory arthritides
15. Major or abdominal surgery
16. Moderately severe or juvenile onset diabetes
17. Multiple sclerosis
18. Osteoporosis, osteomalacia
19. Pregnancy and labor
20. Post-MI
21. Post-CVA
22. Recent head injury

Local (Regional)

1. Acute disk herniation
2. Aneurysm (may be general CI depending on location)

3. Any acute inflammatory condition
4. Any anti-inflammatory infection site
5. Any chronic or longstanding superficial thrombosis
6. Buerger's disease (may be general CI if unstable)
7. Chronic arthritic conditions
8. Chronic abdominal or digestive disease
9. Chronic diarrhea
10. Contusion
11. Endometriosis
12. Flaccid paralysis or paresis
13. Fracture, while casted and following cast removal
14. Hernia
15. Joint instability or hypermobility
16. Kidney infection, stones
17. Mastitis
18. Minor surgery
19. Pelvic inflammatory disease
20. Pitting edema
21. Portal hypertension
22. Prolonged constipation
23. Recent abortion/vaginal birth
24. Trigeminal neuralgia

Other Important Considerations

1. Massage therapists are expected to know how and when to consult with medical doctors and other health professionals.
2. Most emotional or psychiatric conditions will have an impact on massage treatment. Individual decisions must be made according to case circumstances, and in many instances, medical advice. Medications may be a factor.
3. The client may be allergic to certain oils or creams, or to cleansers or disinfectants used on sheets and tables.
4. The presence of pins, staples, or artificial joints may alter treatment indications.

The massage therapist should be aware of the role of common chronic conditions that impact public health (e.g., cardiovascular diseases, cancers, substance abuse, chronic mental diseases).

If additional information is needed regarding public mental health services, environmental hazards, occupational health, or various health care systems available in the community, every community has a health department available to utilize as a resource for such information.

INDICATIONS AND CONTRAINDICATIONS BY BODY SYSTEM: OREGON MODEL

This extensive list was developed by The Oregon Board of Massage. There were no specific recommendations for indications or contraindications. The descriptions for the disease process and the massage recommendations have been added by this author, and a very conservative approach has been taken. If an indication for a disease process is not listed, this means that massage would have no direct benefit. Such indications are designated as N/A. This textbook covers basic massage. Advanced training in the medical application of massage, and direct supervision by a doctor, chiropractor, physical therapist, psychologist, dentist, podiatrist, or other health care professional will greatly expand the application of massage in rehabilitative situations.

Integumentary System

Assessment parameters include color (i.e., pallor, jaundice, cyanosis, erythema, mottling, etc.), texture (i.e., dry, moist, scaly, etc.), scars (normal and keloid), vascularity (i.e., dilated veins, angiomas, varicosities, ecchymosis, petechiae, purpura, etc.), temperature, rashes, lesions, nail condition, hair condition, contour, hydration, and edema.

Deviations suggesting the need for evaluation and referral include lumps or masses, rashes of unknown origin, lesions, burns, urticaria, itching of unknown origin, cyanosis, jaundice, ulcerations, multiple bruises, and petechiae.

Specific disease processes and bacterial conditions:

Acne Symptoms/definition: Inflammation of skin affecting sebaceous gland ducts

Indications: Increased systemic circulation; may assist healing

Contraindications: Regional—avoid the affected area and use of ointments that clog pores

Impetigo Symptoms/definition: Highly infectious bacterial skin infection; occurs most often in children; begins as reddish discoloration and develops into vesicles with yellowish crust

Indications: Increased systemic circulation; massage may assist healing

Contraindications: Regional—refer to a doctor; avoid affected area

Folliculitis Symptoms/definition: Inflammation of hair follicle

Indications: Massage may increase systemic circulation and may assist in healing

Contraindications: Regional—refer to a doctor; avoid affected area

Furuncle (boil) Symptoms/definition: Pus-filled cavity formed by hair follicle infections

Indications: Massage may increase systemic circulation and may assist healing

Contraindications: Regional—refer to a doctor; avoid affected area

Carbuncle Symptoms/definition: Mass of connected boils

Indications: Massage may increase systemic circulation and may assist healing

Contraindications: Refer to a doctor; avoid affected area

Cellulitis Symptoms/definition: Inflammation of subcutaneous tissue with redness and swelling

Indications: Avoid

Contraindications: Regional—may be associated with erysipelas, a contagious condition; referral indicated

Syphilis Symptoms/definition: Primary (canker sore on exposed skin); secondary syphilis appears two months after canker disappears; variety of symptoms including skin rash

Indications: N/A

Contraindications: General; rash; contagious; refer

Viral conditions:

Herpes simplex Symptoms/definition: Acute viral disease marked by groups of watery blisters on or near mucus membranes

Indications: Stress-induced; massage may reduce stress levels

Contraindications: Regional—contagious; avoid affected area

Herpes zoster (shingles) Symptoms/definition: Viral infection that usually affects the skin of a single dermatome; red swollen plaque that ruptures and crusts

Indications: This is a painful condition; general massage may ease pain

Contraindications: Regional—avoid affected area; may need to refer

Bell's palsy Symptoms/definition: Infection of seventh cranial nerve; paralysis of facial features, including the eyelid and mouth

Indications: Relaxation massage may facilitate healing

Contraindications: Regional—refer to a doctor for diagnosis

Warts Symptoms/definition: Usually benign excess cell growth of the skin

Indications: N/A

Contraindications: Regional—avoid affected area; contagious; may become malignant; refer any changes in the wart to a physician

Fungal conditions Symptoms/definition: Tinea, ringworm, athlete's foot, fungal infection of nails; scaly and crusty cracking of skin

Indications: Keep area dry; avoid use of lubricants

Contraindications: Regional—avoid lubricants near area as fungus thrives on moist environment

Allergic reactions:

Contact dermatitis Symptoms/definition: Inflammation occurring in response to contact with an exterior agent

Indications: Use unscented lubricants; scents often cause allergic reaction

Contraindications: Regional—avoid affected area

Urticaria (hives) Symptoms/definition: Red raised lesion caused by leakage of fluid from skin and blood vessels; severe itching

Indications: Avoid scented products; hives may have an emotional component

Contraindications: Regional—avoid affected area

Atopic dermatitis (eczema) Symptoms/definition: Common inflammation of skin with papules, vesicles, and crusts

Indications: Symptom of underlying condition; refer to physician for diagnosis

Contraindications: Regional—avoid affected area

Benign conditions:

Moles Symptoms/definition: A pigmented fleshy growth of skin

Indications: Watch for any change in mole; refer to physician

Contraindications: Regional—avoid mole

Psoriasis Symptoms/definition: Chronic inflammation of the skin; probably genetic; scaly plaque; excessive rate of epithelial cell growth

Indications: May be stress-induced; massage reduces stress

Contraindications: Regional—avoid affected area

Scleroderma Symptoms/definition: Autoimmune disease affecting blood vessels and connective tissue of skin; hard, yellowish skin

Indications: N/A

Contraindications: Regional (except in systemic cases); refer to physician

Malignant conditions:

Skin cancer Symptoms/definition: Squamous cell carcinoma; basal cell carcinoma; melanoma; Kaposi's sarcoma
    Indications: N/A
    Contraindications: Watch for any change in mole or existing skin condition; refer immediately; avoid sun

Skeletal System, Muscular System, and Articulations

Assessment parameters include range of motion, swelling, masses, deformity, pain or tenderness, temperature, crepitus, spasm, paresthesia, pulses, skin color, paralysis, atrophy, and contracture.

Deviations suggesting the need for evaluation and referral include malalignment of an extremity, asymmetry of musculoskeletal contour, progressive or persistent pain, masses or progressive swelling, numbness and/or tingling with loss of function, diminished or absent peripheral pulses, pallor and/or coolness of one extremity, redness and/or increased temperature of one extremity, and asymmetry of the size of one extremity over the other.

Specific disease processes:

Hypertonicity Symptoms/definition: Increased muscle tone
    Indications: Massage and stretch
    Contraindications: Reoccurrence without explanation; refer for diagnosis

Contracture Symptoms/definition: Fixed resistance to passive stretching of muscles; usually resulting from fibrosis or tissue ischemia
    Indications: Massage and stretch
    Contraindications: No stretch past fixed barrier

Atonicity or flaccidity Symptoms/definition: Reduction or inability of the muscle to contract—hypotonicity
    Indications: Massage to tone; relaxation of opposing muscle groups
    Contraindications: Regional—refer to physician for diagnosis before proceeding

Spasms (cramp) Symptoms/definition: Sudden onset of muscle contracture; painful
    Indications: Utilize reciprocal inhibition; push muscle belly together and slow stretch
    Contraindications: If reoccurring and transient, refer to physician

Tic Symptoms/definition: Spasmodic twitching; often occurs in face
    Indications: May be stress-induced; massage beneficial in reducing stress levels
    Contraindications: Refer for diagnosis to rule out serious underlying pathology

Fibrillation Symptoms/definition: A small local contraction of muscle that is invisible under the skin; results from spontaneous activation of single muscle cells synchronously
    Indications: Massage, direct pressure
    Contraindications: If continuous, refer for diagnosis

Convulsion
    Indications: N/A
    Contraindications: Refer immediately

Soft tissue injuries:

Sprains Symptoms/definition: Traumatic injury of ligaments forming a skeletal joint; may involve injury (strain) of muscles or tendon
 Indications: RICE (rest, ice, compression, elevation), first aid, gentle massage and range of motion facilitate healing
 Contraindications: Regional—all traumatic injury should be evaluated by a physician

Strains Symptoms/definition: Traumatic injury from overstretching and/or over-exertion of muscle or tendon tissue
 Indications: RICE first aid, gentle massage and range of motion; may facilitate healing
 Contraindications: Regional—all traumatic injury should be evaluated by a physician

Dislocations Symptoms/definition: Displacement of a bone within a joint
 Indications: N/A
 Contraindications: Refer immediately to a physician

Subluxation Symptoms/definition: Any deviation from the normal relationship where the articular cartilage is still touching any portion of its mating cartilage
 Indications: Massage may help relieve protective muscle spasm
 Contraindications: Refer to a physician

Infectious processes:

Osteomyelitis Symptoms/definition: Bacterial infection of bone; deep pain and fever
 Indications: N/A
 Contraindications: General—Refer immediately to physician; difficult to diagnose and treat

Inflammatory processes:

Rheumatoid arthritis Symptoms/definition: Autoimmune inflammatory joint disease characterized by synovial inflammation that spreads to other tissues
 Indications: Stress-responsive; massage helpful under medical supervision
 Contraindications: General—work closely with physician

Gouty arthritis Symptoms/definition: Metabolic condition where sodium urate crystals trigger chronic inflammatory process
 Indications: Dietary adjustment necessary
 Contraindications: Regional—avoid area of inflammation

Ankylosing spondylitis Symptoms/definition: Chronic inflammatory disease; can be progressive; usually involves the sacroiliac joint and spinal articulations; cause unknown, appears genetic; if progressive, there is calcification of joints and articular surfaces; begins with feelings of fatigue and intermittent low back pain; synovial tissue around the involved joints becomes inflamed; heart disease may also occur
 Indications: Massage may be helpful under direct supervision of a physician
 Contraindications: General; refer; avoid any area of inflammation

Bursitis Symptoms/definition: Inflammation of bursa

Indications: Massage may take pressure off joint by relaxing and normalizing surrounding musculature; ice

Contraindications: Regional—avoid affected area; work above and below jointed area

Tenosynovitis Symptoms/definition: Inflammation of tendon sheath usually from repetitive movement

Indications: Massage may relieve muscle hypertonicity and assist healing of area; ice

Contraindications: Regional—avoid affected area; work above and below the area

Tendinitis Symptoms/definition: Inflammation of tendon and tendon muscle junction

Indications: Massage may assist healing; ice

Contraindications: Regional—avoid affected area; work above and below the area

Lupus erythematosus Symptoms/definition: Chronic inflammatory disease that affects many body tissues; a red rash of the face is often present

Indications: Massage may be beneficial under close supervision of physician

Contraindications: General—systemic disease

Fibromyalgia Symptoms/definition: General disruption in connective tissue muscle component with tender point activity; vague symptoms of pain and fatigue

Indications: Massage may be beneficial; work with physician

Contraindications: General—refer to physician for diagnosis

Osgood-Schlatter disease Symptoms/definition: Osteochondrosis (inflammation of bone and cartilage) of the tuberosity of the tibia

Indications: N/A

Contraindications: Regional—avoid affected area

Compression processes:

Carpal tunnel syndrome Symptoms/definition: Inflammation in tendon sheaths in the carpal tunnel pressing on the median nerve; weakness and tingling in hand

Indications: Symptoms often confused with thoracic outlet syndrome; massage is proving to be beneficial

Contraindications: Regional—refer to physician for diagnosis

Degenerative processes:

Osteoarthritis Symptoms/definition: Degenerative joint disease of the articular cartilage; age and joint damage are risk factors

Indications: Massage is beneficial

Contraindications: Regional—avoid area of inflammation

Muscular dystrophy Symptoms/definition: Group of muscle disorders characterized by atrophy of skeletal muscle without nerve involvement

Indications: Massage beneficial; work closely with supervising physician

Contraindications: General

Osteoporosis Symptoms/definition: Loss of minerals and collagen from bone matrix reducing volume and strength of skeletal bone
   Indications: Gentle massage beneficial; use care and caution
   Contraindications: General

Abnormal spinal curve:

Scoliosis Symptoms/definition: Lateral curve of vertebral column
   Indications: Massage beneficial as part of treatment plan
   Contraindications: Regional—in severe cases proceed after physician's recommendation

Kyphosis Symptoms/definition: Abnormal increased convexity of the thoracic spine
   Indications: Massage beneficial as part of the treatment plan
   Contraindications: Regional—in severe cases proceed after physician's recommendation

Lordosis Symptoms/definition: Abnormal increased concavity in the curvature of the lumbar spine
   Indications: Massage is beneficial as part of the treatment plan
   Contraindications: Regional—in severe cases proceed after physician's recommendation

Disordered muscular processes:

Low back pain Symptoms/definition: May be of many varieties: muscular, nerve entrapment, or disc problem
   Indications: Massage can be beneficial as part of treatment plan
   Contraindications: Regional—important to refer to physician to rule out serious condition of the spine or viscera

Spasmodic torticollis Symptoms/definition: A contracted state of the cervical muscles producing pain and rotation of the head
   Indications: Massage beneficial
   Contraindications: Regional—refer to physician for diagnosis to rule out serious disease

Tempormandibular joint (TMJ) dysfunction Symptoms/definition: Dysfunction in the TMJ; pain and muscle contraction
   Indications: Massage beneficial; work closely with dentist and physician
   Contraindications: Regional—if painful

Neurologic Conditions

Assessment parameters include mental status, the presence of involuntary movements, coordination and balance, and muscle tone and strength, changes in sensory perception (i.e., touch, pain, temperature, vibration, position sense, hearing, visual).

   Deviations suggesting the need for evaluation and referral include inequality of pupil size, diplopia, abnormal Babinski sign (extensor plantar response), seizures (partial or generalized), significant personality changes, changes in sensorium, progressively worsening or persistent headache, temporary loss of function of speech, vision, or motion, triad of fever, headache and nuchal rigidity, headache, vomiting, and alteration in pupil size in client with head injury.

Specific disease processes:

Peripheral neuropathy Symptoms/definition: General functional disturbances and/or pathologic changes in the peripheral nervous system caused from diabetic neuropathy, ischemic neuropathy, traumatic neuropathy, symptoms of numbness, burning, and pain
    Indications: Massage beneficial as part of total treatment plan
    Contraindications: General—refer to physician for diagnosis to determine underlying condition

Vertigo Symptoms/definition: Sensation of movement not to be confused with dizziness
    Indications: N/A
    Contraindications: General—usually symptomatic of underlying condition; physician diagnosis required

Tinnitus Symptoms/definition: Noise in the ear; ringing, buzzing, roaring, or clicking
    Indications: N/A
    Contraindications: Regional—refer for specific diagnosis

Dystonia Symptoms/definition: Disordered random tonicity of muscles
    Indications: Massage beneficial as part of physician-directed treatment plan
    Contraindications: General—refer for diagnosis and treatment plan

Dyskinesia Symptoms/definition: Impairment of the power of voluntary movement resulting in fragmentary or incomplete movement and possible pain
    Indications: Massage beneficial as part of physician-directed treatment plan
    Contraindications: General—refer for diagnosis and treatment plan

Insomnia Symptoms/definition: Inability to sleep or interrupted sleep
    Indications: Massage beneficial
    Contraindications: Regional—refer to physician for specific diagnosis to rule out serious underlying condition

Vascular processes:

Transient ischemic attack (TIA) Symptoms/definition: Episodes of neurologic dysfunction that are usually of short duration (a few minutes) but may persist for twenty-four hours; reversible; symptom pattern same with each attack because the same vessel is involved; small strokes, seizures, migraine symptoms, postural hypotension, and Stokes-Allen syndrome may all be misdiagnosed as TIAs.
    Indications: Massage may be beneficial under supervision of a physician
    Contraindications: Refer for diagnosis

CVA Symptoms/definition: Stroke; a disturbance in cerebral circulation; major causes include atherosclerosis (thrombosis), embolism, hypertensive intracerebral hemorrhage or ruptured saccular aneurysm; symptoms differ depending on where the disturbance in circulation occurs; general symptoms include weakness or paralysis of arm or leg, headache, numbness, blurred or double vision, confusion or dizziness; often only one side is affected; symptoms persist for at least twenty-four hours, usually much longer.

Indications: Massage may be beneficial during recovery with supervision from physician and for continued support during long term care

Contraindications: Refer to physician for diagnosis

Headache Symptoms/definition: Pain or dull ache in head and upper neck; can be from a variety of causes—muscle tension, sinus pressure, pinched nerve, vascular disruption (i.e., migraine, cluster headaches), toxins

Indications: Massage can be beneficial

Contraindications: Refer all persistent severe headaches to physician for specific diagnosis

Head injury Symptoms/definition: Contusion (bump on the head); laceration (cut or break in skin); subdural and epidural (client may be disoriented, or nauseous, with uneven pupil dilation)

Indications: Refer immediately if client shows any signs of concussion

Contraindications: General—all traumatic injury must be evaluated by a physician

Infectious processes:

Poliomyelitis Symptoms/definition: Viral infection of nerves that control skeletal muscles

Indications: Massage beneficial as part of physician-monitored treatment plan

Contraindications: General

Postpolio syndrome Symptoms/definition: Symptoms appear years after poliomyelitis; fatigue and general muscle weakness

Indications: Massage beneficial as part of physician-directed treatment plan

Contraindications: Regional—refer to physician for specific diagnosis

Conjunctivitis Symptoms/definition: Inflammation and/or infection of mucus membranes of the eye

Indications: N/A

Contraindications: Regional—refer; may be contagious; avoid affected area

Parkinson's disease Symptoms/definition: Nervous disorder characterized by abnormally low levels of the neurotransmitter, dopamine, causing involuntary trembling and muscle rigidity

Indications: Massage beneficial as part of physician-directed treatment plan

Contraindications: General

Neuromuscular processes:

Multiple sclerosis Symptoms/definition: Primary disease of the central nervous system; degeneration of myelin

Indications: Massage beneficial as part of physician-directed treatment plan

Contraindications: General

Trigeminal neuralgia (tic douloureux) Symptoms/definition: Compression or degeneration of fifth cranial nerve; recurring episodes of stabbing pain in the face

Indications: Avoid entire area of trigeminal nerve innervation; massage may trigger pain response

Contraindications: Regional

Spinal cord injury Symptoms/definition: Traumatic injury or degenerative process of the spinal cord; may result from compression, cut, or tissue replacement in scarring

Indications: Massage beneficial as part of physician-directed treatment plan

Contraindications: Regional

Miscellaneous disorders:

Sleep apnea Symptoms/definition: Cessation of breathing during sleep

Indications: May have stress component massage beneficial in reducing stress levels

Contraindications: Regional

Thoracic outlet syndrome Symptoms/definition: Compression of brachial nerve plexus radiates pain into shoulder and arm

Indications: Massage beneficial as part of the treatment plan

Contraindications: Regional—refer for specific diagnosis

Seizure disorders Symptoms/definition: Sudden bursts of abnormal neuron activity resulting in temporary changes in brain activity; may vary from mild, affecting conscious motor control or sensory perception, to severe, resulting in convulsion.

Indications: Massage may be beneficial

Contraindications: General—follow physician recommendation for massage

Endocrine System

Assessment parameters include fatigue, depression, changes in energy level, hyper-alertness, sleep patterns, mood; affect skin, hair, and personal appearance.

Deviations suggesting the need for evaluation and referral include cold, clammy skin; numbness of fingers, toes, or mouth; rapid heartbeat, faintness; vertigo; tremors, dyspnea (difficulty breathing), thyroid nodule; unusually warm hands and feet; and lethargy.

Specific disease processes:

Diabetes mellitus Symptoms/definition: Metabolic disorder; Body loses ability to oxidize carbohydrates due to faulty pancreatic activity especially of the islets of Langerhans affecting insulin production; symptoms include thirst, hunger, acidosis; severe symptoms are difficulty breathing and changes in blood chemistry that lead to coma

Indications: Massage under supervision of primary medical care; beneficial for circulation enhancement and stress reduction, exercise is beneficial.

Contraindications: General—work only under the supervision of a physician.

Hypoglycemia Symptoms/definition: Low blood glucose produced by too much blood insulin; Lightheadedness, anxiety, forgetfulness

Indications: Diet; massage helpful; may relieve stress

Contraindications: Client should be referred to determine the reason for low blood sugar

Hyperglycemia Symptoms/definition: High blood sugar levels from too little blood insulin; diabetic symptoms

Indications: See diabetes mellitus

Contraindications: See diabetes mellitus

Neuropathy Symptoms/definition: Functional disturbance or pathologic change in peripheral nervous system; symptoms include numbness, burning, and tingling pain

Indications: Massage beneficial under medical supervision; may calm hypersensitive nerves.

Contraindications: General—work under direction of a physician

Hyperthyroidism Symptoms/definition: Too much thyroid hormone; can be caused by tumor or problems with self-regulatory mechanism in pituitary; symptoms include anxiety, bulging eyes, high metabolic rate, and nervousness

Indications: Massage is beneficial to relax client

Contraindications: General—work within recommendations of physician

Hypothyroidism Symptoms/definition: Low thyroid hormone; Symptoms include cold, weight gain, fatigue, dullness

Indications: Massage beneficial to stimulate metabolic function

Contraindications: General—work with recommendation of physician

Cardiovascular System

Assessment parameters include skin color and appearance, respiratory rate and effort, condition of nails and nail beds (i.e., clubbing, cyanosis), pain or tenderness and points of radiation, swelling, and symmetry of chest cavity.

Deviations suggesting the need for evaluation and referral include pulse over 90 or under 60; dyspnea; pitting edema; distended neck veins; glossy appearance of the skin; positive Homan's sign (calf tenderness upon dorsiflexion of the foot); asymmetry of limb circumference; red, warm, tender, and hard vein; edema, pain and tenderness of extremity; clubbing of nail beds; chest pain (especially if radiating to left arm); central or peripheral cyanosis; pallor; mottling or cyanosis of a limb; stasis ulcers; and splinter hemorrhages (small red to black streaks under fingernails).

Physiologic processes:

Syncope Symptoms/definition: A sudden loss of strength; fainting; may be caused by a cardiac spasm caused by closure of coronary arteries

Indications: N/A

Contraindications: General—refer immediately

Deep vein thrombosis Symptoms/definition: Blood clot in deep veins; risk factor for pulmonary embolism (blood clot in heart); often asymptomatic; swelling and edema, pain described as aching and throbbing

Indications: N/A

Contraindications: Regional to general depending on the severity of symptoms; always refer in unexplained cases of pain; Never massage over such areas

Phlebitis Symptoms/definition: Inflammation of a vein; May be caused by a blood clot; Symptoms include edema, stiffness, and pain; veins may streak red

Indications: N/A

Contraindications: Regional to general—see above.

MI (myocardial infarction) Symptoms/definition: Death of cardiac muscle cells, usually from inadequate blood supply, often from coronary thrombosis or coronary artery disease; Symptoms include severe pain in chest in left arm, difficulty breathing, and weakness

Indications: Massage beneficial in rehabilitation process under supervision of primary care physician

Contraindications: General—refer immediately

Congestive heart failure Symptoms/definition: Left heart failure; inability of the left ventricle to pump effectively; symptoms include body retains fluids

Indications: Massage beneficial in assisting diuretics in removal of excess fluid

Contraindications: General—must work under supervision of a physician; it may be difficult for the client to breath while in a supine position

Angina pectoris Symptoms/definition: Chest pain caused by inadequate oxygen to heart (usually from blocked coronary arteries)

Indications: Massage beneficial as part of total lifestyle change

Contraindications: General—massage performed under supervision of physician

Arteriosclerosis and atherosclerosis Symptoms/definition: Hardening of the arteries; a type of coronary heart disease, symptoms may be mild to severe; may be mistaken for other problems

Indications: Massage beneficial as part of total lifestyle change

Contraindications: General—massage should be performed under supervision of physician.

Aneurysm Symptoms/definition: Abnormal widening of the arterial wall; tends to form thrombi and also to burst; a pulsating bulge and pressure is felt with accompanying symptoms of pain

Indications: N/A

Contraindications: Regional—refer immediately; avoid direct heavy pressure into arterial vessels

Varicose vein Symptoms/definition: Enlarged vein in which blood pools; caused by collapse of valve system; tend to form thrombi

Indications: N/A

Contraindications: Regional—avoid affected area

Raynaud's syndrome Symptoms/definition: Arteriospastic condition produced by vasospasms of the small cutaneous and subcutaneous arteries and arterioles; skin pallor and pain are symptoms; it is usually triggered by cold but is also emotionally reactive

Indications: Care must be taken to avoid triggering the symptoms; interview client carefully; massage may be beneficial for stress reduction

Contraindications: Refer for specific underlying diagnosis; may be symptomatic of serious condition

Hemophilia Symptoms/definition: Blood clotting disorder; spontaneous bleeding due to inability to form clots

Indications: Extremely light energy type of massage only under direction of a physician

Contraindications: General—work only with a physician's supervision

Anemia Symptoms/definition: Reduced red blood cell count or hemoglobin; fatigue and pallor are symptoms

Indications: Massage can be beneficial in complete treatment plan

Contraindications: General—refer to physician for diagnosis; proceed under direction of physician

Mononucleosis Symptoms/definition: Epstein-Barr induced; viral illness; fever, fatigue, swollen glands

Indications: Massage beneficial as part of treatment plan; be careful of contagious conditions

Contraindications: General—refer to physician for specific diagnosis

Lymphatic and Immune Systems

Assessment parameters include skin color and condition, evidence of eye irritation, lymph nodes, and nasal discharge/irritation.

Deviations suggesting the need for evaluation and referral include client history of chronic fatigue or recurrent physical ailments (i.e., skin, respiratory, gastrointestinal) in the absence of general illness; history of food intolerance; failure to gain weight; unexplained weight loss; rashes of unknown origin; urticaria; enlarged, tender nodes; excessive or persistent dryness; and scaliness of skin.

Specific disease processes:

Chronic fatigue syndrome Symptoms/definition: May be viral-induced; symptoms include swollen glands, low grade fever, muscle and joint aches, headache, and fatigue

Indications: Massage beneficial

Contraindications: General—refer to physician for specific diagnosis

Human immunodeficiency virus (HIV) Symptoms/definition: Viral infection transmitted through body fluids; causes immune suppression

Indications: Massage is beneficial with physician recommendations; follow antiviral precautions for control of virus; 10% bleach solution; avoid body fluid contact; see chapter 5 for further information

Contraindications: General—work with physician

Autoimmune disease Symptoms/definition: Process where the body's own immune system attacks itself; inflammation, fatigue, and allergy

Indications: Massage is beneficial with physician recommendation

Contraindications: General—refer for specific diagnosis

Allergy Symptoms/definition: Hypersensitivity of immune system to relatively harmless environmental antigens; increased mucus inflammation, occasionally spastic bladder

Indications: Massage beneficial

Contraindications: Refer for specific diagnosis

Lymphedema Symptoms/definition: Swelling of tissue due to partial or total blockage of lymph vessels

Indications: Massage is beneficial within total treatment plan under supervision of primary care physician

Contraindications: Refer for diagnosis

Respiratory System

Assessment parameters include the rate and pattern of respiration, chest movement, color, nodes, chest configuration, ease of chest excursions, fremitus, and pain.

Deviations suggesting need for evaluation and referral include inspiratory flaring of nostrils; use of accessory muscles; intercostal retractions or bulging; pursed lips on exhalation; splinting; uneven chest movement; altered tactile fremitus/crepitus (increased or decreased); cyanosis or pallor; enlarged, tender nodes; pain with breathing; and a respiratory rate over 20 in absence of exertion or strong emotion.

Specific infectious disease processes:

Upper respiratory infection (including bronchitis, common cold, sinusitis, and pneumonia) Symptoms/definition: viral or bacterial; symptoms of increased mucus production, fever, body aches, headaches

Indications: Light massage may be beneficial to reduce body ache; avoid any heavy pressure; watch for contamination

Contraindications: Refer if symptoms persist for longer than two weeks or if symptoms are severe

Tuberculosis Symptoms/definition: Infectious disease caused by *Mycobacterium tuberculosis;* early stage requires testing to discover; advanced cases show lung destruction, coughing, fatigue, weakness, and weight loss; may be confused with bronchitis and pneumonia

Indications: Droplet transmission; contagious; be aware of sanitation

Contraindications: General—work only if physician recommends and clears for contagious condition

Asthma Symptoms/definition: Recurring muscle spasms in the bronchial wall accompanied by fluid retention and mucus production; stress-specific

Indications: Massage beneficial; monitor breathing closely

Contraindications: Work under direction of primary care physician

Gastrointestinal System

Assessment parameters include skin (see section on integumentary system); contour of abdomen (flat, rounded, concave, protuberant, distended); symmetry; observable masses; palpable masses; movement; tenderness or pain; and location and contour of umbilicus.

Deviations suggesting the need for evaluation and referral include a history of persistent or recurring nausea or vomiting; abdominal pain of unknown origin; rebound tenderness; epigastric pain occurring one to three hours after meals; rigid or boardlike abdomen (not related to calisthenic exercises); persistent or increasing abdominal or epigastric pain; history of blood in stools or vomitus; difficulty swallowing; masses or nodules; enlarged, tender nodes; bulge or swelling in abdomen; change in location or inversion/eversion of umbilicus; and lesions in oral cavity; lips, or tongue.

Specific disease processes:

Halitosis Symptoms/definition: Bad breath may indicate digestive problems or sinus infection

Indications: N/A

Contraindications: Refer for specific diagnosis

Diarrhea Symptoms/definition: Loose bowels; excessive loss of water in stool; can be caused by a virus or bacterium or can be a symptom of other disease processes

Indications: Loose stool not uncommon twenty-four hours after vigorous massage

Contraindications: Refer if symptoms persist or dehydration is present

Constipation Symptoms/definition: Slow movement of bowels; hard compacted dry stool

Indications: Massage beneficial; increase fiber and water consumption and moderate exercise; may be drug-related

Contraindications: Refer if severe or persistent or if a mass is felt in large intestine

Flatulence Symptoms/definition: Intestinal gas

Indications: May be diet or stress related; massage may reduce stress levels

Contraindications: Refer for diagnosis to rule out severe underlying condition or if there is painful distention of the intestinal tract

Inflammatory processes:

Gastritis Symptoms/definition: Inflammation of stomach; acute; common; usually caused from irritant like alcohol or aspirin, leading to pain, nausea, belching

Indications: Massage is beneficial since gastritis is sometimes stress-related; massage may reduce stress

Contraindications: Refer for specific diagnosis

Ulcer Symptoms/definition: Peptic ulcer—break or open sore not covered by protective mucus in the gastrointestinal wall exposed to pepsin and gastric juice often caused by alcohol, pepsin, bile salts, and stress

Indications: Massage beneficial to reduce stress levels; lifestyle and diet changes may be necessary

Contraindications: Refer for specific diagnosis; support physician treatment plan

Duodenal ulcer Symptoms/definition: Hyperacidity in duodenal bulb; burning pain that feels better after eating; stress-related

Indications: Massage beneficial to reduce stress levels; lifestyle and diet changes may be necessary

Contraindications: Refer for specific diagnosis; support physician treatment plan

Stress ulcer Symptoms/definition: Related to severe stress, e.g., trauma, burns, or long-term illness; similar to gastritis symptoms

Indications: Massage is beneficial to reduce stress levels; lifestyle and diet changes may be necessary

Contraindications: Refer for specific diagnosis; support physician treatment plan

Pancreatitis Symptoms/definition: Inflammation of the pancreas; severe abdominal pain; may be present with diabetes; alcohol aggravates

Indications: Painful condition; massage may be helpful in general stress and pain reduction

Contraindications: Refer immediately; work with chronic conditions under direct supervision of physician

Crohn's disease (regional enteritis) Symptoms/definition: Chronic relapsing inflammatory disease of the intestinal tract; intermittent diarrhea; colicky pain in lower abdomen, fatigue; low-grade fever

Indications: Painful condition; massage may be helpful in general stress and pain reduction

Contraindications: Refer immediately; work with chronic conditions under direct supervision of physician

Colitis Symptoms/definition: Inflammatory condition of large intestine; one type of colitis is irritable bowel syndrome brought on by stress

Indications: Painful condition; massage may be helpful in general stress and pain reduction

Contraindications: Refer immediately; work with chronic conditions under direct supervision of physician

Appendicitis Symptoms/definition: Inflammation of mucus lining of the appendix caused by trapped food or fecal matter; more common in people under the age of 25; mild periumbilical pain; nausea and vomiting; pain increases into the lower right quadrant; muscle spasm and rebounding tenderness

    Indications: N/A

    Contraindications: Refer immediately

Diverticulosis Symptoms/definition: Herniation of the mucosa forming small pockets in the large intestine; when inflamed, condition is called diverticulitis; gas, diarrhea, and pain

    Indications: Diet may need adjustment to include more fiber

    Contraindications: Refer if pain or if symptoms persist

Cholelithiasis and cholecystitis Symptoms/definition: Gall stones formed from inflammation; severe pain in upper abdomen radiating to back and right shoulder

    Indications: N/A

    Contraindications: Refer immediately

Cirrhosis of the liver Symptoms/definition: Chronic disease that replaces liver tissue with connective tissue; major cause—alcohol consumption; early symptoms include gas, change in bowel habits, slight weight loss, nausea in morning, dull heavy ache in right upper quadrant of abdomen; advanced symptoms include jaundice, peripheral edema, bleeding, and red palms

    Indications: Massage is beneficial in stress reduction and drug withdrawal

    Contraindications: Refer for diagnosis; work under supervision of physician

Hepatitis Symptoms/definition: Infectious disease; generalized in the body, but has predominant effect on the liver; type A is common in children and institutions; transmitted by fecal matter and orally from contaminated food and water; usual symptoms, mild and flulike; type B and C affect all age groups; transmitted through blood, needles, fecal/oral route and sexual contact

    Indications: Careful use of aseptic procedures

    Contraindications: General—refer and work only under physician recommendation and guidelines concerning contagious condition

Hernia Symptoms/definition: Protrusion of a loop or piece of an organ or tissue through an abnormal opening; hiatal—protrusion of any structure through the hiatus of the diaphragm; usually the esophagus or end of the stomach; inguinal—protrusion through inguinal ring; swelling of scrotum, may become obstructed and become a medical emergency; umbilical—protrusion at the umbilicus; in inguinal and umbilical hernia, weakness may be felt in the abdominal wall

    Indications: N/A

    Contraindications: Refer to physician; avoid the area

Metabolic System

Assessment parameters include eating patterns, skin, hair, nails, weight/height data, and general health status.

    Deviations suggesting the need for evaluation and referral include significant under or overweight, evidence of nutritional deficiencies (e.g., hair, skin, or fatigue), and respiratory problems.

Specific disease processes:

Obesity Symptoms/definition: Excess body fat (over 30% of normal body weight); risks of obesity include diabetes, stroke, heart attack, gallstones, and high blood pressure.

Indications: Morbid obesity—over 60% of normal body fat; difficulty in positioning client; fluid retention; risk of blood pressure fluctuation and interference with breathing; may need to alter massage position

Contraindications: Refer for nutritional and diet consultation

Malnutrition Symptoms/definition: Deficiency of calories in general and often in protein; malnutrition may be caused by increased nutrient demand on the body without sufficient food intake, i.e. severe burns, illness, or simple lack of food, especially protein; symptoms include flaking skin, brittle hair, hair loss, slow-healing sores, bruising, susceptibility to infection; fatigue; more common in children, the aged, and with drug and alcohol abuse; be aware of eating disorders. (Note: malnutrition is also caused by insufficient or improper digestion and absorption or food.)

Indications: In anorexia or bulimia, massage may be beneficial for stress reduction

Contraindications: Refer to a physician to determine the cause and outline treatment care

Cystic fibrosis Symptoms/definition: Inherited disorder that disrupts cell transport and causes exocrine glands to produce thick secretions; thick pancreatic secretions may block the pancreatic duct

Indications: Massage beneficial with specific training to loosen mucus with percussive techniques

Contraindications: General—work under direct care of physician

Genitourinary System

Assessment parameters include pain (groin, periumbilical, flank, abdominal, dysuria), patterns of urination and output, urine consistency (color, concentration, or hematuria), edema (facial, ankle), weight changes, skin changes, discharge, and masses.

Deviations suggesting the need for evaluation and referral include a history of unusual vaginal, urethral, or nipple discharge; breast, penile, scrotal, or inguinal masses or lumps; genital blisters, lesions, or growths; changes in urinary frequency, output, control, or urine characteristics; sudden weight gain, abnormal periods, edema, skin abnormalities, pain or tenderness (costovertebral angle, abdominal, or low back), masses or lumps, and tender or enlarged nodes.

Specific disease processes:

Urinary tract infection Symptoms/definition: Acute pyelonephritis—inflammation of kidney and pelvis; usually woman with abrupt onset of fever, chills, malaise, back pain, tender palpation over the costovertebral region; cystitis—both usually caused by the transmission of bacteria through the urethra due to improper cleansing procedures after bowel movement; may have pain in lower abdomen above pubic bone and low back ache

Indications: N/A

Contraindications: Refer for diagnosis and treatment

Dysmenorrhea Symptoms/definition: Painful menstruation; may be caused by endometriosis (abnormal growth and distribution of uterine lining); heavy periods and clotting

Indications: Massage beneficial for stress reduction and pain

Contraindications: Refer for diagnosis

Premenstrual syndrome Symptoms/definition: Occurs approximately one week before onset of period; breast tenderness, swelling, fluid retention, headache, irritability, anxiety, depression, poor concentration
    Indications: Massage beneficial
    Contraindications: Refer if symptoms are severe

Toxic shock syndrome Symptoms/definition: *Staphylococcus* bacterial infection aggravated by use of tampons; life-threatening; initial flulike symptoms with red rash; preventable with regular changing of tampons several times per day. (Note: this condition has occurred in women who do not use tampons.)
    Indications: N/A
    Contraindications: Refer immediately

Pelvic inflammatory disease Symptoms/definition: Inflammation of the uterus, fallopian tubes, ovaries and surrounding tissue; infection often introduced by intercourse; pain and tenderness in lower abdomen and backache; pain during intercourse, heavy periods and vaginal discharge
    Indications: N/A
    Contraindications: Refer to physician for diagnosis

Breast cancer Symptoms/definition: Abnormal tissue growth on or in breast; malignant; most common cause of cancer in women; encourage monthly self-breast exam and regular check-ups
    Indications: Be aware of changes in tissue around axillary region
    Contraindications: Refer; early diagnosis important

Testicular cancer Symptoms/definition: Malignant growth in testicle; usually slow growing lump
    Indications: N/A
    Contraindications: Refer immediately if there are symptoms

Sexually transmitted diseases:

Gonorrhea Symptoms/definition: Bacterial infection; painful urination, pus or cloudy discharge; may be asymptomatic
    Indications: N/A
    Contraindications: Refer—contagious; follow sanitation requirements

Syphilis Symptoms/definition: Bacterial infection; stage one—red sore or chancre appears; stage two—flulike symptoms; stage three—attacks brain and nervous tissue
    Indications: N/A
    Contraindications: Refer—contagious; follow sanitation requirements

Herpes genitalia Symptoms/definition: Viral-induced; blisterlike lesions
    Indications: N/A
    Contraindications: Refer to physician for treatment; follow sanitation requirements

HIV Symptoms/definition: Viral-induced; blood and body fluid transmitted
    Indications: Massage beneficial with physician recommendations; follow antiviral precautions for control of virus with 10% bleach solution; avoid body fluid contact; immediately wash area thoroughly with antiviral agent should body fluid contact occur
    Contraindications: Refer to physician for treatment; follow sanitation requirements; see Chapter 5.

Psychiatric

Assessment parameters include general appearance and behavior, sensorium, mood and affect, thought content, and intellectual capacity.

Deviations suggesting the need for evaluation and referral include marked changes in posture; dress and hygiene; motor activity; speech and facial expression; lack of orientation to time, place, or person; inappropriate manifestation of anxiety, agitation, anger, euphoria, or depression; presence of hallucinations, delusions, paranoia, illusions; changes in usual intellectual capacity; or suicidal or homicidal ideation.

Specific disease processes:

Symptoms/definition: Anxiety; depression (bipolar or manic/depressive disorders), all types of emotionally erratic or unusual behavior may be symptomatic; listen to conversation carefully; often symptoms are subtle and client may try to hide discomfort; anorexia (self-starvation); bulimia (eating and vomiting and/or laxative abuse); addictive disorders, chemical and compulsive behavior; somatization disorder, manifestation of physical pain or symptoms from emotional causes; posttraumatic stress disorders, often associated with sexual and physical childhood abuse.

Indications: Massage beneficial under direction of psychiatrist or psychologist; always work within treatment parameters of the doctor or counselor.

Contraindications: Refer for counseling care; client will often disassociate from body or be hypersensitive to stimulation; it is important for therapist to be sensitive to psychiatric issues; many times the massage therapist is the first one with whom the client will share these issues; it is important to refer for competent counseling and psychiatric care.

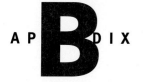

PUBLICATIONS

Bodywork Entrepreneur
584 Castro St.
Suite 373
San Francisco, CA 94114
415-861-4746

Holistic Health Directory
NewAge Journal
342 Western Ave.
Brighton, MA 12135-9907

Massage
Noah Publishing Company
P.O. Box 1500
Davis, CA 95617

Massage Therapy Journal
820 Davis St.
Suite 100 Subscriptions
Evanston, IL 60201-4444
708-864-0123

Touch Therapy Times
13407 Tower Rd.
Thurmont, MD 21788

The Journal of Alternative and Complementary Medicine
Green Library LTD.
Mariner House, 53a High St.
Bagshot Surrey, GU195AH, UK

The Journal of Soft Tisue Manipulation
(An International Journal Sponsored by the Ontario Massage
Therapist Association—OMTA)
950 Yonge St.
Suite 1007
Toronto, ON M4W 2J4
416-968-6818

BOOKS

Massage: A Career at Your FingerTips
Martin Ashley, J.D., L.M.T.
Stanton Hill Press, Inc., Barrytown, New York 12507
Distributed by The Talman Company
ISBN 0-88268-135-4

Business Mastery
Cherie Sohnen-Moe
Sohnen-Moe Associates
3906 W. Ina Rd. #200-348
Tucson, AZ 85741

The Insurance Reimbursement Manual
Christine Rosche
1-800-888-1516
10441 Pharlap Dr.
Cupertino, CA 95014

PROFESSIONAL ORGANIZATIONS IN EXISTENCE FIVE YEARS OR LONGER:

ABMP (Associated Bodywork and Massage Professionals)
28677 Buffalo Park Road
Evergreen, CO 80439-7347
800-458-ABMP or 303-674-8478

AMTA (American Massage Therapy Association)
820 Davis St.
Suite 100
Evanston, IL 60201-4444
708-864-0123

IMF (International Myomassethics Federation)
17172 Bolsa Chica #60
Huntington Beach, CA 92649
800-433-4IMF (4463)

OTHER ORGANIZATIONS

NANMT (National Association of Nurse Massage Therapists)
P.O. Box 67
Tuckahow, NY 10707
914-961-3251

Physical Medicine Research Foundation
#510-207 West Hastings St.
Vancouver, BC Canada V6B 1H7
604-684-6247

National Certification Examination for Therapeutic Massage
and Bodywork
1-800-622-3231

BUSINESS SERVICES

Service Corps of Retired Executives (SCORE)
1825 Connecticut Avenue NW
Suite 503
Washington, DC 20009
800-368-5855
202-653-6279

U.S. Chamber of Commerce
1615 H Street NW
Washington, DC 20062
800-638-6582
202-659-6000

U.S. Small Business Administration (SBA)
1441 L Street NW
Washington, DC 20062
800-368-5855
202-653-6822

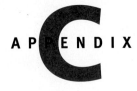

APPENDIX C

WORKS CONSULTED

The following works have been used by the author in the development of this text. They are listed by chapter in alphabetical order.

* – denotes a recommended reading for further study

** – denotes a recommended companion textbook and/or reference

CHAPTER 1

Arvedson J: *Medical Gymnastics and Massage in General Practice* London, 1930, J.A.Churchill.

Arvedson J: *The Techniques, Effects, and Uses of Swedish Medical Gymnastics and Massage.* London, 1931, J.A. Churchill.

Baumgartner AJ: *Massage in Athletics,* Minneapolis, 1947, Brugess Publishing Company.

Benjamin, P: Massage Therapy in the 1940s and the College of Swedish Massage in Chicago *Massage Therapy Journal* Fall 32 (4):56, 1993.

Beard G: A history of massage technic, *Phy Ther Rev* 32:613–624, 1952.

Cantu RI and Grodin AJ: *Myofascial Manipulation Theory and Clinical Application,* Gaithersburg, Md, 1992, Aspen Publishers, Inc.

Chaitow L: Massage moves mainstream into a UK university *International Journal of Alternative and Complementary Medicine,* 1993.

Chaitow L: *Soft Tissue Manipulation,* Rochester Vermont, 1988, Healing Arts Press.

Despard LL: *Text-Book of Massage and Remedial Gymnastics,* ed 3, New York, 1932, Oxford University Press.

Graham, D: The history of massage *The Medical Record* approximately 1874.

Graham D: Massage, *Med Surg Rep* XXXL (10), 1874.

Graham D: *A Treatise on Massage Its History, Mode of Application and Effects,* ed 3, Philadelphia, 1902, Lippincott.

Greenman, PE: *Principles of Manual Medicine,* Baltimore, 1989, Williams and Wilkins, 1989.

Gurevich D: *Historical Perspective,* unpublished article, 1992.

Johnson W: *The Antriptic Art and Medical Rubbing,* London, 1866, Simpkin, Marshall and Co.

Kellogg JH: *The Art of Massage,* Battle Creek, MI, 1929, Modern Medicine Publishing Co.

Knott M and Voss DE: *Proprioceptive Neuromuscular Facilitation: Patterns and Techniques,* ed 2, New York, Harper and Row, 1968.

Kleen E: *Massage and Medical Gymnastics,* ed 2, New York, 1921, William Wood Co.

Lewit K: *Manipulative Therapy in Rehabilitation of the Locomotor System,* ed 2, Oxford, 1991, Butterworth-Heinemann Ltd.

McMillian M: *Massage and Therapeutic Exercise,* ed 3, Philadelphia, 1932, W.B. Saunders.

Norstrom G: *Handbook of Massage,* New York, 1896, The Faculty of Stockholm.

Post SE: *Massage: A Primer for Nurses,* New York, 1891, Nightingale Publishing.

Roth M: *Hand-book of the Movement Cure,* London, 1856, Groombridge and Sons.

Tappan FM: *Massage Techniques: A Case Method Approach,* New York, 1961, Macmillian.

Tappan FM: *Healing Massage Techniques, Holistic, Classic, and Emerging Methods,* ed 2, Norwalk, CN, 1988, Appleton and Lange.

Taylor CF: *Theory and Practice of the Movement Cure by the Swedish System,* Philadelphia, 1861, Lindsay and Blakiston.

van Why R: *History of Massage and Its Relevance to Today's Practitioner,* The Bodywork Knowledgebase, 1992.

van Why R: *Lecture on the History of Massage in Four Parts,* The Bodywork Knowledgebase, 1992.

van Why R: *Notes Toward a History of Massage,* ed 2, The Bodywork Knowledgebase, 1992.

CHAPTER 2

Administrative Rules of Michigan Occupational Regulations Department of Licensing and Regulation. Michigan Department of Commerce, Lansing, MI, 1994.

American Massage Therapy Association: *American Massage Therapy Association Code of Ethics,* Chicago, IL, The Association.

*Ashley M: *Massage: A Career at Your Fingertips,* New York, 1992, Station Hill Press.

Bass E and Davis L: *The Courage to Heal: A Guide for Women Survivors of Child Sexual Abuse,* New York, 1988, Harper and Row.

Blanchard K and Peale NV: *The Power of Ethical Management,* New York, 1988, William Morrow and Company, Inc.

Carlson K, Barbara RA, Schatz A: Is state regulation of massage illegal? *Massage and Bodywork Quarterly* Fall: 42–52, 1993.

Denny NW and Quadagno D: *Human Sexuality,* ed 2, St. Louis, 1992, Mosby-Year Book.

Guidelines for Core Curriculum For Massage Therapy School, Board of Directors of Masseurs-Province of Ontario, 1992. *Regulated Health Professions Act and the Massage Therapy Act.* Ontario, Canada, Standards of Practice. June 1992.

Guidelines for Core Curriculum For Massage Therapy School, Board of Directors of Masseurs-Province of Ontario, 1992. *Therapeutic Massage Curriculum Guidelines,* Toronto, Ontario.

International Myomassethics Federation, Inc: *Code of Ethics,* Huntington Beach, CA, 1993.

In Touch with the Future Massage Therapy in the 90's: Issues of Professional Development, Chicago, IL, 1990, American Massage Therapy Association.

Kohn A: Shattered innocence, *Psychology Today.* Feb: 54–58, 1987.

Legislative updates, Touch Therapy Times October 1993.

National Certification Examination for Therapeutic Massage and Bodywork: Candidate Handbook, Lansing, MI, 1993, The Psychological Corporation.

Occupational Regulation Section of the Michigan Public Health Code, Articles 1, 7, 15, and 19 of Act 368 of 1978. Michigan Department of Licensing and Regulation, Lansing, Michigan.

Oregon Administrative Rules, Board of Massage Technicians Chapter 334 Division 10 Massage Licensing, Portland, OR, July 1991, Oregon Board of Massage Technicians.

Palmer D: *Defining our profession: strategies for inventing the future of massage, Massage and Bodywork Quarterly* Summer: 28–32, 1993.

Pearson JC and Spitzberg BH: *Interpersonal Communication: Concept, Components, and Contexts,* ed 2, Dubuque, IA, 1987, Wm. C. Brown.

Sohnen-Moe C: Business ethics, *Massage.* Jan-Feb: 44–46, 1994.

Sorrentino SA: *Mosby's Textbook for Nursing Assistants,* ed 3, St. Louis, 1992, Mosby-Year Book.

State Medical Board of Ohio: *4731-1-05 Scope of Practice of Massage.* January 1992.

State of Florida. Massage Practice Act, Chapter 480. No. 1993.

**Successful Business Handbook,* Evergreen, CO, 1993, Associated Bodywork and Massage Professionals.

Texas Public Health Act. 4512K, Title 71. *Regulation of Massage Therapists and Massage Establishments.* Chapter 141 Jan. 1990.

**Thibodeau GA and Patton K: *The Human Body in Health and Disease,* St. Louis, 1992, Mosby–Year Book.

Touch Training Directory. Evergreen, CO, 1993, Associated Bodywork and Massage Professionals.

Waites E: *Trauma and Survival: Post-Traumatic and Dissociative Disorder in Women.* New York, 1993, W. W. Norton and Co.

Warren DM: An analysis of existing law governing licensed and unlicensed health practices, *American Holistic Medicine,* vol. 1, 1979.

Washington State. *The Law Relating to Massage Therapy,* 18.108 RCW, 1991.

Williams KM: Taking the "parlor" out of massage, *Zoning and Planning News* 7; 6–13, 1989.

**Yates J: *A Physician's Guide to Therapeutic Massage: Its Physiological Effects and their Application To Treatment,* Vancouver, B.C. Massage Therapists Association of British Columbia, 1990.

CHAPTER 3

**Birmingham JJ: *Medical Terminology: A Self-Learning Text,* ed 2, St. Louis, 1990, C.V. Mosby.

**Brooks ML: *Exploring Medical Language, A Student-Directed Approach,* ed 3, St. Louis, 1994, Mosby Lifeline.

Sorrentino SA: *Mosby's Textbook for Nursing Assistants,* ed 3, St Louis, 1992, Mosby–Year Book.

Thomas CL: *Taber's Cyclopedic Medical Dictionary,* ed 16, Philadelphia, 1985, F.A. Davis.

**Thibodeau GA and Patton K: *The Human Body in Health and Disease.* St. Louis, 1992, Mosby–Year Book.

CHAPTER 4

Bulluck BL and Rosendahl PP: *Pathophysiology Adaptations and Alterations in Function,* ed 3, Philadelphia, 1992, Lippincott.

Dean BZ and Geiringer SR: Physiatric therapeutics, 5. pain, *Arch Phys Med Rehabil* 71: S-271-274, 1990.

*Cantu RI and Grodin AJ: *Myofascial Manipulation Theory and Clinical Application,* Gaithersburg, Md, 1992, Aspen Publishers, Inc.

Chaitow L: *Osteopathic Self-Treatment,* London, 1990, Thorsons.

*Chaitow L: *Palpatory Literacy.* London, 1991, Thorsons.

*Chaitow L: *Soft-Tissue Manipulation.* Rochester Vermont, 1988, Healing Arts Press.

*Chaitow L: *Soft Tissue Manipulation and Neuromuscular Techniques: Improving Palpatory Literacy and Treatment Efficiency.* Soft Tissue Manipulation Seminar, 1991.

deGroot J and Chusid JG: *Correlative Neuroanatomy*, ed 20, San Mateo, CA, 1985, Appleton and Lange.

Ganong WF: *Review of Medical Physiology*, ed 13, Norwalk, CN, 1987, Appleton and Lange.

*Greenman PE: *Principles of Manual Medicine*, Baltimore, 1989, Williams and Wilkins.

Hahn DB and Payne WA: *Focus on Health*, ed 2, St. Louis, 1994, Mosby–Year Book.

Melzack R: TP Relationship to mechanisms of pain, *Arch Phys Med Rehabil*. 62: 114–117, 1981.

Nimmi ME: *Collagen Vol I Biochemistry*, Boca Raton, 1988, CRC Press.

Ontario, Canada Therapeutic Massage Curriculum Guidelines, Toronto, Ontario, Board of Directors of Masseurs-Province of Ontario, 1992.

Oregon Board of Massage Technicians: Sanitation Requirements for the State of Oregon, Portland, OR, Oregon Administrative Rules, 1991.

Scull CW: Massage—physiological basis, *Arch Phys Med* 159-167, 1945.

*Selye H: *The Stress of Life*, ed 2, New York, 1978, McGraw-Hill.

Shealy NC: The neurochemical substrate of behavior, *Psychol Health Immun Dis* B: 434–456, 1992.

*Sheridan CL and Radmacher SA: *Health Psychology: Challenging the Biomedical Model*, New York, 1992, John Wiley and Sons, Inc.

Tate P, Seeley RR, Stephens TD: *Understanding the Human Body*, St Louis, 1994, Mosby–Year Book.

**Thibodeau GA and Patton K: *The Human Body in Health and Disease*, St. Louis, 1992, Mosby–Year Book.

**Thibodeau GA: *Structure and Function of the Body*, St Louis, 1992, Mosby–Year Book.

Thomas CL, ed: *Taber's Cyclopedic Medical Dictionary*, Philadelphia, 1985, F.A. Davis.

**Thompson CW: *Manual of Structural Kinesiology*, ed 10, St. Louis, 1985 Times Mirror/Mosby College Publishing.

Timms R and Connors P: *Embodying Healing: Integrating Bodywork and Psychotherapy in Recovery from Childhood Sexual Abuse*. Orwell, VT, 1992, The Safer Society Press.

Waites EA: *Trauma and Survival: Post-traumatic and Dissociative Disorders in Women*. New York, 1993, Norton.

Yates J: *Physiological Effects of Therapeutic Massage and their Application to Treatment*. British Columbia, 1989, Massage Therapist Association.

CHAPTER 5

Bulluck BL and Rosendahl PP: *Pathophysiology Adaptations and Alterations in Function*, ed 3, Philadelphia, 1992, Lippincott.

**Hamann B: *Disease: Identification, Prevention and Control*. St. Louis, 1994, Mosby–Year Book.

Ontario, Canada Therapeutic Massage Curriculum Guidelines, Toronto, Ontario, Board of Directors of Masseurs-Province of Ontario, 1992.

Sanitation Requirements for the State of Oregon, Oregon Board of Massage Technicians. Portland, OR, Oregon Administrative Rules, 1991.

Sorrentino SA: *Mosby's Textbook for Nursing Assistants*, ed 3, St. Louis, 1992, Mosby–Year Book.

**Thibodeau GA and Patton K: *The Human Body in Health and Disease*, St. Louis, 1992, Mosby–Year Book.

CHAPTER 6

Alcock J: *Animal Behavior: An Evaluatory Approach,* Sunderland, MA, 1989, Sinawer Assoc.

**Anderson LE and Glanze WD, eds: *Mosby's Medical, Nursing, and Allied Health Dictionary,* ed 4, St. Louis, 1990, Mosby–Year Book.

*Baldry PE: *Acupuncture, Triggers Points and Musculoskeletal Pain.* New York, 1989, Churchill Livingstone.

Bullock BL and Rosendahl PP: *Pathophysiology Adaptations and Alteration in Function,* ed 3, Philadelphia, 1992, Lippincott.

*Cailliet R: *Soft Tissue Pain and Disability,* Philadelphia, 1977, FA Davis.

*Cantu RI and Grodin AJ: *Myofascial Manipulation Theory and Clinical Application,* Gaithersburg, Md, 1992, Aspen Publishers, Inc.

*Chaitow L: *Soft-Tissue Manipulation,* Vermont, 1988, Healing Arts Press.

Dean BZ and Geiringer SR: Physiatric Therapeutics. 5. Pain, *Arch Phys Med Rehabil* 71:S-271-S-274, 1990.

deGroot J and Chusid JG: *Correlative Neuroanatomy,* ed 20, San Mateo, CA, 1985, Appleton & Lange.

Ernst M and Lee MHM: Sympathetic effects of manual and electrical acupuncture of the Tsusanli knee point: comparison with the Huko hand point sympathetic effects, *Exp Neurol* 1986.

Ganong WF: *Review of Medical Physiology,* ed 13. Norwalk, CN, 1987, Appleton & Lange.

Gewirtz D: Touchpoints Vol 1. No. 1 Edited by Miami Touch Research Institute, 1993.

*Greenman PE: *Principles of Manual Medicine,* Baltimore, 1989, Williams & Wilkins.

Gunn, CC: *Reprints on Pain, Acupuncture and Related Subjects,* Seattle, 1992, University of Washington.

Gunn CC: Clinical Research Unit, Rehabilitation Clinic. J Acupuncture 6. 1978.

*Hooper J and Teresi D: *The Three Pound Universe,* New York, 1986, Dell Publishing.

Levin SR: Acute Effects of Massage on the Stress Response, thesis, Greensboro, 1990, University of North Carolina.

Longworth J: Psychophysiological effects of slow stroke back massage in normotensive females, *Adv Nursing Sci* 44–61, 1982.

*Manheim CJ and Lavett DK: *The Myofascial Release Manual,* Thorofare, NJ, 1989, Slack.

Marieb E: *Human Anatomy and Physiology,* ed 2, 1992, The Benjamin/Cummings Publishing, Redwood City, CA.

McArdle WD, et al.: *Exercise Physiology Energy Nutrition and Human Performance,* ed 3, Philadelphia, 1991, Lea and Febiger.

NNIH Funds Massage Studies. *Hands On, The Newsletter of the American Massage Therapy Association,* Vol IX NO 4, Winter, 1993.

Research at TRI. *Touch Therapy Times,* vol 5, no 5, May 1994.

*Selye H: *The Stress of Life,* ed 2, New York, 1978, McGraw-Hill.

Selye H: *The Healing Brain: Understanding Stress, Stress Without Distress,* BMA Series: Stress and Behavior Medicine, edited by Gary Swartz, Ph.D. Biomonitoring Application, Inc., New York, (cassette), Los Altos, CA, ISHK Paperbacks.

Shealy NC: The neurochemical substrate of behavior. *Psychol Health Immun Dis* B: 434–456, 1992.

Thomas CL, ed: *Taber's Cyclopedic Medical Dictionary,* ed 16, Philadelphia, 1985, FA Davis.

**Thibodeau GA and Patton KT: *The Human Body in Health and Disease,* St. Louis, 1992, Mosby–Year Book.

Tortora GJ and Grabowski SR: *Principles of Anatomy and Physiology*, ed 7, New York, 1992, Harper Collins College Publishers.

Touch Research, Int J Alternative and Complementary Med 11: 7, 1993.

*Travell JG and Simons DG: *Myofascial Pain and Dysfunction: The Trigger Point Manual*, Baltimore, 1984, Waverly Press, Williams and Wilkins.

*Travell JG and Simons DG: *Myofascial Pain and Dysfunction: The Trigger Point Manual: The Lower Extremities*, vol 2, Baltimore: 1992, Williams and Wilkins.

van Why R: History of massage and its relevance to today's practitioner, 1992 (self-published).

Wale JO: *Tidy's Massage and Remedial Exercises*, 1968, ed 11, rev England, 1987, John Wright & Sons Ltd.

Work Modification, Work Hardening, and Work Rehabilitation (Cassette #22), Physical Medicine Research Foundation 3rd. International Symposium, 1990 Vancouver, British Columbia.

Yates J: *Physiological Effects of Therapeutic Massage and their Application to Treatment*. British Columbia, 1989, Massage Therapists Association.

CHAPTER 7

Bliss E: *Getting Things Done*, Boulder, CO, 1986 (cassette series).

Calano J and Salzman J: *Success Shortcuts, 25 Career Skills You Were Never Taught, But Must Know*, Chicago, Career Track Publications, Boulder, CO (cassette series).

*Capo M: *The Business of Massage: a Manual for Students and Professionals*. New York, 1992, Ten Plus Ten.

Jordan DM: An analysis of existing law governing licensed and unlicensed health practices, *Am Holistic Med* 1, 1979.

Ornstein R and Ehrlich P: *New World New Mind: Moving Toward Conscious Evolution*. New York, 1989, Doubleday.

Successful Business Handbook. Evergreen, CO, 1993, Associated Bodywork and Massage Professionals.

Touch Training Directory. Evergreen, CO, Associated Bodywork and Massage Professionals, 1993.

Tracy B: *The Psychology of Achievement*, Chicago, Brian Tracy Learning Symposium, Solana Beach, CA (cassette series).

Verbury K: *Managing the Modern Michigan Township*. Lansing, MI, 1990, Community Development Publishers, Michigan State University.

CHAPTER 8

Birnbaum JS: *The Musculoskeletal Manual*, ed 2, Philadelphia, 1986, W.B. Saunders.

Kreighbaum E and Barthels KM: *Biomechanics: A Qualitative Approach for Studying Human Movement*, ed 2, New York, 1985, Macmillan.

Lehmkuhl LD and Smith LK: *Brunnstrom's Clinical Kinesiology*, ed 4, Philadelphia, 1983, F.A. Davis.

Norkin CC and Levangie PK: *Joint Structure and Function: a Comprehensive Analysis*, ed 2, Philadelphia, 1992, F.A. Davis.

Sorrentino SA: *Mosby's Textbook for Nursing Assistants*, ed 3, St Louis, 1992, Mosby–Year Book.

CHAPTER 9

Sorrentino SA: *Mosby's Textbook for Nursing Assistants*, ed 3, St Louis, 1992, Mosby–Year Book.

Small C: *A Handbook for the Holistic Health Practitioner.* Irving, TX 1983, (self-published).

CHAPTER 10

Arvedson J: *Medical Gymnastics and Massage in General Practice.* London, 1930, J.A. Churchill.

Arvedson J: *The Techniques, Effects and Uses of Swedish Medical Gymnastics and Massage.* London, 1931, J.A. Churchill.

*Basmajian JV, ed: *Manipulation Traction and Massage,* ed 3, Baltimore, 1985, Williams and Wilkins.

Baumgartner AJ: *Massage in Athletics,* Minneapolis, 1947, Brugess Publishing Company.

Beard G: A history of massage technic, *Phys Ther Rev* 32: 613–624, 1952.

Breakey BM: An overlooked therapy you can use ad lib, *Registered Nurse* July: 50-54, 1982.

Bishop B: Vibratory stimulation, *Phys Ther* 54:1273-1281, 1974.

Carpenter IC. *A Practical Guide to Massage,* Baltimore, 1937, William Wood and Co.

*Chaitow L: *Osteopathic Self-Treatment,* London, 1990, Thorsons.

*Chaitow L: *Palpatory Literacy,* London, 1991, Thorsons.

*Chaitow L: *Soft-Tissue Manipulation,* Rochester, VT, 1988, Healing Arts Press.

*Chaitow L: *Soft Tissue Manipulation and Neuromuscular Techniques: Improving Palpatory Literacy and Treatment Efficiency,* Soft Tissue Manipulation Seminar, Lapeer, MI, 1991.

Cyriax E: Some misconceptions concerning mechano-therapy, *Br J Phys Med* 92–94, 1938.

Cyriax J: Treatment by movement, *Bri Med J* 1944.

*Danials L and Worthingham C: *Muscle Testing Techniques of Manual Examination,* ed 5, Philadelphia, 1986, W.B. Saunders.

Darian-Smith I: Touch in primates, *Ann Rev* 157–186, 1982.

De Puy CE: Remarks on the efficacy of friction in palsy and apoplexy, Oct. 1817.

Despard LL: *Text-Book of Massage and Remedial Gymnastics,* ed 3, New York, 1932, Oxford University Press.

Eccles AS: *The Practice of Massage: Its Physiological Effects and Therapeutic Uses,* ed 2, London, 1898, Bailliere, Tindall, and Cox.

Frank LK: Tactile communication, *Genet Psychol Monographs* 56: 209-225, 1957.

Gammon GD and Starr I: *Studies on the Relief of Pain by Counterirritation,* Hospital of the University of Pennsylvania, Philadelphia: July, 1940.

Grafstrom AV: *Medical Gymnastics Including the Schott Movements,* London, 1899, The Scientific Press Ltd.

Graham D: The history of massage, *The Medical Record* approximately 1874.

Graham D: Massage, *Med Surg Rep* XXXL 1874.

Graham D: *A Treatise on Massage Its History, Mode of Application and Effects,* ed 3, Philadelphia, 1902, J.B. Lippincott.

*Greenman PE: *Principles of Manual Medicine,* Baltimore, 1989, Williams and Wilkins.

Hough T: *A Review of Swedish Gymnastics,* Boston, 1899, George Ellis.

Jensen K: *Fundamentals in Massage for Students of Nursing,* New York, 1936, Macmillan.

Johnson W: *The Antriptic Art and Medical Rubbing,* London, 1866, Simpkin, Marshall and Co.

Kellogg JH: *The Art of Massage,* Battle Creek, MI, 1929, Modern Medicine Publishing Co.

Kisner CD and Taslitz N: Connective tissue massage: influence of the introductory treatment on autonomic functions, *Phys Ther* 48: 107–119, 1967.

Kleen E: *Massage and Medical Gymnastics,* ed 2, New York, 1921, William Wood Co.

Knapp ME: Massage, physical medicine and rehabilitation. *Postgrad Med* 192-195, 1968.

Lewit K: *Manipulative Therapy in Rehabilitation of the Locomotor System,* ed 2, Oxford, 1991, Butterworth-Heinemann Ltd.

Melzack R: Hyperstimulation analgesia, *Clin Anesthesiol* 3: 81–91, 1985.

Mennell JB: *Physical Treatment by Movement, Manipulation, and Massage,* London, 1940, J.A. Churchill.

McMillian M: *Massage and Therapeutic Exercise,* ed 3, Philadelphia, 1932, W.B. Saunders.

McNaught AB and Callander R: *Illustrated Physiology,* ed 4, New York, 1983, Churchill Livingstone.

Mulliner MR: *Mechano-Therapy,* Philadelphia, 1929, Lea and Febiger.

Norstrom G: *Handbook of Massage,* New York, 1896, The Faculty of Stockholm.

Post SE: *Massage: A Primer for Nurses,* New York, 1891, Nightingale Publishing.

Preuss' J: In Fred Rosner, editor, *Biblical and Talmudic Medicine,* New York, Sanhedrin Press.

Roth M: *Hand-book of the Movement Cure,* London, 1856, Groombridge and Sons.

Scull CW: Massage–physiological basis, *Arch Phys Med* 159–167, 1945.

Tappan FM: *Massage Techniques: A Case Method Approach,* New York, 1961, Macmillan Company.

Taylor CF: *Theory and Practice of the Movement Cure by the Swedish System,* Philadelphia, 1861, Lindsay and Blakiston.

Taylor GH: *An Illustrated Sketch of the Movement Cure: Its Principle Methods and Effects,* New York, 1866, (self-published).

The Elements of Kellgren's Manual Treatment, New York, 1901, William Wood and Co.

**Thibodeau GA and Patton K: *The Human Body in Health and Disease,* St. Louis, 1992, Mosby–Year Book.

**Thibodeau GA: *Structure and Function of the Body,* St Louis, 1992, Mosby–Year Book.

Wall PD: Pain, itch, and vibration, *Arch Neurol* 2: 365-374, 1960.

CHAPTER 11

Alfaro R: *Applying Nursing Diagnosis and Nursing Process: A Step-by-Step Guide,* ed 2, Philadelphia, 1990, Lippincott.

*Basmajian JV, ed. *Manipulation Traction and Massage,* ed 3, Baltimore, 1985, Williams and Wilkins.

Birnbaum JS: *The Musculoskeletal Manual,* ed 2, Philadelphia, 1986, W.B. Saunders.

**Cailliet R: *Soft Tissue Pain and Disability,* Philadelphia, 1988, F. A. Davis.

**Chaitow L: *Palpatory Literacy,* Hammersmith, London: 1991, Thorsons Harper Collins.

**Chaitow L: *Osteopathic Self-Treatment.* 1990, Thorsons Harper Collins.

**Chaitow L: *Soft Tissue Manipulation,* Rochester, VT, 1988, Healing Arts Press.

Clark J, ed: *The Human Body*, New York, 1989, Arch Cape Press.

**Daniels L and Worthingham C: *Therapeutic Exercise for Body Alignment and Function*, ed 2, Philadelphia, 1977, W.B. Saunders.

**Daniels L and Worthingham C: *Muscle Testing Techniques of Manual Examination*, ed 5, 1986.

deGrout J and Chusid JG: *Correlative Neuroanatomy*, ed 12, East Norwalt, Connecticut, 1985, Appleton and Lange.

**Greenman PE: *Principles of Manual Medicine*, Baltimore, 1989, Williams and Wilkins.

**Gunn CC: *Treating Myofascial Pain*, Seattle, 1989, Health Services Center for Educational Resources University of Washington.

Hall-Craggs ECB: *Anatomy as a Basis for Clinical Medicine*, Baltimore, 1985, Urban and Schwarzenberg.

Kapit W and Elson M: *The Anatomy Coloring Book*, New York, 1977, Harper Collins.

Kreighbaum E and Barthels KM: *Biomechanics: A Qualitative Approach for Studying Human Movement*, ed 2, New York, 1985, Macmillan.

Lehmkuhl LD and Smith LK: *Brunnstrom's Clinical Kinesiology*, ed 4, Philadelphia, 1983, F.A. Davis.

LeVay D: *Human Anatomy and Physiology*, Binge Suffolk, 1974, Hodder and Stoughton Ltd.

*Lewit K: *Manipulative Therapy in Rehabilitation of the Locomotor System*, ed 2, Oxford, 1991, Butterworth-Heinemann Ltd.

Memmler RL and Wood DL: *Structure and Function of the Human Body*, ed 3, Philadelphia, 1983, Lippincott.

**Mennell J: *The Musculoskeletal System Differential Diagnosis from Symptoms and Physical Signs*, Gaithersburg, MO, 1992, Aspen.

McNaught AB and Callander R: *Illustrated Physiology*, ed 4, New York, 1983, Churchill Livingstone.

Norkin CC and Levangie PK: *Joint Structure and Function: a Comprehensive Analysis*, ed 2, Philadelphia, 1992, F.A. Davis.

Sorrentino SA: *Mosby's Textbook for Nursing Assistants*, ed 3, St. Louis, 1992, Mosby–Year Book.

Sparks SM and Taylor CM: *Nursing Diagnosis Reference Manual*, ed 2, Springhouse, PA, 1993, Springhouse.

The Academy of Traditional Chinese Medicine. *An Outline of Chinese Acupuncture*, Peking, 1975, Foreign Language Press.

Tate P, Seeley RR, Stephens TD: *Understanding the Human Body*, St. Louis, 1994, Mosby–Year Book.

**Thibodeau GA and Patton KT: *The Human Body in Health and Disease*, St. Louis, 1992, Mosby–Year Book.

**Thibodeau GA: *Structure and Function of the Body*, ed 9, 1992.

*Travell JG and Simons DG: *Myofascial Pain and Dysfunction the Trigger Point Manual*, Baltimore, 1883, Williams and Wilkins.

Wale JO, ed. *Tidy's Massage and Remedial Exercises*, ed 11, Bristol, England, 1987, John Wright & Sons Ltd.

Walther DS: *Applied Kinesiology Synopsis*, Pueblo, CO, 1988, SDC Systems.

CHAPTER 12

Allison TG: How to counsel patients with chronic fatigue syndrome, *Psychol Health Immun Dis* A: 5-21, 1992.

Bandler R and Grinder J: *Patterns of the Hypnotic Techniques of Milton H. Erickson, M.D*, vol 1, Cupertino, CA, 1975, Meta Publications.

Bass E and Davis L: *The Courage to Heal: A Guide for Women Survivors of Child Sexual Abuse,* New York, 1988, Harper and Row.

Calvert R: Dolores Krieger, PhD and her therapeutic touch, *Massage.* Jan/Feb 47: 56–60, 1994.

Cunningham AJ: The healing journey: how to organize healing efforts at the psychological, social, and spiritual levels, *Phych Health Immun Dis* A: 63–72, 1992.

Denny NW and Quadagno D: *Human Sexuality,* ed 2, St. Louis, 1992, Mosby–Year Book.

Doore G, ed. *Shaman's Path: Healing, Personal Growth and Empowerment,* Boston, 1988, Shambhala Publications.

Hahn DB and Payne WA: *Focus on Health,* ed 2, St. Louis, 1994, Mosby–Year Book.

Hammerschlag CA: *The Dancing Healers: A Doctor's Journey of Healing with Native Americans,* San Francisco, 1988, Harper.

Jevne R: Enhancing hope in the chronically ill, *Phychol Health Immun Dis* A: 127-150, 1992.

Kohn A: Shattered innocence, *Psychol Today,* Feb: 54–58, 1987.

Kubler-Ross E: *To Live Until We Say Goodbye.* Englewood Cliffs, New Jersey, 1978, Prentice-Hall.

Lee D: Amplifying the power of visualization techniques with neuro-linguistic programming, *Phychol Health Immun Dis* A: 215–248, 1992.

Ludhman R: *The Sociological Outlook,* ed 3, San Diego, 1992, Collegiate Press.

McArdle WD, et al.: *Exercise Physiology: Energy Nutrition and Human Performance,* ed 3, Philadelphia, 1991, Lea and Febiger.

McGladrey and Pullen. *The Americans With Disabilities Act* (Rev), New York, 1994, Panel Publishers.

Mower MB: An interview with Tiffany Field, Ph.D. Director of the Touch Therapy Research Institute, *Massage* Jan/Feb: 76, 1994.

Mower MB: An interview with Clyde Ford, author of *Compassionate Touch, Massage* Jan/Feb: 77, 1994.

Pearson JC and Spitzberg BH: *Interpersonal Communication: Concept, Components, and Contexts,* ed 2, Dubuque, IA, 1987, Wm. C. Brown.

*Sheridan CL and Radmacher SA: *Health Psychology: Challenging the Biomedical Model,* New York, 1992, John Wiley and Sons, Inc.

*Selye H: *The Stress of Life,* ed 2, New York, 1978, McGraw-Hill.

Shaughnessy J, ed: *The Roots of Ritual,* Grand Rapids, MI, 1973, William B. Eerdmans Publishing.

Shealy NC: The neurochemical substrate of behavior, *Psych Health Immun Dis* B: 434–456, 1992.

Siegal BS: *Peace, Love and Healing,* New York, 1989 Harper and Row.

Sorrentino SA: *Mosby's Textbook for Nursing Assistants,* ed 3, St. Louis, 1992, Mosby–Year Book.

Tate DA: Health, hope, and healing: a survivor's perspective, *Psychol Health Immun Dis* A: 304–321, 1992.

Tate P, Seeley RR, Stephens TD: *Understanding the Human Body,* St. Louis, 1994, Mosby–Year Book.

**Thibodeau GA and Patton K: *The Human Body in Health and Disease,* St. Louis, 1992, Mosby–Year Book.

Timms R and Connors P: *Embodying Healing: Integrating Bodywork and Psychotherapy in Recovery from Childhood Sexual Abuse,* Orwell, VT, 1992, The Safer Society Press.

Upledger JE: Tissue memory, energy cysts and somatoemotional release, *Phychol Health Immun Dis* A: 323–336, 1992.

*Wade C and Tavris C: *Psychology,* ed 2, New York, 1990, Harper.

Waites E: *Trauma and Survival: Post-Traumatic and Dissociative Disorder in Women,* New York, 1993, W. W. Norton and Co.

Work Modification, Work Hardening and Work Rehabilitation, Physical Medicine Research Foundation 3rd International Symposium, 1990, Vancouver, BC, 1990 (cassette #22).

CHAPTER 13

*Baldry PE: *Acupuncture, Triggers Points and Musculoskeletal Pain,* New York, 1989, Churchill Livingstone.

*Basmajian JV, ed: *Manipulation Traction and Massage,* ed 3, Baltimore, 1985, Williams and Wilkins.

Berube R: *Evolutionary Traditions: Unique Approaches to Lymphatic Drainage and Circulatory Massage Techniques.* Hudson, NH, 1988 (self-published).

Buchman DD: *The Complete Book of Water Therapy: 500 ways to Use our Oldest Natural Medicine,* New York, 1979, E.P. Dutton.

Bugaj R: The cooling analgesic, and rewarming effects of ice massage on localized skin, *Phys Ther* 55: 11–19, 1975.

*Cailliet R: *Soft Tissue Pain and Disability,* Philadelphia, 1977, FA Davis.

*Cantu RI and Grodin AJ: *Myofascial Manipulation: Theory and Clinical Application,* Gaithersburg, Md, 1992, Aspen Publishers, Inc.

*Chaitow L: *Soft-Tissue Manipulation,* Vermont, 1988, Healing Arts Press.

Chaitow L: Workshop Notes, Lapeer, MI, 1988, 1991, 1992, 1993.

Chaitow L: Extremely light manipulative methods: time for research, *Int J Alternative Complementary Med* 10: 12-13, 1992.

Ciolek J: Cryotherapy: Review of Physiological Effects on Clinical Application, *Cleveland Clinic Quarterly* 52: 193-201, 1985.

Coulter J: Interview with Hildegard Wittlinger, *J Soft Tissue Manipulation* 1: 12–15, 1993.

Cyriax J and Coldham M: *The Textbook of Orthopaedic Medicine Treatment by Manipulation Massage and Injection,* vol 2, ed 11, East Sussex, England, 1984, Bailliere Tindall.

Ewig J and Provost STP: *An Inaugural Essay on the Effects of Cold upon the Human Body,* Philadelphia, 1797, Joseph Gales.

Gunn CC: *Reprints on Pain, Acupuncture and Related Subjects,* Seattle, 1992, University of Washington. Clinical Research Unit, Rehabilitation Clinic. *J Acupuncture* 6: 1978.

Gunn CC: *Treating Myofascial Pain: Intramuscular Stimulation (IMS) for Myofascial Pain Syndromes of Neuropathic Origin.* Seattle, 1989, University of Washington Medical School.

Harris R: Edema and its treatment in massage therapy, *J Soft Tissue Manipulation* 1:4–6, 1993-94.

Hayden CA: Cyrokinetics in an early treatment program, *J Am Phys Ther Assoc* 44, 1964.

Holmes G: Hydrotherapy and spa treatment, *The Practitioner* CXLI, 1938.

Ingham ED: *Stories the Feet Have Told,* St. Petersburg, FL, 1982, Ingham Publishing Inc.

Kreighbaum E and Barthels KM: *Biomechanics: A Qualitative Approach for Studying Human Movement,* ed 2, New York, 1985, Macmillan.

*Manheim CJ and Lavett DK: *The Myofascial Release Manual,* Thorofare, NJ, 1989, Slack.

Segal M: *Reflexology,* North Hollywood, CA, 1976, Hal Leighton.

Singer E: *Fasciae of the Human Body and their Relations to the Organs The Envelop,* Baltimore, 1935, Williams and Wilkins.

*Travell JG and Simons DG: *Myofascial Pain and Dysfunction: The Trigger Point Manual,* Baltimore, 1984, Waverly Press, Williams and Wilkins.

*Travell JG and Simons DG: *Myofascial Pain and Dysfunction The Trigger Point Manual: The Lower Extremities,* vol 2, Baltimore, 1992, Williams and Wilkins.

Walther DS: *Applied Kinesiology Synopsis,* Pueblo, CO, 1988, SDC Systems.

Yao JH: *Acutherapy.* Acutherapy Postgraduate Seminars, Libertyville, IL 1984.

CHAPTER 14

Allard N and Barnett G: The Power of the Breath Part II *Massage and Bodywork Quarterly* Summer: 47–50, 1993.

Chaitow L: *The Body/Mind Purification Program.* New York, 1991, Fireside.

Hahn DB and Wayne PA: *Focus on Health.* ed 2, St Louis, 1994, Mosby–Year Book.

Lippert L: *Clinical Kinesiology for Physical Therapist Assistants,* Portland, OR, 1991.

Sacks O: An Anthropologist on Mars, *The New Yorker,* Dec: 106–125, 1993.

Selye H: *The Stress of Life,* ed 2, New York, 1978, McGraw-Hill.

Shealy NC: The Neurochemical Substrate of Behavior *The Psychology of Health Immunity and Disease,* vol B, CT, 1992

Sheridan CL and Radmacher SA: *Health Psychology: Challenging the Biomedical Model,* New York, 1992, John Wiley and Sons, Inc.

Tate P, Seeley RR and Stephens TD: *Understanding the Human Body,* St Louis, 1994, Mosby–Year Book.

Travis JW and Ryan RS: *Wellness Workbook,* ed 2, Berkeley CA, 1998, Ten Speed Press.

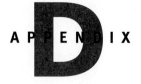

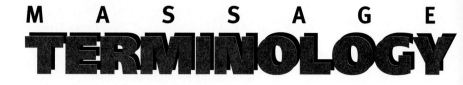

Active joint movement: The client produces the movement of a joint through its range of movement.

Acupressure: Methods used to tone or sedate acupuncture points without the use of needles.

Acupressure point: Eastern term for a specific point that correlates with a neurological motor point.

Acute pain: A symptom of a disease condition, or a temporary aspect of medical treatment. It acts as a warning signal, as it can activate the sympathetic nervous system. It is usually temporary, of sudden onset, and easily localized. The client can frequently describe the pain, which often subsides with or without treatment.

Adaptation: A response to a sensory stimulation in which nerve signalling is reduced or ceases.

Allied health: A division of medicine in which the professional receives training in a specific area of medicine to serve as support for the doctor.

Antagonists: The muscles that oppose the movement of the prime movers.

Application: A record of what was done during the session. A general list of methods used, record of any specific work, and what the response was to the work is recorded during S.O.A.P. note charting.

Applied kinesiology: Methods of evaluation and bodywork that use a specialized type of muscle testing and various forms of massage and bodywork for corrective procedures.

Arterial circulation: Movement of oxygenated blood under pressure from the heart to the body through the arteries.

Arthrokinematic movement: Accessory movements that occur as a result of inherent laxity or joint play that exist in each joint. The joint play allows the ends of the bones to slide roll or spin smooth on each other. These essential movements occur passively with movement of the joint, and are not under voluntary control.

Assessment: The collection and interpretation of information provided by the client, the client's family and friends, the massage practitioner, and referring medical professionals.

Asymmetrical stance: Position in which the body weight is shifted from one foot to the other during standing.

Autonomic nervous system: Regulates involuntary body functions using sympathetic "fight/flight/fear response" and the restorative parasympathetic "relaxation response." Sympathetic and parasympathetic systems work together to maintain homeostasis through a feedback loop system.

Autoregulation: Control of homeostasis by alteration of tissue or function.

Barrier: A restriction of joint or tissue movement. There are two types. Anatomical barriers are from the fit of the bones at the joint. Physiological barriers are from the limits of range-of-motion from protective nerve and sensory function.

Beating: Form of heavy tapotement that uses the fist.

Body mechanics: Use of the body in an efficient and bio-mechanically correct way.

Body/mind: The interaction between thought and physiology connected to the limbic system, hypothalamus influence of the autonomic nervous system, and the endocrine system.

Body segment: Area of the body located between joints that provide movement during walking and balance.

Body supports: Pillows, folded blankets, designed foam, or commercial products that help contour the flat surface of a massage table or mat.

Bodywork: Term describing all of the various forms of massage, movement, and other touch therapies.

Boundary: Personal space located within an arms length perimeter. Personal emotional space is designated by morals, values, and experience.

Centering: The ability to focus on a specific circumstance through screening sensation.

Certification: Voluntary credentialing process usually requiring education and testing, administered either privately or by government regulatory bodies.

Chemical effects: Results from massage due to the release of chemical substances within the body. These may be substances released locally from the massaged tissue, or hormones released into the general circulation.

Chronic pain: Pain that persists or recurs for indefinite periods, usually for more than six months. It frequently has an insidious onset, and the character and quality of the pain changes over time. It frequently involves deep somatic and visceral structures. The pain is usually diffused and poorly localized.

Client information form: Document used to obtain information from the client about health, pre-existing conditions, and expectations of the massage.

Client outcome: The desired results from the massage and the massage therapist.

Client practitioner agreement and policy statement: A detailed written explanation of all rules, expectations, and procedures for the massage.

Coalition: A group formed for a particular purpose.

Cognitive: Conscious awareness and perception, reasoning, judgment, intuition, and memory.

Communicable disease: A disease caused by pathogens that are easily spread; a contagious disease.

Compression: Pressure into the body to spread tissue against underlying structures. (This massage manipulation is sometimes classified with petrissage.)

Compressive force: Amount of pressure against the surface of the body to apply pressure to the deeper body structures; pressure directed in a particular direction.

Concentric isotonic contraction: The massage therapist applies a counterforce but allows the client to move, bringing origin and insertion of the target muscle together against the pressure.

Connective tissue: The most abundant tissue of the body. Its functions include support, structure, space, stabilization, and scar formation.

Contamination: The process by which an object or area becomes unclean.

Contraindication: Any condition that renders a particular treatment improper or undesirable.

Counterirritation: Superficial stimulation that relieves deeper sensation by stimulation of different sensory signals.

Counterpressure: The force applied to an area which is designed to match exactly (isometric contraction) or partially (isotonic contraction) the effort, or force, produced by the muscles of that area.

Cranial sacral and myofascial approaches: Methods of bodywork that work both reflexively and mechanically with the fascial network of the body.

Cream: Type of lubricant that is in a semi-solid or solid state.

Credential: Designation earned by completing a process that verifies a certain level of expertise in a given skill.

Cross-directional stretching: Tissue stretching that pulls and twists connective tissue against its fiber direction.

Cryotherapy: Therapeutic use of ice.

Cupping: Type of tapotement that uses a cupped hand and is often used over the thorax.

Cutaneous sensory receptors: Sensory nerves in the skin.

Depth of pressure: Compressive stress that can be light, moderate, deep, and variable.

Dermatome: Cutaneous (skin) distribution of spinal nerve sensation.

Direction: Flow of massage strokes from the center of the body out (centrifugal), or from the extremities in toward the center of the body (centripetal). Direction can be circular motions; it can be from origin to insertion of the muscle following the muscle fibers, or transverse to the tissue fibers.

Direction of ease: The position the body assumes with postural changes and muscle shortening or weakening depending upon how it has balanced against gravity.

Disclosure: Acknowledging and informing the client of any situation that interferes with or impacts upon the professional relationship.

Disinfection: The process by which pathogens are destroyed.

Drag: The amount of pull (stretch) on the tissue (tensile stress).

Drape: Fabric used to cover the client and keep the client warm while the massage is given.

Draping: The procedures of covering and uncovering areas of the body and turning the client during the massage.

Duration: The length of time the method lasts or stays in the same location.

Eccentric isotonic contraction: The massage therapist applies a counterforce but allows the client to move the jointed area to let origin and insertion separate. The muscle lengthens against the pressure.

Effleurage: (Gliding stroke) Horizontal strokes applied with the fingers, hand, or forearm that usually follow the fiber direction of the underlying muscle, fascial planes, or a dermatome pattern.

Electrical-chemical: Physiological functions of the body that rely on or produce body energy. Often called chi, prana, and meridian energy.

Endangerment site: Area of the body where nerves and blood vessels surface close to the skin and are not well protected by muscle or connective tissue; therefore, deep sustained pressure into these areas could damage these vessels and nerves. The kidney area is included because they are loosely suspended in fat and connective tissue and heavy pounding is contraindicated in that area.

Endogenous: Made in the body.

Endorphin: Part of the endogenous opioid peptides which are a group of more than 15 substances present in the brain, certain endocrine glands, and gastrointestinal tract, that have morphine-like analgesic properties, behavioral affects, neurotransmitter, and neuromodulator functions. Chemical that is released in response to stimulation that reduces the sensation of pain and lifts the mood.

Energetic approaches: Methods of bodywork that work with subtle body responses.

Essential touch: Vital, fundamental, and primary touch crucial to well being.

Ethics: Standards, ideals, morals, values, and principles of honorable, decent, fair, responsible and proper conduct.

Exemption: A situation in which a professional is not required to comply with an existing law because of educational or professional standing.

External sensory information: Stimulation that is detected by the body with its origin exterior to the surface of the skin.

Facilitation: A state of a nerve when it is stimulated, but not to the point of threshold where it will transmit a nerve signal.

Fascial sheaths: Flat sheet of connective tissue used for separation, stability, and muscular attachment points.

Feedback: A method of autoregulation to maintain internal homeostasis that interlinks body functions.

Frequency: The number of times a method repeats itself in a time period.

Friction: Specific circular or transverse movements that do not glide on the skin and are focused on the underlying tissue.

Gait: Walking pattern.

Gate control theory: Hypothesis that painful stimuli may be prevented from reaching higher levels of the central nervous system by stimulation of larger sensory nerves.

General contraindications: Those that require a physician's evaluation to rule out serious underlying conditions before any massage is indicated. If a massage is recommended by the physician, then the physician will need to help develop a comprehensive treatment plan.

Gestures: The way a client touches their body as they explain a problem. Their movements may indicate if the problem is a muscle problem, joint problem, or visceral problem.

Golgi tendon receptors: Receptors in the tendons that sense tension.

Hacking: Type of tapotement that alternately strikes the surface of the body with quick snapping movements.

Hardening: A method of teaching the body to deal more effectively with stress.

Heavy pressure: Compressive force that extends to the bone under the tissue.

Histamine: A chemical produced by the body which dilates the blood vessels.

History: Information from the client about past and present medical conditions, and patterns of symptoms.

Homeostasis: Dynamic equilibrium of the internal environment of the body through processes of feedback and regulation.

Hydrotherapy: The use of various types of water applications and temperatures for therapy.

Hygiene: Practices and conditions for the promotion of health and the prevention of disease.

Hyperstimulation analgesia: Reduction of perception of a sensation by stimulation of large diameter nerve fibers. Examples of methods used are ice, heat, counter irritation, acupressure, acupuncture, rocking, music, and repetitive massage strokes.

Indication: A therapeutic application that promotes health or assists in a healing process.

Inflammatory response: A normal mechanism that usually speeds recovery from an infection or injury characterized by pain, heat, redness, and swelling.

Informed consent: Client authorization for any service from a professional based on adequate information provided by the massage professional.

Inhibition: To decrease or cease a response or function.

Insertion: The muscle attachment point that is closest to the moving joint.

Integrated approaches: Combined methods of various forms of massage and bodywork styles.

Inter-competition massage: Massage provided during an athletic event.

Intimacy: A tender, familiar, and understanding experience between beings.

Intuition: Knowing something by using subconscious information.

Isokinetic contraction: A multiple isotonic movement where the client moves their joint through a full range of motion using full muscle strength, against partial resistance supplied by the massage therapist.

Isometric contraction: Contraction in which the effort of the muscle, or group of muscles, is exactly matched by a counterpressure, so that no movement occurs, only effort.

Isotonic contraction: The effort of the target muscle, or group of muscles, is partially matched by the counterpressure, allowing a degree of resisted movement to occur.

Joint kinesthetic receptor: Sensory nerve in the joint that detects position and speed of movement.

Joint movement: The movement of the joint through its normal range-of-motion.

Lengthening: The assuming of a normal resting length by a muscle through the neuromuscular mechanism.

License: A type of credential required by law to regulate the practice of a profession to protect the public health, safety and welfare.

Longitudinal stretching: A stretch applied along the fiber direction of the connective tissues and muscles.

Lubricant: Substance that reduces friction on the skin during massage movements.

Lymphatic drainage: Specific type of massage that enhances lymphatic flow.

Manipulation: Skillful use of the hands in a therapeutic manner. Massage manipulations focus on the soft tissues of the body and are not to be confused with joint manipulation using a high velocity thrust.

Manual lymph drainage: Methods of bodywork that influence lymphatic movement.

Massage chair: Specially designed equipment that allows the client to sit comfortably during the massage.

Massage environment: An area or location where a massage is given.

Massage equipment: Tables, mats, chairs, and other incidental supplies and implements used during the massage.

Massage mat: A cushioned surface that is placed on the floor.

Massage procedures: Activities that prepare for the massage such as client history, how to get on the massage table, how drapes are used.

Massage routine: Step-by-step protocol and sequence used to give a massage.

Massage table: Specially designed equipment that allows massage to be done with the client laying down.

Mechanical: Response that is based on structure change of tissue. The change in the tissue results directly from the application of the technique.

Medical rehabilitative massage: Level of professional responsibility based on extensive education that prepares the massage therapist to develop, maintain, rehabilitate, augment physical function, relieve or prevent physical dysfunction and pain, and to enhance the well being of the client. Methods include assessment of the soft tissue and joints, treatment by soft tissue manipulation, hydrotherapy, remedial exercise programs, actinotherapy, and client self care programs.

Moderate pressure: Compressive pressure that extends to the muscle layer but does not press the tissue against the underlying bone.

Motor point: Point at which a motor nerve enters the muscle it innervates and causes a muscle to twitch if stimulated.

Movement cure: Term used in the 19th and early 20th centuries for a system of exercise and massage manipulations focused to treat a variety of ailments.

Muscle energy techniques: (Neuromuscular facilitation) Specific use of active contraction in individual or groups of muscles to initiate a relaxation response. Activation of the proprioceptors to facilitate muscle tone, relaxation, and stretching.

Muscle testing procedures: Assessment process using muscle contraction. Strength testing seeks to discover if the muscle being tested is responding with sufficient strength to perform the required body functions. Another type of muscle testing seeks to discover if the neurological interaction of the muscles is working smoothly. The third type of muscle testing is of the applied kinesiology type that uses muscle strength or weakness as an indicator of body function.

Muscular tendinous junction: Where muscle fibers end and the connective tissue continues to form tendon. Major site of injury.

Myofascial release: A system of bodywork that affects the connective tissue of the body through various methods that elongate and alter the plastic component and ground matrix of the connective tissue.

Nerve impingement: Pressure against a nerve by skin, fascia, muscles, ligaments, and joints.

Neuromuscular: The interaction between the control of the nervous system of the muscles and the response of the muscles to these nerve signals.

Neuromuscular approaches: Methods of bodywork that influence the reflexive responses of the nervous system and its connection to muscular function.

Neuromuscular mechanism: The interplay and reflex connection between sensory and motor neurons and muscle function.

Objective assessment: Measurable information and defined goals that the massage therapist gathers from the assessment process.

Oil: Type of liquid lubricant.

Open-ended question: Stating a question so that the answer cannot be a simple one word response.

Oriental approaches: Methods of bodywork that have developed from the ancient Chinese.

Origin: attachment point of a muscle at the fixed point during movement.

Osteokinematic movements: Flexion, extension, abduction, adduction, and rotation. Also referred to as physiological movements.

Pain-spasm-pain cycle: Steady contraction of muscles causing ischemia and stimulating pain receptors in muscles. The pain, in turn, initiates more spasms, setting up a vicious circle.

Palpation: Assessment through touch.

Parasympathetic autonomic nervous system: The restorative part of the autonomic nervous system. The parasympathetic response is often called the relaxation response.

Passive joint movement: The massage practitioner moves the jointed areas without the assistance of the client.

Petrissage: (Kneading) Rhythmic rolling, lifting, squeezing, and wringing of soft tissue.

Phasic muscles: The muscles that move the body.

Physical assessment: Evaluation of body balance, efficient function, basic symmetry, range of motion, and ability to function.

Piezoelectricity: The production of an electric current by application of pressure to certain crystals such as mica, quartz, Rochelle Salt, and connective tissue.

Placebo: A treatment for an illness that influences the course of the disease even if the treatment is not specifically validated.

Plan/Progress: Information about what the next massage may include, things to remember to look for, and reevaluation of the progress, what seems to be working and not working, any self help that is shared, and other information that will influence future sessions.

Positional release: A method of moving the body into the direction of ease (the way the body wants to go out of the position that causes the pain), the proprioception is taken into a state of safety and may stop signally for protective spasm.

Positioning: Placing the body in such a way that specific joints of muscles are isolated.

Post-event massage: Massage provided after an athletic event.

Post Isometric Relaxation (PIR): Occurs after an isometric contraction of a muscle, results from the activity of minute neural reporting stations called the golgi tendon bodies.

Postural muscles: Muscles that support the body against gravity.

Powder: Type of lubricant that consists of a finely ground substance.

Pre-massage activities: Any activity that is involved in preparation for a massage including, setting up the massage room, obtaining supplies, and determining the temperature of the room.

Pressure: Compressive force.

Prime movers: The muscles responsible for movement.

Prone: Laying face down.

Proprioceptive Neuromuscular Facilitation (PNF): Specific application of muscle energy techniques that uses strong contraction combined with stretching and muscular pattern retraining.

Proprioceptors: Sensory receptors that detect joint and muscle activity.

Pulsed muscle energy: Procedures that involve engaging the barrier and using minute, resisted, contractions (usually 20 in 10 seconds) which introduces mechanical pumping as well as PIR or RI.

Range-of-motion: Movement of joints.

Rapport: The development of a relationship based on mutual trust and harmony.

Reciprocal Inhibition (RI): Occurs when a muscle contracts, obliging its antagonist to relax in order to allow normal movement to take place.

Referral: Sending a client to a health care professional for specific diagnosis and treatment of a disease.

Referred pain: Pain felt in an area different than the source of the pain.

Reflex: An involuntary response to a stimulus. Reflexes are specific, predictable, adaptive, and purposeful. Reflexive methods work by causing a stimulation of the nervous system (sensory neurons) and the tissue changes in response to the body's adaptation to the neural stimulation.

Reflexology: A massage system directed primarily to the feet and hands.

Refractory period: Amount of time that a muscle will be unable to contract after a contraction of the muscle has occurred.

Regional contraindications: Contraindications that relate to a specific area of the body.

Resting stroke: First stroke of the massage. The simple laying on of hands.

Rhythm: The regularity of the application of the technique. If the method is applied at regular intervals, it is considered even or rhythmical. If the method is choppy or irregular, it is considered uneven or not rhythmic.

Right of refusal: The entitlement of both the client and the professional to stop the session.

Rocking: Rhythmical movement of the body.

Safe touch: Secure, respectful, considerate, sensitive, responsive, sympathetic, understanding, supportive, and empathetic contact.

Sanitation: The formulation and application of measures to promote and establish conditions favorable to health, specifically public health.

Science: The intellectual process to understand by observation, measurement, accumulation of data, and analysis of the findings.

Scope of practice: The where, when, and how a professional may provide their service or function as a professional.

Sexual misconduct: Any behavior that is sexually oriented in the professional setting.

Shaking: The body area is grasped and shaken in a quick loose movement. This is sometimes classified as rhythmic mobilization.

Shiatsu: Acupressure and meridian focused bodywork system from Japan.

Side-lying: Position of the client on their side.

Skin-rolling: A form of petrissage that lifts skin.

Slapping: Form of tapotement that uses a flat hand.

S.O.A.P Notes: A method of charting and record keeping. The acronym for S.O.A.P stands for Subjective assessment, Objective assessment, Application, and Plan/Progress.

Soft tissue: The skin, fascia, muscles, tendons, joint capsules, and ligaments of the body.

Somatic: Pertaining to the body.

Somatic pain: Arises from stimulation of receptors in the skin, this is called superficial somatic pain; or from stimulation of receptors in skeletal muscles, joints, tendons, and fascia, this is called deep somatic pain.

Speed: Rate of application that is fast, slow, or variable.

Spindle cells: Sensory receptors in the belly of the muscle that detect stretch.

Stabilization: Holding the body in a fixed position during joint movement, lengthening, and stretching.

State dependent memory: The encoding and storing of a memory based on the autonomic nervous system and the resulting chemical levels of the body. The memory is only retrievable during a similiar physiological experience in the body.

Sterilization: The process by which all microorganisms are destroyed.

Stimulation: Excitation that activates the sensory nerves.

Stress: Any substantial change in routine, or any activity which causes the body to have to adapt.

Stretching: Mechanical tension applied to lengthen the myofascial unit (muscles and fascia). Longitudinal and cross-directional are two types of stretching.

Stroke: A technique of therapeutic massage that is applied with a movement on the surface of the body whether superficial or deep.

Structural and postural integration approaches: Methods of bodywork derived from biomechanics, postural alignment, and the importance of the connective tissue structures.

Subjective assessment: Information the client provides during the interview and history taking process and the client's goals and outcome for the session.

Subtle energies: Weak electrical fields that surround the body and run through the body.

Superficial fascia: Connective tissue layer just under the skin.

Superficial pressure: Pressure that stays on the skin.

Supine: Position with the client laying face up.

Symmetrical stance: Position in which the body weight is distributed equally between the feet.

Sympathetic autonomic nervous system: Part of the autonomic nervous system that is energy using and where the fight of flight response is activated.

Systemic massage: Massage structured to primarily effect one body system. This approach is usually used for lymphatic and circulation enhancement massage.

Tapotement: Springy blows to the body at a fast rate to create rhythmical compression to the tissue. Also called percussion.

Tapping: Type of tapotement using the finger tips.

Target muscles: The muscle or groups of muscles that the response of the methods is specifically focused upon.

Techniques: Methods of therapeutic massage that provide sensory stimulation or mechanical alteration of the soft tissue of the body.

Therapeutic massage: The scientific art and system of assessment, and manual application to the superficial soft tissue of the skin, muscles, tendons, ligaments, fascial, and the structures that lie in the superficial tissue using the hand, foot, knee, arm, elbow, forearm through the systematic external application of touch, stroking (effleurage), friction, vibration, percussion, kneading (petrissage), stretching, compression, passive and active joint movements within the normal physiological range of motion, and adjunctive external applications of water, heat, and cold. Therapeutic massage is a way to establish and maintain good physical condition and health through normalizing and improving muscle tone, promoting relaxation, stimulating circulation, and producing therapeutic effects on the respiratory, nervous system, and the subtle interactions between these systems through the energetic and mind/body connections, in a safe, nonsexual environment that respects the client's self determined outcome for the session.

Tone: State of causing the muscle to contract or strengthen.

Tonic vibration reflex: Reflex that tones a muscle with stimulation through vibration methods at the tendon.

Touch: Contact with no movement.

Traction: Gentle pull on the joint capsule to increase the joint space.

Treatment plan: A total program for patient/client care developed by a doctor or other supervisory personnel.

Trigger point: An area of local nerve facilitation resulting in hypertonicity of a muscle bundle and referred pain patterns.

Universal precautions: Procedures developed by the Centers for Disease Control (CDC) to prevent the spread of contagious diseases.

Vibration: Fine or coarse tremulous movement that creates reflexive responses.

Wellness: The efficient balance of body, mind, and spirit all working in a harmonious way providing for quality life.

Wellness personal service massage: The assessment procedures focused to determine contraindications to massage and need for referral to other health care professionals, and the development of a health enhancing, nonspecific approach to massage. The massage session plan is developed by combining information received from the client, desired results and directions from the client, and skill levels of the massage practitioner. The massage practitioner develops an individualized massage session focused on normalization of the body systems through external manual stimulation of the nervous system, connective tissue, muscle, circulatory, and respiratory systems providing generalized stress reduction, reduction of muscle tension, symptomatic relief of pain related to soft tissue dysfunction, increased circulation, and other benefits similar to exercise or other relaxation methods produced by therapeutic massage to increase the well-being of the client.

Yang: The portion of the whole realm of function of the body, mind, spirit of eastern thought that corresponds with sympathetic autonomic nervous system functions.

Yin: The portion of the whole realm of function of the body, mind, spirit of eastern thought that corresponds with parasympathetic autonomic nervous system functions.

INDEX

A

Abdomen
  assessment of, 320
  palpation of, 309
  quadrants of, 55f
Abdominal pattern sequence,
    234–238
Abdominals, 253
Abduction, 62
Abductor, 63t, 264
Abductor digiti minimi pedis,
    65t
Abuse
  during critical time, 329
  re-enactment of, 331
  survivors of, 21
Abuse victim, 328–331
  adult, 329
  child, 328–329
Accessory movement, 263
Achilles tendon reflex, 363
Aching pain, 94
Acquired immunity, 72t
Acquired immunodeficiency
    syndrome (AIDS), 72t
  misunderstanding about
    spread of, 107
  transmission of, 116–117
  understanding and
    preventing, 115–117
Active assisted range of motion,
    266–267
Active movement
  joint, 225, 264
  purpose of, 259–260
Active muscle energy
    techniques, 138–139
Active range of motion, 265–268
Acupressure, 13–14, 20, 21,
    372–374
  instructions for, 352f
Acupressure points, 319, 373,
    375
  compression on, 247
  stimulation of, 373–374
Acupuncture, 372–374
  in ancient China, 4–5
  for depression, 138–139
  inhibitory effects of, 140
  in pain relief, 129
Acupuncture points, 86
  instructions for stimulating,
    352f
  motor points and, 130–131f
Acute illness, 89, 335
Adaptation, 92–93
Adder, Robert, 387
Addictive behavior, 387–388
Adduction, 62
Adductor, 63t
Adductor longus, 65t
Adductor magnus, 65t
Adolescents, 334
Adrenaline release, 137
Adrenocorticotropic hormone,
    90
Advertising, 155–159
  honest, 39
  sample of, 158f
Aerobic activity, 181
Afferent nerves, 67t
African medicine, 5
Age factors, 89
Aging population, 336–337
Agonist-antagonist strength
    assessment, 311
Agonists, 63
AhShi, 372
Alcohol consumption, 108
Allergy, 72t
  to lubricant, 202
All-or-none law, 125

American Association of
  Masseurs and Masseuses,
    12
American Massage Therapy
    Association, 12
American Massage Therapy
    Association (AMTA),
    liability insurance
    through, 167
Americans with Disabilities Act,
    339, 343
Amma, 20
Amputations, 342
Analgesia
  hyperstimulation, 14, 129–132,
    138, 257
  stimulation-produced,
    130–132
Anatomic barrier, 264, 308
Anatomic position, 54
Anatomical benefits, 87–88
Anatripsis, 5
Ankle
  in gait, 301–302
  movement of, 262f, 267f
Anmo, 4
Antagonists, 63, 311
Antigen, 72t
Anxiety
  breathing and, 384
  as drug side effect, 99
  with excessive sympathetic
    stimulation, 137
Apocrine sweat gland, 76
Aponeuroses, 246
Application, 292
Appointment hours, 35
Approximation, 278
Arm movements, 48
Arndt-Schultz law, 127
Art, 121
Arterial flow, 80–81, 361
  benefits to, 87
Arteries, 361
  principal, 70f
  pulse points and, 310f
Arthrokinematic movement, 263
Articular system, 61–62
  diagnostic terms for disease
    of, 62
Articulation, 59
Asclepiades, 4
Aseptic techniques, 110
Asian methods, 20, 21
Assessment, 290, 291–295, 322
  gait, 300–302
  interpretation of, 314–321
  with palpation, 302–310
  physical, 295–313
  posture, 295–299
Associated Bodywork and
    Massage Professionals, 15
Associated Massage and
    Bodywork Professionals
    (AMBP), liability
    insurance through, 167
Asymmetrical stance, 298f
Asymmetry, 316; *See also* Balance;
    Symmetry
Athletes, 332–333
Attitudes, responsibility for,
    28–29
Auras, 86
Auricularis superior, 64
Autism, 389
Autonomic approach, 14
Autonomic functions, 138t
Autonomic nervous system, 68
  effects on, 127–129, 138–140
  massage effects on, 343–344
  physiologic effects on, 82–84
  stress effects on, 122
  traditional energy centers and,
    85f
  yin/yang and, 372–374
Autonomic plexuses, 68
Axillary area, 97

B

Bacteria, 109
Balance
  body quadrants and, 313
  dynamic, 296
  in joint function, 307
  mechanical, 297
Balance points, 180, 183
Balloon vibration exercises, 252f
Banking accounts, 167–168
Barnes, John, 21
Barrier-free access, 342
Bathroom facility, 112, 204
  cleaning of, 115
Battle Creek Sanatorium, 8
Baumgartner, Albert, 13, 240
Beard, Gertrude, 13, 226
Beating, 256
Becker, Robert, 123–124
Behavior
  modification of, 336
  in wellness, 387–388
Belief, 151
Bell's law, 125
Bending, inappropriate, 178
Beta-endorphins, 139; *See also*
    Endorphins
Biceps brachii, 65t
Biceps muscles
  isolation of, 272f
  shaking of, 253
Bindegewebsmassage, 20
Bio-chemical benefits, 87–88
Bioenergetics, 11
Biofeedback mechanism, 311
Biomechanics, 20, 87
Bland, Jeffrey, 379
Bleach, 113–114
Blood
  contact with, 113
  in skin, 317–318
  sugar cycles of, 383
Blood vessels, 69
  palpation assessment of,
    304–305
  principal, 70f
Boards, 42
Body
  muscle strength as indicator of
    function, 311
  nutrition of, 383
  planes of, 54
  positioning of, 186; *See also*
    Positionings; Positions
  quadrants of, 313
  rhythms of
    assessment of, 302, 320
    palpation assessment of, 309
  structure of, 55–56
  sway of, 297
  system of, 27
  terminology of, 56–57
  wellness of, 381–382
  in wellness training, 383–386
Body cavities, 56, 57f
Body fluids, 113
  spills of, 113–114
Body hair, excessive, 246
Body language, 34
  closure, 35f
  code of, 315
Body mechanics, 177
  basic principles of, 179–180
  considerations in, 181–183
  correct *vs.* incorrect, 182f
  improper, 177–179
  in side-lying massage position,
    234
  while giving massage, 184–195
Body supports, 198–200
  positioning of, 212
  size and shapes of, 201f
Body weight
  positioning of, 184
  shifting of, 179
Body/mind connection, 128–129

Body/mind effect, 137–141
Body-righting reflex, 129
Bodywork, 19
  research on, 124
  rhythmic, 138
  tree for, 22f
Bodywork Knowledgebase, 15
Bohm, Max, 12
Bone
  in elderly, 336–337
  palpation assessment of, 309
  terminology of, 58
Bookkeeping, 167–168
Boundaries
  in abuse victim, 330–331
  client, 30
  defining, 30–31
  personal, 28–29
Bowditch's law, 125
Brachial plexus impingement,
    134
Brachialis muscle isolation, 272f
Breath odor, 108
Breathing, 139, 383–384; *See also*
    Deep breathing
  interpretation of, 320
  patterns of
    assessment of, 302
    palpation assessment of, 309
  retraining of, 385
British Institute for Massage by
    the Blind, 12
Broadening contraction, 365
Brochures, 156–157
Burn patients, 342
Burning pain, 94
Burnout, 151–152
Bursae, 62
Business
  banking accounts for, 167–168
  client-practitioner agreement
    in, 170–173
  development of, 152–155
  issues of, 146–174
  legal structure of, 166
  location of, 166
  management of, 165–169
  marketing of, 155–162
  plan for, 152–154
  structure of, 162–165
Business cards, 159f

C

Cancer, warning signs of, 90–91
Candles, 207
Cannon's law of denervation,
    127
Capillary system, 317–318
Carbon dioxide
  improved elimination of, 87
  removal of, 73
Cardiovascular system, 70f
  managing disease of, 13–14
  organs of, 56
  terminology of, 69
Career resource directory, 149f
Caregiver-child relationship, 124
Carpal tunnel syndrome, 132, 134
Cartilage, 58–59
Catheters, 342
Celsus, Aulus Cornelius, 6, 354
Centering, 197, 212
Centers for Disease Control
    (CDC)
  standards of, 107
  Universal precautions of,
    113–115
Central nervous system, 67, 68,
    127
Centrifugal direction, 227
Centripetal direction, 227
Cerebellum, 128–129
Cerebral cortex, 128
Cerebral spinal fluid circulation,
    82

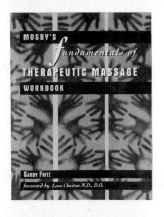
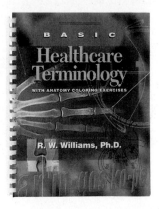
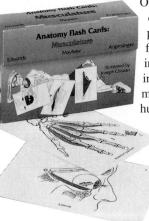
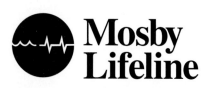